Sacred Lives:
an account of the history, cultural associations and social impact of epilepsy

Ian Bone

The Book Guild Ltd

First published in Great Britain in 2022 by
The Book Guild Ltd
9 Priory Business Park
Wistow Road, Kibworth
Leicestershire, LE8 0RX
Freephone: 0800 999 2982
www.bookguild.co.uk
Email: info@bookguild.co.uk
Twitter: @bookguild

Copyright © 2022 Ian Bone

The right of Ian Bone to be identified as the author of this
work has been asserted by him in accordance with the
Copyright, Design and Patents Act 1988.

All rights reserved. No part of this publication may be
reproduced, transmitted, or stored in a retrieval system, in any form or by any means,
without permission in writing from the publisher, nor be otherwise circulated in
any form of binding or cover other than that in which it is published and without
a similar condition being imposed on the subsequent purchaser.

Typeset in 12pt Adobe Garamond Pro

Printed and bound by CPI Group (UK) Ltd, Croydon, CR0 4YY

ISBN 978 1913913 991

British Library Cataloguing in Publication Data.
A catalogue record for this book is available from the British Library.

This publication has been made possible with financial support from Sir Boyd Tunnock of Thomas Tunnock Ltd, and Bill Scott, Patron of the William Quarrier Scottish Epilepsy Centre.

*This volume is dedicated to my wife Isabel and our daughters
Clare and Sarah, in recognition of their constant support, and to our son Tim, whose
own journey with epilepsy has been the inspiration and reason for this book.*

Ian Bone is a retired neurologist with 40 years of professional and personal experience of caring for people with epilepsy. He is currently an Honorary Senior Research Fellow at the Institute of Cardiovascular and Medical Sciences, University of Glasgow. He has co-authored three textbooks, including *Neurology and Neurosurgery Illustrated*, which has run to five editions and been translated into seven languages. He has edited and authored many scientific papers and still lectures widely.

For more information visit **www.sacredlives.co.uk** or contact **ianbone@sacredlives.co.uk**

Jo Hargreaves is a development editor with a background in life sciences research and medical publishing.

Contents

Foreword	vii
Introduction	ix

Part I: History, classification, and causes of epilepsy — 1

Chapter 1: Epilepsy from ancient times to the eighteenth century	3
Chapter 2: Epilepsy from the nineteenth century to the present	22
Chapter 3: The investigation, classification, and causes of epilepsy	50

Part II: Epilepsy in the arts — 65

Chapter 4: Epilepsy in literature and in authors	67
Chapter 5: Epilepsy in works of art and in artists	98
Chapter 6: Epilepsy on the moving screen	123
Chapter 7: Epilepsy in music and the theatre	156

Part III: Epilepsy in the media — 181

Chapter 8: Epilepsy in print, online, and social media	183
Chapter 9: Famous people with epilepsy	205

Part IV: Epilepsy in society   225

Chapter 10: Epilepsy, laws, and officialdom   227
Chapter 11: Epilepsy, behaviour, violence, and criminal law   248
Chapter 12: Stigmatization, discrimination, and social isolation   275

Part V: Epilogue   311

A personal account of living with epilepsy   313
Figures and tables   335
Illustration credits   341
Acknowledgments   342
Index   343

Foreword

Epilepsy can be a devastating condition. Whether receiving the diagnosis yourself or being told your child has epilepsy, the news is life changing.

The effects can be accompanied by shame and embarrassment, and the aftermath of the loss of control as a result of seizures can include guilt, loss of confidence, and low mood.

A clinician's primary aim is to support people to manage their condition by reducing their seizures at the same time as minimising the negative effects of the medication. For many, this results in seizure control and reduces the impact of the condition on day to day life.

So why do we still hear directly that the impact of having epilepsy goes beyond that of living with, or controlling, seizure activity? For some people, their seizures can't be controlled and the effects of medication can be disabling. It can affect every aspect of life including relationships, education, employment and opportunity, compounded by a lack of understanding around the condition which can lead to discrimination with social attitudes, fears and mistruths which impact negatively on the quality of lives of those with epilepsy.

In Scotland, we have internationally recognised Clinical Guidelines for Epilepsy and whilst this provides vital support for clinicians, Professor Bone highlights the literature to date focusses on informing and educating the clinical community. There can be an unintentional divide created where the expert is informed in medical matters and they become conversant in a language that does not translate readily to common interpretation. We also have a third sector voice where charities have a developed a representative position and aims to inform and translate the lived experience to the wider community.

Sacred Lives offers an opportunity for professionals and public's awareness and knowledge to be developed by using common language and interest. It delivers a unique insight into epilepsy as a condition, its historical, cultural and social impact.

The author has a rare combination of professional and personal experience. He has been both a treating neurologist and the father of a son with epilepsy, with a background of innovation, service development and education of a generation of clinicians to inform him. He encapsulates and delivers a unique exploration and story of the subject.

Sacred Lives is a compelling narrative, which builds the reader's understanding of a complex condition, societal influences and the experience and impact on the individual.

Professor Bone has dedicated his professional life to improving the landscape for people with neurological conditions in Scotland and further afield. His relentless focus, expertise and leadership have given us a unique contribution to support our understanding of epilepsy and take a critical step in bringing it out of the shadows.

Professor Jason Leitch
National Clinical Director
Scottish Government

Introduction

It may come as a surprise to the reader that at one time, before the religious demonization of epilepsy, people with the condition were believed to have unique powers, even to be geniuses, and were regarded as having a sacred disease and leading sacred lives. It is from this perception of the illness that this book takes its title.

I have been motivated to write this book by my personal experience of my son Tim having epilepsy, an experience that, for 40 years, has run almost in parallel with my career as a neurologist treating many patients with the condition. It is the insights that have resulted from learning about epilepsy from 'both sides of the fence' that form the basis of this personal account of the condition and society's reaction to it.

There are already a number of authoritative books on epilepsy, including Owsei Temkin's *The Falling Sickness*,[1] Michael Eadie and Peter Bladen's *A Disease Once Sacred*,[2] and Jeannette Stirling's *Representing Epilepsy*.[3] However, these are targeted at an academic professional readership, and do not make easy reading for the more general reader. Similarly, the many articles about epilepsy that have been published in medical and scientific journals are intended to communicate advances in scientific knowledge to informed experts, rather than to provide a more widely accessible understanding of the condition. In contrast, much of what the general public does hear about epilepsy depends on what is deemed newsworthy

---

1   Temkin O (1971) *The Falling Sickness: A History of Epilepsy from the Greeks to the Beginnings of Modern Neurology*, 2nd edition. Johns Hopkins University Press, Baltimore, MD.
2   Eadie MJ and Bladen PF (2001) *A Disease Once Sacred: A History of the Medical Understanding of Epilepsy*. John Libbey & Company Ltd, London.
3   Stirling J (2010) *Representing Epilepsy: Myth and Matter*. Liverpool University Press, Liverpool.

by the popular media. A more modest contribution is provided by epilepsy charities, whose websites include information about recent advances in treatment and care. Consequently, despite the increasingly well-informed support provided by healthcare professionals for people living with epilepsy, the majority of the general population still have a very limited and often erroneous understanding of the condition. This is clearly a recipe for the perpetuation of myths about epilepsy.

My hope is that by offering an accessible text that bridges the gap between expert and public knowledge, I can in some small way address this situation. The intended readership is broad, encompassing people with epilepsy and their families, those who encounter the condition through friends, work colleagues, or acquaintances, and those who simply wish to have a better understanding of this highly stigmatized condition and the effect that it has on people's lives. It is also my earnest wish that healthcare professionals themselves may find something in these pages that will help them to better understand and support their patients with epilepsy.

It is the unpredictable and repeated, albeit short-lived, loss of self-control that accompanies seizures which sets epilepsy apart from other long-term conditions. The embarrassment and shame caused by being 'out of control' are accompanied by fear and anxiety about what might have been said or done during a seizure episode. The emotions that are experienced after a seizure can include guilt, loss of confidence, and low mood. Being in control of our thoughts and actions is central to our self-image and the manner in which we and society believe we should behave, and failure to conform to such norms, for whatever reason, is deemed antisocial and dismissed as unacceptable. An appreciation of this is central to understanding the mindset of people with epilepsy. Finally, the condition is regarded as a 'hidden disability', as during the periods between seizures there are no visible clues to its presence. This results in less public empathy for people with epilepsy, despite the ongoing social and medical effects of the condition, than for those with a visible physical disability.

Chapters 1 and 2 of this book review the history of epilepsy from ancient times to the present, exploring why the condition became so stigmatized and how people with epilepsy have been persecuted, demonized, and socially rejected. Chapter 3 examines the investigation, classification, and causes of epilepsy in relation to the major scientific advances that have been made in the last 100 years or so, while at the same time social understanding and acceptance of epilepsy has lagged far behind. The depiction of epilepsy in the arts is then discussed in detail. Chapter 4 focuses on the portrayal of epilepsy in works of literature, and examines the evidence that a significant number of writers were affected by the condition. Chapter 5 considers the depiction of seizures in works of art, and discusses artists of the past who had epilepsy themselves. Chapter 6 examines the positive and negative ways in which epilepsy has been depicted on the moving screen, and Chapter 7 covers similar ground in relation to music and the theatre.

Raising awareness of the many misconceptions about epilepsy is the key to bringing about widespread social acceptance of the condition by the general public. Chapter 8 evaluates the impact of print, online, and social media as a tool for education, communication, and support for people with epilepsy. Chapter 9 considers a number of famous people whose epilepsy has been established with certainty, claimed, or disputed. The lack of modern-day 'celebrities' who are willing to be open about their epilepsy and become role models for others with the condition is also discussed.

Society still treats people with epilepsy differently from the rest of the population by adversely affecting their quality of life, limiting their life opportunities, and eroding their human rights. Epilepsy in society is examined in relation to laws and officialdom in Chapter 10, with regard to behaviour, violence, and criminal law in Chapter 11, and in terms of stigmatization, discrimination, and social isolation in Chapter 12. The book concludes with a personal account of my experience from a parent's perspective as my son's life with epilepsy has slowly unfolded. My hope is that this epilogue will allow others who are on a similar path both to learn how to approach problems and challenges differently, and to be reassured that they are not alone in their feelings of anxiety and the constant dilemmas that they face. However, the subjective experiences and emotional and physical challenges that Tim himself has faced are his story to tell, as indeed he has done in his forthcoming eBook.

My aim in writing *Sacred Lives* has been to bring epilepsy out of the shadows and challenge the reader to think afresh both about the condition itself, and about the lives of those for whom epilepsy is a daily reality. Inevitably the book represents my own personal experience, is eclectic in its content, and largely reflects a western European perspective. However, despite these limitations I hope that it may engage and inform a diverse non-professional readership. If even a few people who would not normally have considered reading a book on epilepsy gain a greater understanding of the condition and empathy with those who live with it, this project will have achieved its objective.

Finally, we should consider who the real experts are. We owe a huge debt of gratitude to those who have dedicated their professional lives to exploring the science of epilepsy. However, the people who have the widest and deepest experience of the condition are those whose lives are directly affected by it – that is, people with epilepsy and their families. This book is dedicated to my own family, for their constant support, and to my son Tim, who has shown such courage.

In 1906 the William Quarrier 'Colony for the Mercy of Epileptics' opened in the West of Scotland. Its ethos was that the country air, companionship and pleasant rural surroundings would, by helping to reduce anxiety and stress among its residents, improve their quality of life. Now an independent hospital known as the William Quarrier Scottish Epilepsy Centre (quarriers.org.uk/epilepsy), it is run by the health and social care charity Quarriers to provide epilepsy assessment and treatment services for patients across Scotland. Funds raised by the sales of *Sacred Lives* will be donated to this centre.

Ian Bone
Helensburgh, Scotland, July 2021
www.sacredlives.co.uk

PART I

History, classification, and causes of epilepsy

CHAPTER 1

Epilepsy from ancient times to the eighteenth century

Cassius: *But soft, I pray you. What, did Caesar swoon?*
Casca: *He fell down in the market-place, and foamed at mouth, and was speechless.*
Brutus: *Tis very like: he hath the falling sickness.*
                              (William Shakespeare, *Julius Caesar*, Act 1, Scene 2)

To understand why epilepsy remains the most stigmatized of all illnesses, it is necessary to go back in time to the early myths and beliefs that enshrouded it. The term 'epilepsy' is derived from the ancient Greek word *epilepsia*, meaning 'to seize, or take hold of'. This accurately conveys the idea of being seized by forces that are beyond an individual's control, and thus being taken hold of, attacked or even 'possessed' by an alien force.

Ancient civilizations

Of the many accounts of the history of epilepsy that are available, by far the most comprehensive is Owsei Temkin's *The Falling Sickness*.[1] Written in 1945 and revised in 1971, it explores both attitudes to and treatments for the condition from ancient to modern times. Temkin suggests

---

1   Temkin O (1971) *The Falling Sickness: A History of Epilepsy from the Greeks to the Beginnings of Modern Neurology*, 2nd edition. Johns Hopkins University Press, Baltimore, MD.

that ancient civilizations considered diseases to be either the result of possession by gods or demons, or a consequence of natural causes. Treatments therefore focused either on the casting out of demons by magicians or priests, or on measures designed to counter what were believed to be the physical causes, and administered by physicians.

One of the first descriptions of epileptic seizures can be found in an ancient Akkadian text from Mesopotamia around 2000 bce. The author describes how the patient's 'neck turns left, his hands and feet are tense and his eyes wide open, and from his mouth froth is flowing without having any consciousness.' The condition is termed *antasubbû* (meaning 'the hand of sin'), is believed to be brought on by the god of the moon, and is treated by exorcism.

The *Code of Hammurabi* (*c.* 1790 bce), a well-preserved Babylonian record of the laws of ancient Mesopotamia, lists epileptic seizures as one of the reasons for which a purchased slave may be returned for a refund: 'If a man buys a male or female slave and before one month has passed *bennu* [epilepsy] falls upon him, he [the buyer] will return the slave to his seller, and the buyer will take back the silver that he had paid.'[2] The code also states that an individual with epilepsy cannot marry or testify in court. Discovered by archaeologists in 1901, it is one of the oldest preserved interpretable writings in the world, now kept on display at the Louvre Museum in Paris.

The term 'falling disease' first appears in the *Sakikku*, a Babylonian cuneiform medical text compiled between 1067 and 1046 bce. Cuneiform is a system of writing that was first developed by the ancient Sumerians of Mesopotamia around 3500–3000 bce. The word *antasubba* is used to refer to falling disease, and the translation by Kinnier Wilson and Reynolds describes how an individual 'clenches his hands as though rigor had seized him, and, with legs extended, is greatly convulsed; if then the seizure abates ... he begins to regain consciousness.'[3]

The observational details in the original text describe with uncanny accuracy a range of different types of seizure, including what we now call complex partial or temporal lobe epilepsy. It is here too that the attribution of epilepsy to demonic possession first makes an appearance in literature: 'if epilepsy falls once upon a person it is the result of possession by a demon or departed spirit.' Babylonian physicians believed that such possession was at its most extreme at the height of the seizure, and then dissipated as the attack resolved.

Around 900 bce, **Atreya**, regarded as the father of Indian medicine as well as a great Hindu sage, provided descriptions of episodes of loss of consciousness with convulsions, and subsequent loss of memory. He also recognized four different types of epilepsy, with dribbling saliva, spasms, and other symptoms. Similar accounts of epilepsy can be found in early Chinese medical writings.

---

2   Bryant T (2005) *The Life and Times of Hammurabi*. Mitchell Lane Publishers, Hallandale, FL.
3   Kinnier Wilson JV and Reynolds EH (1990) Texts and documents. Translation and analysis of a cuneiform text forming part of a Babylonian treatise on epilepsy. *Medical History* 34, 185–198.

Ancient Greek and Roman period

The ancient Greeks had conflicting views about epilepsy, as they considered it to be a form of spiritual possession, but also associated the condition with genius and the divine. They believed that epilepsy was a consequence of sinning against Selene, the goddess of the moon. The conflict between magical beliefs and physical explanations for epilepsy dominated the early literature on the condition. Around 400 bce, the famous Greek physician **Hippocrates** rejected the idea that the disease was caused by spirits. In his landmark work entitled *On the Sacred Disease* he proposed that epilepsy was not divine in origin, but rather that it was a medically treatable problem that originated in the brain: 'Men regard its nature and cause as divine from ignorance and wonder, because it is not at all like to other diseases. ... Men being in want of the means of life, invent many and various things, and devise many contrivances for all other things, and for this disease, in every phase of the disease, assigning the cause to a god. ... Neither truly do I count it a worthy opinion to hold that the body of man is polluted by god, the most impure by the most holy.'[4] He postulated that the disease began with an accumulation of phlegm (one of the 'four humors') in the veins of the brain, and that once the disease had become established, speech was lost and foaming of the mouth and choking ensued. He believed that cosmic factors such as rain and wind released the phlegm, thereby altering the constituency of the brain and triggering the attack.

Hippocrates observed that children usually died as a result of their attacks, whereas the elderly tended to survive. He suggested that this was due to the small size of the veins within children's brains. He also made the astute observation that many people affected by epilepsy seemed to know when an attack was imminent, and would immediately make efforts to withdraw from human company due to feelings of shame. Intended for a lay readership, *On the Sacred Disease* was a strong written attack on the magicians and charlatans who had originally introduced the term 'sacred' in relation to epilepsy, and it emphasized the need to treat the condition not by magical cures but with drugs and dietary regimens. At that point in history all diseases were considered to be hereditary, and epilepsy had now been added to that category. The divine influence of the elements (including the wind, sun, and cold temperatures) on disease continued to be accepted, and to that extent the course of illness was considered to be subject to 'divine' influence. However, the underlying causes of illness and susceptibility to the forces of nature were now established as physical. Hippocrates described many of the manifestations of epilepsy, and his successors introduced the term

---

4   Temkin O (1971) *The Falling Sickness: A History of Epilepsy from the Greeks to the Beginnings of Modern Neurology*, 2nd edition. Johns Hopkins University Press, Baltimore, MD. p. 33.

aura (derived from the Greek word for 'breeze') to refer to the subjective onset that occurs before some seizures.

The Romans replaced the expression 'Sacred Disease' with the term 'Great Disease' (*morbus major*), which in French translation became *grand mal* – a term that is still used today to describe major tonic–clonic seizures (where the body becomes rigid in the tonic phase, and there is uncontrolled jerking in the clonic phase). The Romans also frequently used the term *morbus comitialis* to indicate how witnessing an epileptic attack could ruin the day for a crowd or public assembly (*comitia*). They considered individuals with epilepsy to be unclean, and they also believed that the condition was contagious, so would avoid eating and drinking from the same dish and cup used by persons with epilepsy. **Pliny**, a Roman writer, made the frank admission that 'in cases of epilepsy we spit, that is, we throw back contagion'. One of his contemporaries described the following behaviour of a superstitious individual: 'When he sees a madman or an epileptic person, he shudders and spits on his bosom.'[5] A contemporaneous account of an epileptic slave describes how his peers would spit on him and refuse to eat with him, in order to avoid becoming contaminated by him.

The treatments documented during ancient Greek and Roman times are too numerous to list here, but mostly involve cleansing the unclean or casting out evil. Meanwhile the early physicians used a range of bizarre therapies, including camel hair, sea-tortoise blood, crocodile faeces, and ram or boar testes. Over time these became replaced by less extreme treatments. Herbal remedies, such as peony root, were worn in an amulet, and there was a continuing belief in the importance of the stages of the moon in influencing seizures and insanity. **Galen** (*c.* 130–210 ce), a Turkish-born Greek physician and philosopher of the Roman Empire, noted that in women there was a relationship between fits, periods, and pregnancy. He also suggested that the aura that preceded an attack might indicate where in the brain a seizure might start. Galen's 'advice to an epileptic boy', a letter written to the boy's father around 190 ce, has been translated from the Greek by Oswei Temkin.[6] This letter is remarkable in outlining Galen's views on the causes of epilepsy, factors that need to be avoided, and possible treatments. He recommends the avoidance of sleeplessness, whirling wheels, thunder and lightning, strenuous baths, and emotional upset. Measures that he suggests should be taken following a seizure include rest and quiet. Lifestyle advice is also given, including the need for early rising, light exercise, study, and regular routines. He advises against swimming, and recommends a diet that provides regular intake of vinegar-honey, capers, and fresh fish. He also refers to a drug made from squills (a lily-like medicinal

---

5 Temkin O (1971) *The Falling Sickness: A History of Epilepsy from the Greeks to the Beginnings of Modern Neurology*, 2nd edition. Johns Hopkins University Press, Baltimore, MD. p. 8.
6 Temkin O (transl.) (1934) Galen's 'Advice for an epileptic boy'. *Bulletin of the Institute of the History of Medicine* 2, 179–189.

plant) to be taken over a period of 40 days, and he suggests the drinking of wormwood after vigorous evacuation of the bowels by means of a purgative, and before using the squill remedy.

Galen witnessed the visible manifestations of seizures and described them in meticulous detail. For example, he documented the progression of a seizure from onset to loss of consciousness, as well as the aura ('breeze'), as follows: 'I heard the boy say that his condition began in his lower leg and then moved up through the thigh, the groin and side of the chest above the affected thigh up to the neck and then to the head. As soon as [the condition] reached this part, he said that he was no longer aware of himself. When the doctors asked what the movement into the head was like, [another] boy said the movement upwards was like a cold breeze (aura).' Galen suggested that a typical case of chronic epilepsy would begin in childhood, and that if it did not disappear at puberty it would become more severe and worsen with age. Other authors described the effect of climate and the need to avoid certain foods and alcohol. Injuries to the skull were also reported to result in seizures that tended to affect the opposite side of the body to the site of injury. Galen was the first philosopher to speculate about the seat of the mind or soul, believing that the brain was the rational seat of the latter and that the heart was the spiritual seat. We echo this today when we tell people who are facing a difficult decision to follow their head and not their heart.

Theodorus Priscianus, a physician at Constantinople during the fourth century ce, wrote two textbooks on medicine, describing epilepsy in both of them. He provided one of the earliest descriptions of a grand mal seizure, with stiffening (tonic) and jerking (clonic) movements followed by deep sleep, and amnesia on recovery.[7] Other writers noted arching of the body, redness of the face, and biting of the tongue, and emphasized prolonged memory loss and confusion on recovery. These early descriptions were very variable, reflecting what we know today, namely that there are many different types of epilepsy.

Aretaeus of Cappadocia, a Greek physician who studied in Alexandria and practised in Rome in the second century ce, was considered second in importance only to Hippocrates, and revived many of the latter's teachings. He published two four-volume manuscripts, entitled *On the Causes and Symptoms of Acute and Chronic Diseases* and *On the Cure of Acute and Chronic Diseases*. He was among the first to describe diabetes and he also gave it its name, from the Greek word *diabetes* (meaning 'siphon', referring to the associated symptom of thirst). He noted that epilepsy could follow a chronic course after the first attack, becoming a lifelong condition. Aretaeus described tongue biting, clenched teeth, and incontinence during seizures, as well as commenting that 'lowness of spirits' could precede an attack.[8]

---

7   Stol M (1993) *Epilepsy in Babylonia*, Cuneiform Monographs 2. Styx Publications, Groningen.
8   Adams F (ed.) (1856) On epilepsy. In: *The Extant Work of Aretaeus*. The Sydenham Society, London. pp. 244–246.

The Roman encyclopaedist **Aulus Celsus** (*c.* 25 bce to *c.* 50 ce), in his eight-volume treatise *De Medicina* (*On Medicine*), was the first to introduce the term 'insanity' and to consider the possibility that listening to music might be therapeutic.[9] He cautioned against trying to arouse someone with epilepsy during a seizure, and he did not believe that bloodletting, a common practice at that time, served any useful therapeutic purpose. He recommended that emetics should be used, and that the sufferer's head should be shaved and then doused in vinegar. He advised avoiding both consumption of too much wine and exposure to extremes of temperature, and he advocated massage, exercise, and measures to reduce stress. Much of this lifestyle advice remains applicable in the twenty-first century, but in Celsus' day, if the seizures persisted the treatments would become more drastic, involving cautery, burning the nape of the neck, and bleeding the legs from above the ankles. His most dramatic treatment, which was used as a last resort, was based on his observation that 'some have freed themselves from such a disease [epilepsy] by drinking the hot blood from the cut throat of a gladiator: a miserable aid made tolerable by a malady still more miserable.'[10] Other authors suggested that the person having an epileptic seizure should be made to vomit during the attack (in order to get rid of excess phlegm) by tickling the back of the throat with a feather. Alternative remedies, among many others, included rubbing the limbs with particular ointments, or the application of oils to the scalp.

The ancient Greeks and Romans believed that once epilepsy was established and chronic there was little likelihood of complete recovery. They also highlighted the risk of sudden death in epilepsy, which is known today as sudden unexpected death in epilepsy (SUDEP). The followers of Hippocrates noted similarities between hysteria and epileptic attacks. The increased frequency of the former in women led those authors to suggest that the cause was related to the uterus. The use of the Greek word *hystera* (meaning 'uterus') strengthened this ancient belief that hysterical behaviour occurred only in women. Over time, the theory that uterine epilepsy was a discrete condition in which epilepsy and hysteria coexisted gained support, only to be dismissed later on. These early descriptions of hysteria are consistent with what is now known as non-epileptic attack disorder (NEAD) or pseudo-seizures. Celsus and his colleagues also noted a tendency in some women for epileptic attacks to occur most frequently around the time of menstruation, and today we refer to this as catamenial epilepsy (derived from the Greek word *katamēnios*, meaning 'monthly').

Although the theories of the ancient Greeks and Romans about the cause and treatment of epilepsy were wide of the mark, one can only marvel at the detailed accuracy and comprehensiveness of their clinical observations, and the value of these to understanding

---

9   Prioreschi P (1996) *A History of Medicine*. Horatius Press, Omaha, NE.
10 *De Medicina*; www.wdl.org/en/item/11618/

epilepsy. Aretaeus of Cappadocia in particular was a champion of the power of observation in the practice of what he termed 'the Art of Medicine', which allowed him to provide detailed and accurate descriptions of disorders as diverse as asthma and tetanus.

The medieval period (c. 500 to 1500 ce)

During the medieval period (also known as the Middle Ages), physicians inherited not only the detailed clinical observations of epilepsy made by the ancient Greeks and Romans, but also their misconceptions with regard to mysticism and demonic possession. Although a belief in the divine or sacred nature of epilepsy was still held by some, it had now been largely replaced by fear and prejudice. The scientific basis of illness remained a mystery, and was dominated by religious beliefs that diseases may reflect punishment for misdemeanours in an earlier life.

The scientific alternative to this view was the humoral theory of disease (also known as humorism), which dated back to the ancient Greeks and Romans, but was to continue to influence European medical thinking up until the nineteenth century. It was central to the teachings of both Hippocrates and Galen. According to this theory, the four humors existed as internal body fluids: sanguine (blood), choleric (yellow bile), melancholic (black bile), and phlegmatic (phlegm). The humors represented the elements and could be externally influenced by them. Blood represented air, phlegm represented water, yellow bile represented fire, and black bile represented earth. Each humor was associated with a season (for example, blood was linked with spring). All four of these humors, or vital fluids, were believed to be present in the bloodstream in varying quantities, and their balance within the body was considered to determine illness and personality. In medieval times the equilibrium of the four humors was considered to be critical to the understanding of disease and its treatment. This concept of 'humoral constitutionalism' dating back to the time of Galen resulted in the use of cleansing treatments such as purgation and bloodletting, and dominated medical practice for centuries to come.

(We still use the terms 'phlegmatic', 'sanguine', and 'melancholic' to describe a person's personality. The influence of this legacy from our Greek forebears can also be seen in English literature, especially in Shakespeare's moulding of the characters in his plays, which are dominated by sanguine, melancholic, and choleric personalities.)

Epilepsy was believed to be caused by the phlegmatic humor, which was described as cold and wet, and included not only phlegm, but also all the other clear fluids of the body (mucus, saliva, plasma, lymph, and interstitial fluids). This humor was considered to have an expulsive force that flushed out impurities, transported essential nutrients, and eliminated waste, and it was thought to reside in the veins and lymphatics of the body. The notion that epilepsy could be attributed to an imbalance of phlegm is interesting when one considers the contrast between the phlegmatic personality type and the so-called 'epileptic personality'. The former is characterized by an even temperament without emotional outbursts, anger, bitterness, or an unforgiving nature. The latter has been described by some twentieth-century writers as an impulsive and egocentric temperament, and will be discussed in Chapter 11.

Medieval physicians maintained the Babylonian and early Jewish belief that demonic possession was the main cause of all epilepsy. This inevitably led to prejudice, social isolation, and treatment by exorcism. A religious treatment for an irreligious state of being seemed logical, and as well as the adoption of ritualistic measures such as exorcism, incarceration, and even execution, terms such as 'witch' and 'warlock' were widely used to describe the 'epileptic'. In the Christian world, views about the nature, treatment, and disposal of people with epilepsy were now strongly influenced by the domination of the Catholic Church.[11] This led to the superstitious and discriminatory belief that epileptics could be universally regarded as 'possessed', and that the Church alone could cure them, by whatever means necessary. The Catholic Church perceived seizures as the 'rod of Christ' or the 'shaking punishment of God' being inflicted upon those who had sinned.

The early eleventh-century scholar and Benedictine abbess **St Hildegard of Bingen** (1098–1179) gained her medical knowledge from a monastery library and became skilled at healing, as well as an influential scientific writer and observer of illness.[12] In 2012 she was honoured as Doctor of the Church by Pope Benedict XV1. In her book *Causae et Curae* she described two forms of epilepsy. In the first form a 'vengeful wrath sets the blood in motion', whereas the second form occurs in those 'with unstable or low morals'. She accepted the humoral theory of disease, but regarded sin as an external factor that could disrupt and precipitate specific illnesses. Therefore she appears to be saying that her first type of epilepsy was caused by internal forces beyond the individual's control, whereas the second type was a deserved punishment.

Arnald of Villanova (1240–1311), a Spanish physician, alchemist, and religious reformer, was forced to escape the Spanish Inquisition because of his writings. He produced the most influential medieval text on epilepsy, entitled *De Epilepsia*, in which he stated that the diet was the most important aspect of the treatment of epilepsy, and he emphasized the significance of the stars and the moon in predicting the timing of seizures. He advocated the application of leeches and a poultice consisting of ravens' eggs, precious stones and pigeon dung as treatments. He believed that physical treatments alone were required, and that the use

---

11 Diamantis A, Sidiropoulou K and Magiorkinis E (2010) Epilepsy during the Middle Ages, the Renaissance and the Enlightenment. *Journal of Neurology* 257, 691–698.
12 Flanagan S (1989) *Hildegard of Bingen: A Visionary Life*, 2nd edition. Routledge, London.

of magic, divine symbols, and prayers should be discouraged, and he denounced conjurors and augurs or fortune tellers. He divided epilepsy into two categories, namely what he called 'true epilepsy', caused by phlegm, and 'spurious epilepsy', caused by a mixture of black bile and phlegm. Although he did not look to religion as a possible form of treatment, he did make an appeal to Jesus Christ to show compassion for those with this 'unfortunate disease'.

John of Gaddesden (1280–1361) was the most famous English physician of the early fourteenth century. In his book *Rosa Medicinae*, the leading medical textbook of its time, he made many astute observations on epilepsy.[13] He described flickering lights and loud noises as triggers of seizures, and noted that childhood epilepsy can often resolve over time. The treatments he suggested for epilepsy ranged from fasting to the wearing of a cuckoo's beak around the neck to draw out the seizure. Like Galen, whose writings he had studied, he recognized three different types of epilepsy, which he termed 'minor', 'medium' and 'major' according to whether they were due to obstruction of the arteries, nerves, or ventricles (cavities) within the brain. In order to rid people with epilepsy of their (presumed) excessive phlegm, he concocted a prescription that consisted of a large number of herbs mixed with honey; this was expensive and almost certainly ineffective. Despite his generally advanced views about epilepsy, the few hospitals that existed at that time would not generally admit people with epilepsy, as it was believed that only the clergy could treat the condition. The predominant approach involved casting out the demon by prayer: 'Howbeit this kind goeth not out but by prayer and fasting' (Matthew 17:21, King James Version).

From the mists of confusion as to whether epilepsy had a physical or demonic cause emerged **Joan of Arc** (1412–1431), the 'Maid of Orléans'. From the age of 13 she experienced visions and voices that have since been widely viewed as symptoms of temporal lobe epilepsy. Records of her trial provide a detailed description of the episodes, during which she experienced voices and visions, which were felt to give her a sense of divine mission. Her accounts of these experiences resulted in her being accused of witchcraft and heresy, and she was eventually burned at the stake.[14] Her name was later cleared, she went on to become the patron saint of France, and she was canonized in 1920. The cases for and against Joan of Arc having epilepsy will be discussed in detail in Chapter 9.

In 1487, *Malleus Maleficarum* ('The Hammer of Witches'), regarded for several centuries as the standard text on witchcraft, was written by the German clergyman Johann Sprenger and the German theologian and inquisitor Heinrich Kraemer, who persisted in linking witchcraft and disability. Pope Innocent VIII had denounced the spread of what he perceived as witchcraft in Germany, and had authorized Sprenger and Kraemer to eradicate

---

13 Lennox WG (1939) John of Gaddesden on epilepsy. *Annals of Medical History* 1, 283–307.
14 Nicastro N and Picard F (2016) Joan of Arc: Sanctity, witchcraft or epilepsy? *Epilepsy & Behavior* 57, 247–250.

it. Kraemer had already been denounced by his local bishop because of his methods of interrogating women standing trial for witchcraft. *Malleus Maleficarum* described how to identify witches and warlocks, based on their impairments and their ability to pass these on to others or by giving birth to a disabled child. It recommended torture as a means of obtaining confessions, and the death penalty as the appropriate punishment for witchcraft. The book referred to epilepsy several times, and suggested that witches spread epilepsy to others rather than necessarily having it themselves: 'But there is no bodily infirmity, not even leprosy or epilepsy, which cannot be caused by witches. … For we have often found that certain people have been visited with epilepsy or the falling sickness by means of eggs which have been buried with dead bodies, especially the dead bodies of witches, together with other ceremonies of which we cannot speak, particularly when these eggs have been given to a person either in food or drink.'[15] At the height of the witch hunts, between 1490 and 1680, the 'Hammer of Witches' went through 70 editions in 14 languages, and was second only to the Bible in its sales.

Medieval and Renaissance paintings, altarpieces, and frescos abound with illustrations of exorcisms or the 'casting out' of demons or unclean spirits by Jesus Christ and numerous saints. It is unclear whether this iconography was depicting epilepsy or a whole host of physical illnesses, such as leprosy, as the characteristics of an evolving seizure cannot be captured in the single frame of a painting. However, some works of art, such as Raphael's *Transfiguration*, portray an image that does suggest an epileptic attack, whereas others that depict individuals in a state of collapse or loss of consciousness are open to many different medical interpretations. In this Christian art, the beneficiary of the 'casting out' is usually depicted in rags and of inferior social status. By now, in line with the Church's changing religious interpretation of epilepsy, the descriptive term 'sacred illness' had been replaced by 'falling evil'.

Over subsequent years, a more caring attitude towards those with epilepsy gradually emerged. **St Valentine**, a medieval saint, was said to have treated the condition. His name was probably derived from the similarity between the sounds of the words for 'Valentine' and 'fallen' in the German language, and in 1486 his followers established an isolation hospital in Upper Alsace, due to the continuing belief that the condition was contagious. There in the Cloister of St Valentine at Rufach the inmates were denied the Eucharist because it was feared they would infect the communion cup and plate. The link between the moon and epilepsy still prevailed, and the term 'lunacy' became synonymous both with this association and with madness. Even today some people believe that seizures are more likely to occur at full moon.

---

15   Mackay C (2009) *The Hammer of Witches: A Complete Translation of the Malleus Maleficarum*. Cambridge University Press, Cambridge.

A late fifteenth-century woodcut, currently in the National Gallery of Art in Washington, shows St Valentine praying for two people who are lying on the ground (see Figure 1), echoing accounts in the Bible of similar behaviour by Jesus. It is now believed that it is possible there was more than one St Valentine. Another saint who is thought to have helped those suffering from epilepsy was St Vitus. His name gave rise to the term 'St Vitus' dance', which was used to describe epilepsy, or possibly another neurological disorder characterized by involuntary movements, now known as chorea.

Much of the background to the perception of people with epilepsy as being somehow tainted can be found in religious writings. No book in the Christian world had a greater impact on public perception than the King James Bible, and epilepsy and its 'casting out' make several appearances in three of the four Gospels of the New Testament:

'Teacher, I brought you my son; he has a spirit that makes him unable to speak; and whenever it seizes him, it dashes him down; and he foams and grinds his teeth and becomes rigid; and I asked your disciples to cast it out, but they could not do so.' He [Jesus] answered them, 'You faithless generation, how much longer must I be among you? How much longer must I put up with you? Bring him to me.' And they brought the boy to him. When the spirit saw him, immediately it threw the boy into convulsions, and he fell on the ground and rolled about, foaming at the mouth. Jesus asked the father, 'How long has this been happening to him?' And he said, 'From childhood. It has often cast him into the fire and into the water, to destroy him; but if you are able to do anything, have pity on us and help us.'

(Mark 9:17–22, New Revised Standard Version)

Towards the end of the sixteenth century, no longer so bound by the dogmas of the church, physicians began to view epilepsy as a disease rather than some form of supernatural curse, and they then started to explore possible causes and appropriate treatments. Up until that time, European medicine had been dominated by 'humoral constitutionalism', with illness considered to be caused by an imbalance of the four humors. This preoccupation with humoral balance had dominated medical practice and impeded progress in understanding the pathogenesis of disease.

Philippus von Hoenheim (1493–1571), a Swiss physician, alchemist, and astrologer of the German Renaissance, better known as **Paracelsus**, wrote about the pathology and treatment of epilepsy and devoted a whole book to what he termed the 'divine evil', entitled *On Diseases that Deprive Man of his Reason* (1525). Not without controversy, as his beliefs were often wildly inconsistent, he nevertheless advanced chemistry from alchemy into a science, and he formulated theories on the universe and its formation. He introduced into medicine the theory of Hermeticism, in which sickness and health were attributed to the balance between the person, nature, and the environment. At last an alternative to the humoral theory started to emerge. Paracelsus believed that epilepsy was a physical disease and not an unnatural, mystical experience, and to support this view he cited the fact that other animals could also have seizures. He commented that 'Doctors who thrive on slight diseases which cure themselves, but pretend that epilepsy is incurable, are frauds.' However, he also noted that it was not always possible to cure the cause ('root') of the disease, but in such cases the symptoms could be treated (that is, it was possible to 'prevent the root from growing'). In today's terminology he was expounding the principles of symptomatic therapy. He also emphasized the need for a more compassionate approach to the 'unfortunate disease' than had previously been offered, and recommended that the physician should seek divine help when treating epilepsy. He concluded that 'God has provided remedies for all diseases, including epilepsy.'[16]

Despite his enlightened views about the condition, Paracelsus also held many erroneous beliefs about epilepsy. He suggested that it originated in the liver, heart, intestines, or limbs, rather than in the brain. He also believed that earthquakes had an epileptic nature: 'earthquakes and the falling sickness have the same causes'. He suggested that something that boiled internally produced vapours that affected the whole body, and that the type of attack or the way in which it manifested was influenced by the specific location in the body where the boiling had originated.

The rationale for many of Paracelsus' proposed treatments for epilepsy was based on his interest in chemistry and his theory of spontaneous boiling within the body (*spiritus vitae*) as the cause of the condition. As well as inorganic substances such as oil of vitriol that would soothe and quell the symptoms, he also suggested opium (*Papaver somniferum*), autumn mandrake (*Mandragora*), and nightshade (*Hyoscyamus*). Although opium may have had some effect, it is doubtful whether this would have been true of any of the other treatments mentioned.

The Italian physician and botanist **Andrea Cesalpino** (1519–1603) attempted to distinguish between the features of epilepsy and demonic possession so that the treatments advocated by Paracelsus could be applied to the former, and divine intervention to the latter. This significant and undervalued contribution resulted in accusations of heresy, of which he was acquitted. Cesalpino's interest in classifying seeds and his work as director of the Botanical Garden in Pisa inevitably led him to study the medicinal properties of plants in relation to many conditions, including epilepsy.

---

16 Jacobi J (ed.) (1951) *Paracelsus: Selected Writings*. Princeton University Press, Princeton, NJ.

In the seventeenth century a number of treatises were produced on the mechanisms of epileptic seizures, and also on the occurrence of seizures in various medical conditions that were known to affect the brain directly, such as tumours and syphilis. **Jean Taxil** (1564–1618), a French physician, conducted post-mortem examinations of children who had died as a result of epilepsy. In his two-volume book *Traicté de l'épilepsie* he listed possible causes of death, among which he included toxins and poisons.[17] However, he was a deeply religious man and remained convinced that demonic processes were also implicated. He believed that any person who was possessed by a demon would also be epileptic, and that by drilling a hole in the skull using simple surgical tools (a procedure known as trepanning or trephining) it was possible to release the demon from the brain. This is probably the oldest surgical procedure for which there is archaeological evidence, dating back to 6500 bce, and Galen, Hippocrates and others cited it as a way of releasing vapours, or even devils, from the brain. Taxil also claimed that the skull itself had curative powers, and that shavings from it placed over the sutures of the skull of a person with epilepsy, or even a potion made from skull scrapings, could be curative. He based his treatment on the observation that in Neolithic times it was common practice to wear bones around the neck to ward off evil spirits. Skull shavings continued to be used as an epilepsy treatment for many years.[18] As a growing number of seventeenth-century physicians began to claim that irritation of the brain by vapours or poisonous substances could cause epilepsy, this treatment approach gained increasing support.

Thomas Willis (1621–1675), a physician and anatomist, is regarded as the founder of neurology, the specialty that now provides medical care for people with epilepsy. After studying medicine, he served as a Royalist soldier during the English Civil War,[19] but he was to become widely known as a result of the extraordinary case of Anne Green. The bodies of executed criminals were commonly used for anatomical dissection during the education of medical students. When the hanged body of Anne Green, a servant girl who had been executed for concealing her own stillborn child, was presented to Thomas Willis and William Petty, an anatomist. At Petty's lodgings, Willis noticed that she was still alive and he resuscitated her. She was subsequently pardoned and went on to have three children, and Willis's reputation spread far and wide. It was then cemented by his written works.[20]

In his book *Cerebri Anatome* ('The Anatomy of the Brain') (1664) he provided a detailed description of the internal structure of the brain, and was the first writer to use the word 'neurology' (which appeared in the English translation of the Greek term *neurologia*) to refer

---

17 Taxil J (1602) *Traicté de l'épilepsie*. Robert Renaud libraire, Lyon.
18 Arnott R, Finger S and Smith CUM (eds.) (2003) *Trepanation: History, Discovery, Theory*. Swets & Zeitlinger, Lisse, The Netherlands.
19 Hughes JT (1991) *Thomas Willis, 1621–1675: His Life and Work*. Royal Society of Medicine, London.
20 Rose FC (2012) *The History of British Neurology*. Imperial College Press, London.

to the study of the function and disorders of the nervous system. *Pathologiae Cerebri et Nervosa* ('On the Pathology of the Brain and Nerves') (1667) was an essay on convulsive disorders, and *De Anima Brutorum Quae Homine Vitalis ac Sensitiva est* ('On the Soul of Brutes Which is That of the Vital and Sensitive of Man') (1672) outlined the clinical picture of various illnesses. Through these three books Willis firmly established epilepsy as a disorder of the brain, and classified the condition into different types of seizure, according to the part of the brain in which they originated. He also distinguished between hereditary and non-hereditary epilepsy, noted that loss of consciousness does not always occur, and speculated as to whether the post-mortem finding of a 'heap' of blood within the brain was the cause or the result of the fatal seizure.

Willis wrote in Latin, and his works were translated into readable English by the poet Samuel Pordage, who collected all of Willis's writings on the treatment of illnesses in a book entitled *The London Practice of Physick* (1685). Willis advocated a two-step approach to the treatment of epilepsy – to limit the current attack, and to prevent the next one. These principles of epilepsy treatment, namely acute management and prevention (prophylaxis), still apply today.

Willis believed that during the seizure the use of bloodletting and emetics was required, together with strong smelling salts (such as ammonia) to aid recovery of consciousness. His prophylactic treatments for prevention of future attacks aimed to remove the source or cause of the seizure, and involved further bloodletting, purging, cauterizing, and 'specific' remedies such as peony, castor oil, and assorted minerals. The aim of these specific remedies was to strengthen the brain as well as to purify animal spirits that Willis believed might be moving in and out of the brain through what he described as 'gaping pores'. The use of bleeding, cauterizing, and purging with various additional medicines remained the mainstay of treatment well into the eighteenth century.

Despite the published works of Willis and the evolving medical literature of that time, the public perception that seizures represented demonic forces persisted. The Salem Witches Trial is believed to have been initiated when several young girls had convulsions that were thought to be a manifestation of magic, and then other people started to exhibit similar behaviour. Clearly it was no longer believed that witches passed on epilepsy but did not have the condition themselves. The epilepsy-like attacks engendered fear and repulsion among the population of Salem, Massachusetts, and between 1692 and 1693 more than 200 people were accused of witchcraft, 19 of whom were found guilty and hanged. The cause of the attacks that led to the accusation of witchcraft remains a mystery, although hysteria, epilepsy, or even poisoning through crop failure resulting in the consumption of rye infected with ergot, are the most likely explanations.

The Convulsionists of Saint Médard were a curious eighteenth-century religious sect. In a similar manner to events in Salem, one member of the sect would start to exhibit body shaking, grimacing, and foaming at the mouth, and others then displayed similar behaviour. A large number of sect members who had seizures were unmarried adolescent girls. Lindsay Wilson points out that the physicians of the time attributed the convulsions to female hysteria, sexual frustration, and menstrual irregularities, as well as the inherent moral inferiority of women.[21] However, the attacks attracted hostility among the wider public, with punishment by imprisonment in the Bastille, and the stigmatization of epilepsy through association.

The Enlightenment

The Age of Enlightenment (also known as the Age of Reason) was an intellectual movement that dominated Western Europe from the mid seventeenth century to the late eighteenth century. It encompassed a range of ideas on philosophy, science, art, and politics that centred on reason, and it marked the beginning of the age of free speech and thought. Scientific academies and societies were formed, links with universities were established, and scientific advancement was widely associated with the overthrow of established religion and orthodoxy. In this era, physicians had still not completely abandoned the idea that epilepsy was the devil's work. The belief that Christ had cured an epileptic boy possessed by an unclean spirit supported the view that supernatural forces must be implicated. **Jonathan Harle**, an English minister and physician, stated 'that there were some actually possessed by the devil is a truth as plain as words can make it.'[22] Although the idea of demonic possession gradually disappeared from many of the more advanced medical writings of the time, it was still championed by some, and such a belief was almost universally held among the poorly educated. Then, as now, the education of an uninformed public about epilepsy was a major challenge.

Justinus Kerner (1786–1862) was a German physician and poet famous for his interest in inkblots (long before Rorschach's inkblot test) and the eccentric poems that he wrote about them. He made a major effort to revive belief in demonic possession, emphasizing that it was the sole cause of epilepsy. However, by now he was in a minority, as the Enlightenment rejected the occult with its superstitions and beliefs in witches and warlocks. The idea that a person could be possessed by a spirit was no longer considered reasonable by the scientific community, even if the public were not yet on board.

The theory that the moon exerted some influence on epilepsy persisted right up until the end of the seventeenth century. Isaac Newton had shown that the moon had a gravitational effect on the Earth and the oceans' tides, so it was considered not unreasonable to suppose that

---

21 Wilson L (1993) *Women and Medicine in the French Enlightenment.* Johns Hopkins University Press, Baltimore, MD.
22 Temkin O (1971) *The Falling Sickness: A History of Epilepsy from the Greeks to the Beginnings of Modern Neurology*, 2nd edition. Johns Hopkins University Press, Baltimore, MD. p. 71.

it could also affect human health. Some physicians believed that the stars could have physical effects on the human body and on the animal kingdom in general. **Richard Mead** (1673–1754), an English physician, described seizures occurring at the new or full moons around the spring or autumn equinox. The scientists and philosophers of the Enlightenment became increasingly sceptical about the ever more unlikely claims that were being made for the power of the moon, and eventually the notion of a lunar influence on physical illness was dismissed.

The Dutch physician **Gerald van Swieten** (1700–1772) argued against superstitious views, particularly in relation to vampires, and wrote a discourse that claimed to disprove the existence of ghosts. He became personal physician to Maria Theresa, the Austrian Empress, and was also renowned in the field of medical education. He commented that it was not surprising that a disorder with such variable and alarming symptoms as epilepsy had been linked to the supernatural. He also provided a description of the clinical features of epilepsy, and a comparison of these with stroke (apoplexy) and hysteria.

The Swiss physician **Samuel-Auguste Tissot** (1728–1787), who held the position of Calvinist Protestant adviser to the Vatican, made both positive and negative contributions to our understanding of epilepsy in his *Treatise on Epilepsy* (1770). At that time it was widely believed that most epilepsy was hereditary, reflecting the 'taint' of the mother, father, or earlier generations. It was also thought that the shock of witnessing a seizure while pregnant could pass epilepsy on to the baby, and that either this or questionable paternity would account for cases where there was no family history of the condition. Tissot acknowledged that hereditary factors were important, to the extent that he recommended that people with epilepsy should not have children. However, he refuted the idea that witnessing a seizure during pregnancy could pass epilepsy on to the offspring.

For the next 100 years, Tissot's main legacy was his erroneous belief that sexual excess was the cause of many diseases, including epilepsy, and that masturbation had an even greater effect than debauchery. This view led to clitoridectomy, castration, or (in pre-pubertal boys) circumcision being regarded as suitable treatment options in extreme cases. Although his book *On Masturbation* became one of the medical best-sellers of that era, he admitted that the cause of seizures was very often unknown, and he introduced the term 'essential epilepsy' to describe cases in which there was no obvious cause. He recognized that disruption of the brain itself might sometimes be a cause of epilepsy, and he cited the case of a young man whose headaches and seizures were shown by post-mortem findings to have been caused by a brain tumour.

Tissot also recommended trepanning or trephining (the drilling of a hole in the skull using simple surgical tools) as a treatment for epilepsy, particularly in cases where there was a skull fracture or deformity, or if it was suspected that there was an accumulation of fluid on the brain. This represents one of the earliest suggestions that brain surgery, targeted at a specific site and condition, might alleviate seizures. The procedure continued to be used as a treatment for epilepsy right up until the early twentieth century.[23]

The drug and physical treatments provided by the physicians of the Enlightenment have overtones of therapeutic nihilism. In an age of reason, if the cause of epilepsy was not known it was considered unreasonable to suggest a cure. It was recognized that if seizures could be prevented or controlled a cure might be possible, but apart from recommending a healthy lifestyle free from stress, little other advice could be offered. However, there was a growing awareness of the pathology of epilepsy, a greater understanding of the different types of seizure, and the emergence of experimental or animal models of the condition.

During the late seventeenth and early eighteenth centuries there was little progress in the search for the cause of epilepsy, until the Swiss anatomist and naturalist **Albrecht von Haller** (1708–1777), often referred to as the 'father of modern physiology',[24] introduced the concept of 'irritability'. He defined this as a sudden contracture or jerk, normally confined to muscles, that was the property of the sensibility of nerves in response to a stimulus. He noted that neither the brain nor the membranes and tissues that surrounded it had the property of movement, and thus movement of the brain alone could not account for seizures. He knew that muscles contracted when the nerves that supplied them were stimulated, and he suggested that such stimulation arising in the brain and then travelling down nerves accounted for the shaking of limbs that was observed during seizures. Haller believed that the irritability that caused epilepsy originated deep within the brain, in the medulla, rather than on its surface or cortex.

However, the cause of the irritability remained elusive, although various implausible suggestions were offered by other writers, including compression, animal spirits, and vapours. Indeed it was not until the late eighteenth century that the doctrine of animal spirits disappeared from the lexicon of epilepsy causes. Haller had stumbled close to the truth by suggesting that abnormal energy within the brain resulted in seizures, but in the absence of a credible explanation for this, the search for the cause of epilepsy was diverted to the exploration of what we would now call 'risk factors' in people with epilepsy.

By the second half of the eighteenth century, the Scottish physician **William Cullen** (1712–1790) had become a renowned medical teacher in Europe and further afield. As Professor of Medicine in Edinburgh he was a central figure in the Scottish Enlightenment, and a friend of such luminaries of the movement as David Hume, Adam Smith, Joseph Black, and Adam Ferguson.[25] Cullen was heavily influenced by the work of Haller. He

---

23 Munro JC (1904) Report of cases of trephining for epilepsy. *Boston Medical and Surgical Journal* 150, 109–115.
24 Frixione E (2006) Albrecht von Haller (1708–1777). *Journal of Neurology* 253, 265–266.
25 Doig A, Ferguson JPS, Milne LA et al. (eds.) (1993) *William Cullen and the Eighteenth Century Medical World*. Edinburgh University Press, Edinburgh. pp. 40–55.

defined illnesses as being due to an excess or deficiency of irritability, and he considered disorders of the nervous system to be the result of stimulation or sedation. He applied this concept to epilepsy in his writings entitled *First Lines of the Practice of Physic* (1777), in which he classified causes as either proximate (the basic underlying physiological process) or remote (factors that trigger the process, such as penetrating head injury, violent emotions, or unpleasant painful challenges such as renal colic and stomach ulcers). His writings contain no mention either of hereditary factors or of devils, demons, and animal spirits.

Taking his lead from Tissot, Cullen attempted to produce a classification of the epilepsies, which he based on two main categories – idiopathic and symptomatic. The term 'idiopathic' is used in medicine to denote any disease or condition that appears to have no obvious cause or explanation, whereas the term 'symptomatic' indicates that there is a known cause, such as a head injury. Cullen defined three further subdivisions: epilepsia cerebralis, which has a sudden onset with no warning; epilepsia sympathetica, in which the attack is preceded by a warning or aura; and epilepsia occasionalis, in which removal of an 'irritating factor' causes the seizures to cease. His list of such irritating factors was extensive, and included head injury, poisoning, and unspecified mental conditions. Remnants of Cullen's classification persist to this day, despite the fact that many of his contemporaries were extremely critical of it.

Haller's concept of the irritability and sensitivity of the nervous system was carried forward into the nineteenth century by the Italian toxicologist and physicist **Abbé Felice Fontana** (1730–1805), who conducted experiments on the nerves and brains of animals. These studies demonstrated that seizures could be reproduced by stimulating the surface (cortex) of the brain with electricity. This indicated that seizures could arise from the surface of the brain, not just from deep within the medulla or brainstem as had previously been believed. Fontana described the differences between the grey matter (nerve cell bodies) and the white matter (nerve axons) of the brain, and also demonstrated that the retina (the part of the eye that senses light and creates nerve impulses) is connected to the brain.[26]

Conclusion

The first 2000 years or so of the history of epilepsy have taken us a long way down the path towards understanding the condition. However, by the end of the Enlightenment there was still no known treatment, the mechanism underlying seizures remained obscure, and despite the fact that medical science had refuted the notion that demons and animal spirits were

---

26 Garrison FH (1935) Felice Fontana: A forgotten physiologist of the Trentino. *Bulletin of the New York Academy of Medicine* 11, 117–122.

involved, beliefs about demonic possession and madness were still widespread among the general population. Prejudice, stigma, and rejecting attitudes prevailed, and there was still little prospect of hope for those with a 'Sacred Disease' that had to be endured without respite.

The Age of Enlightenment in Europe allowed physicians and scientists to abandon the religious dogmas without fear of persecution. The humoral theory of illness was beginning to be discredited, and the scientific community was dismissing beliefs that epilepsy was a punishment for misdemeanours in an earlier life, a curse passed down within a family, or a condition dispensed by witches and warlocks. However, these beliefs were still harboured by the general population. The theory that seizures were caused by vapours and poisons was losing support, and the emergence of pathological and experimental studies was beginning to allow the development of a better understanding of epilepsy. The brain was now considered to be the site of origin of seizures, and irritation of the brain was regarded as the mechanism involved. In some cases, head injuries and tumours were accepted as causal factors. The ancients had passed on their clinical observations on seizures, giving their successors the scientific basis needed to further their understanding of epilepsy and thus to develop logical and effective treatments for the condition. Throughout this period, the voice of those with epilepsy had been silenced, as it would continue to be for a long time to come.

CHAPTER 2

Epilepsy from the nineteenth century to the present

By the early nineteenth century, scientific advances were gathering pace and it was increasingly being recognized that epilepsy was a physical disorder. We shall first look at the epilepsy treatments that were developed in the nineteenth century, and consider the effect of public perceptions of epilepsy during the Victorian period, when the huge stigma that had once surrounded the condition resurfaced. We shall then examine the major advances that have been made over the last 120 years.

The early nineteenth century

In the early years of the century, people with severe epilepsy began to be hospitalized, rather than being sent to prison, the poorhouse, asylums for the insane, or hospices for the incurable, as had previously been their destiny. In England, France, and Italy, people with epilepsy were starting to receive medical care in institutions that had been established for their welfare as well as for enabling them to learn basic occupational skills.

The French psychiatrist **Jean-Étienne Esquirol** (1772–1840) had a major role in establishing hospital- or colony-based accommodation specifically for people with epilepsy, thus separating them from those deemed insane. He worked at the famous Salpêtrière Hospital in Paris, a building that had previously been used to house beggars and outcasts, and which derived its name from the fact that it was built on the site of a former gunpowder factory. Esquirol envisaged a role for psychiatrists in caring for people accused of crimes for which they were not responsible by reason of insanity, as well as for those with epilepsy. In 1805 he published his views in his seminal work *Mental Maladies: A Treatise on Insanity*. As a teacher he established his reputation in 1817 by giving the first formal tutorials in psychiatry, in the Salpêtrière Hospital dining hall. In view of the fact that he was considered to be the father of French psychiatry, Esquirol's reasons for separating those with epilepsy from those who were deemed insane are somewhat surprising. His rationale was to protect those who were mentally ill from those who had epilepsy, based on his continued belief that epilepsy might be contagious, or that the sight of a seizure might trigger epilepsy in those who witnessed it, as he pointed out that the mentally deranged were impressionable and easily given to mimicry.

Esquirol began to experiment with various treatments, and every year would conduct a clinical trial involving the treatment of a group of around 30 patients with bloodletting, cold baths, and herbal remedies such as mistletoe. The predictable failure of each of these approaches reinforced the negative beliefs about the treatability of epilepsy.

The French physician **Jacques Gilles Maisonneuve** (1745–1826) studied at the Salpêtrière Hospital around the time that Esquirol was working there, and in 1805 published his key work *Recherches et Observations sur l'Épilepsie*. He had been schooled to believe that epilepsy was best studied in the favourable environment of residential care. Introducing the concept of clinical investigation, he stated that 'first of all epilepsy, like all chronic diseases, can be studied only in the hospitals; there alone is it possible to find all its varieties together, to see it in all its nuances and to acquire in a short time more experience of the disease than in the whole course of ordinary practice.'[27] This was a clarion call for specialist care for people with epilepsy, and it comes as no surprise that for many years thereafter the most valuable studies on epilepsy were conducted in asylum and hospital wards for epileptic patients.

Esquirol was among those early epilepsy specialists who made important clinical observations on the nature and form of epilepsy. In *Des Maladies Mentales* he introduced the terms *grand mal* and *petit mal* to differentiate between severe and milder attacks, and he illustrated these with line drawings. Other clinical investigators at the Salpêtrière Hospital and elsewhere introduced the term *status epilepticus* to describe a series of seizures, with progression from one to the next without interruption or the regaining of consciousness. They re-defined the epileptic aura (or 'breeze') that had been first recognized by the ancient Greeks, and they identified the various different forms of aura. The categorization of the

---

27 Temkin O (1971) *The Falling Sickness: A History of Epilepsy from the Greeks to the Beginnings of Modern Neurology*, 2nd edition. Johns Hopkins University Press, Baltimore, MD. p. 257.

many different types of epilepsy would lay the foundations for future studies of the incidence, causes, outcomes, and treatments of the condition.

Esquirol was also one of the first to attempt to determine the incidence of epilepsy – that is, the frequency with which seizures occurred. In his book *Des Maladies Mentales* he describes how he counted 389 epileptic women at Salpêtrière Hospital and 162 epileptic men at Bicêtre Hospital in Paris. The latter had originally been a prison, and then an asylum (the many inmates of which included the notorious Marquis de Sade), before it became a men's hospital. The link between Salpetrière and Bicêtre Hospitals had attracted some notoriety in the eighteenth century when the mentally ill patients from each hospital had been forcibly married and then sent out to populate the French colonies of the Americas.

The use of such large patient numbers in medical studies was leading to the dawn of medical statistics, and Esquirol's information on these 551 patients provided demographic data that are still relevant today. The gender imbalance would tend to suggest not that epilepsy was twice as common among women as in men, but rather that men under-reported the condition. The data on the marital status of the men (no such data were available for the women) revealed that the vast majority (119 out of 162) were unmarried. Investigations of these and other hospital populations found histories of both epilepsy and mental illness in the families of sufferers. Data on age of onset revealed an association between the first seizure and menstruation in young girls. The search for causes addressed everything from bad teeth to skin complaints, as well as the usual suspects relating to mental state and lifestyle, particularly drunkenness, debauchery, and masturbation; head injury and childbirth were also regarded as likely candidates.

The social consequences of epilepsy were also starting to be documented. **Jacques-Louis Doussin-Dubreuil** (1762–1831), a French physician, focused on the morality of the individual as a potential cause of epilepsy. In his book *On Epilepsy in General and Particularly that Determined by Moral Causes* (1825) he revised the theory that epilepsy was caused by the moral state and emotions of the individual and arose from the heart. Sadness, isolation, anger, and misery were considered to be the major causative factors, and it was believed that they gave rise to what became known as the 'epileptic personality'. The promotion of the concept of such a personality owes much to the French psychiatrist **Bénédict Augustin Morel** (1809–1873). His own experience of abandonment as a small child almost certainly gave rise to his theory that the mental problems of adulthood could all be traced back to childhood traumas. With regard to epilepsy he noted that irritability, anger, and fury were characteristic of the personality that accompanied it. He believed that epileptic fury could be related to the timing of seizures, being evident either just before or immediately afterwards, or it could be unrelated. This led to the belief in 'epileptic insanity', a state that was thought to occur immediately before or after a fit. Morel, as director of an asylum for those deemed to be insane, regularly encountered people with chronic uncontrolled epilepsy, and based his views about the personality of people with epilepsy on this population. However, the anger and irritability that he identified could have been entirely due to the effect of being institutionalized. He also introduced the term 'masked epilepsy' to denote insanity in those who had no visible features of the condition, but whose mental symptoms resembled those that he had documented in patients with obvious epilepsy.

Although most of the early-nineteenth-century theories and observational studies of epilepsy had originated from continental Europe, and from France in particular, Britain had its own early investigators who were following in the footsteps of Thomas Willis and William Cullen. **James Cowles Prichard** (1786–1848) was a British physician and anthropologist with an interest in psychiatry. He became a Medical Commissioner in Lunacy, and was responsible for the introduction of the term 'senile dementia'. Prichard came from a Hertfordshire-based Quaker family, and benefited from the Scottish Enlightenment in that when he studied at Edinburgh University, his membership of the Society of Friends did not exclude him from a medical training. However, being a Quaker would eventually prevent him from becoming a member of the Royal College of Physicians of London.

The Commissioners in Lunacy replaced the former Metropolitan Commissioners in Lunacy, which were established by the Madhouses Act 1774. Like all such commissioners, Prichard had the remit of overseeing asylums and guarding the welfare of the mentally ill throughout London. From this position he would have observed at first hand many people with epilepsy as well as a host of psychiatric conditions, enabling him in 1837 to publish *A Treatise on Insanity and Other Disorders Affecting the Mind*.[28] He dedicated this book to Jean Étienne Esquirol, with whose observations on epilepsy he was well acquainted. In it he gave a detailed account of what is now called an automatism, but which at that time he described as 'epileptic ecstasy', 'during which the patient is in an undisturbed reverie, and walks about, fancying himself occupied in some of his customary amusements. … This takes place during the waking as well as the sleeping hours.' We shall discuss the legal implications of automatisms in Chapter 11 when we consider epilepsy and criminal law. Prichard also documented the progression, from onset to completion, of what we now call a 'Jacksonian seizure': 'the attack seems to commence in some extreme part, as in a foot or hand; a convulsive tremor, or sometimes a rigid contraction of the muscles, takes place, first at the extremity of the limb, and gradually ascends towards the head: when it reaches the head the paroxysm of coma and convulsion ensues.' Meticulous observations such as these were the forerunners of

---

28 Prichard JC (1835) *A Treatise on Insanity and Other Disorders Affecting the Mind.* Sherwood, Gilbert, and Piper, London.

the mapping of brain function, which would enable future generations to localize symptoms and target brain surgery. At the time when Prichard was describing what we might now call a focal seizure (one that starts at a specific location in the brain cortex), the idea of localizing function to different brain regions was still in its infancy. Based on the limited information that was available, it was believed that insanity was caused by some kind of impairment of the grey matter of the brain, and that some superficial areas of the brain might be responsible for intellectual functions.

The Victorian era

The English physician **Sir John Russell Reynolds** (1828–1896) was an eminent and influential figure in the Victorian era. In 1855 he published his *Diagnosis of Diseases of the Brain, Spinal Cord, Nerves, and Their Appendages*, and in 1861 his treatise *Epilepsy: Its Symptoms, Treatment, and Relation to other Chronic, Convulsive Diseases*, in which he re-introduced Cullen's idea of idiopathic epilepsy as a brain condition that has no obvious causes. He dismissed the widely held belief that other parts of the body, such as the uterus, could be the source of seizures (what had up until then been referred to as 'uterine epilepsy'). Russell Reynolds' other important contributions to the understanding of epilepsy included his attempts to distinguish it clinically from hysteria, and to consider treatments with opium, belladonna, and chloroform for acute attacks.[29] He also introduced a system of classification of neurological disorders that (in a modified form) is still often used, in which he described all neurological symptoms as involving either the absence of movement (e.g. paralysis) or the presence of abnormal or excessive movement (e.g. seizures).[30] His notion of inhibition and excitation within the nervous system was to become more pertinent to epilepsy as the condition became better understood.

The Victorian era was a time of conflicting influences, with a re-embracing among the wider public of the old beliefs, along with increasing levels of social isolation, and the emergence of the eugenics movement. These were to a large extent counterbalanced by the work of some of the great medical scientists and their major contributions to our modern understanding of epilepsy and its treatments. The Victorian period also heralded the portrayal of the 'epileptic' character in literature.

There was little improvement in the wider public's understanding of the causes of epilepsy, and feelings of blame and shame were experienced by those who suffered from the condition,

---

29 McHenry LC (1969) *Garrison's History of Neurology*. Charles C Thomas, Springfield, IL.
30 Eadie MJ (2007) The neurological legacy of John Russell Reynolds (1828–1896). *Journal of Clinical Neuroscience* 14, 309–316.

due to the stigma that remained associated with it. As beliefs in demonic possession, witches, and sorcerers dwindled, there was an increasing preoccupation with the view that epilepsy could be caused by excessive masturbation, self-strangulation, and sexual promiscuity, among many other misdemeanours. The myth that epilepsy arose from the genitals and was therefore impure had many adherents among the Victorians. Consequently it was believed that epilepsy could be avoided if one adopted a 'moral' Christian lifestyle, and that people who suffered from the condition were degenerates and had brought their affliction on themselves.

Prosperous middle-class people with epilepsy were usually able to conceal their condition in order to avoid public disgrace. As a result, epilepsy soon became regarded as a disease that only affected the poor and the destitute. It was now closely associated with prisons, asylums, debt, the workhouse, drunkenness, madness, and violence. By 1827 there were only nine asylums in England and Wales, and people with epilepsy were generally housed alongside criminals in prisons. In Britain the Lunacy Reform in 1845 (Lunacy/Lunatics Act 1845) ensured that the institution of choice for housing people with epilepsy had become the insane asylum, so a small step forward had been made.

However, epilepsy had by now become regarded as the very antithesis of Victorian standards and morals. It was firmly established in the public mind that people with epilepsy were burdens on society, and that social engineering was required to deal with this perceived problem, either by deporting the 'undesirables' to the colonies, or through the emerging concept of eugenics. Many had argued that in order to rid society of epilepsy, individuals with the condition should not be allowed to marry, have children, or participate in any way in 'normal' society. **Francis Galton** (1822–1911), a cousin of Charles Darwin, was a talented polymath. He coined the phrase 'nature versus nurture', and his book *Hereditary Genius* (1869), which was the first scientific attempt to study how what he regarded as 'superior' and 'inferior' human qualities were genetically transmitted from one generation to the next, led to the emergence of the eugenics movement. Galton believed that 'degenerates', 'idiots', and people with conditions such as epilepsy were a threat to the British nation and therefore should not be allowed to have children. From that position it was but a short step to the recommendation of sterilization and ultimately death. The legacy of the eugenicists was the extermination of people with any kind of disability, including epilepsy, in Nazi Germany in the 1930s and early 1940s. It is salutary to note how many distinguished Victorians supported the eugenics movement, and this will be discussed later.

Dedicated epilepsy hospitals and the epilepsy colony movement

By the mid-nineteenth century a more compassionate approach to epilepsy was starting to emerge. **Anthony Ashley-Cooper** (Seventh Earl of Shaftesbury), who was Chairman of the

Lunacy Commission from 1845 to 1885, believed that epilepsy would be best managed in sanatoriums or in separate wards within asylums. The National Hospital for the Paralysed and the Epileptic opened in London in 1860 as a result of the remarkable fundraising efforts of **Johanna Chandler** (1820–1875). Chandler and her sister Elizabeth had cared for their paralysed grandmother and, from small beginnings and by enlisting the help of the influential, including the Lord Mayor of London (who was also paralysed), they helped to found the hospital, which initially had just eight female inpatients. In its early years the majority of the inpatients had epilepsy.

The philanthropist **John Passmore Edwards** (1823–1911), the son of a carpenter, had made his fortune in the newspaper business as an editor of the *London Echo*, before he became a Liberal Member of Parliament. After selling his newspaper to the Scottish American industrialist Andrew Carnegie, he embarked upon a journey of philanthropy that involved the support of hospitals, libraries, and schools. He paid £4000 towards the purchase of farmlands on which one of the first 'colonies', established to provide care and employment for people with epilepsy, was built near Chalfont St Peter in Buckinghamshire. The Chalfont Epileptic Colony was supported by a group of industrialists known as the National Society for the Employment of Epileptics, and the first patients were admitted in 1894.

William Quarrier (1829–1903), a Scottish shoe retailer and philanthropist, had been born into poverty in the town of Greenock in west Scotland. A devout Christian, he used the money from his chain of shoe shops to open a night refuge and eventually to found the Orphan Homes of Scotland in Renfrewshire. Around 13,000 children passed through the homes during that organization's first 30 years. In 1901, Quarrier visited the Chalfont Epileptic Colony and resolved to set up a similar establishment in Scotland. At that time it was estimated that there were around 4000 people with epilepsy living in Scotland, many of whom were housed in the poorhouse or local insane asylum. Quarrier named his establishment the Colony for Mercy of Epileptics, and at a cost of £20,000 he built six cottages (two for men, two for women, and two for children). In 1902, in an article in 'Narrative of Facts', he stated that 'our aim is to provide this open door where afflicted ones may be sent with the assurance that all that medical skill and sanctified common sense can do for them will be lovingly rendered'.[31] The establishment opened in 1906, and 90 years later 140 people with epilepsy were still residing there.

In 1888, **Henry Cox**, a wealthy Liverpool merchant, and **Dr William Alexander**, a medical officer at a workhouse where there were many epileptic patients, established the centre for people with epilepsy known as the Maghull Home for Epileptics. Based in Liverpool, it was established for 'sane epileptics' who were unable to find employment because of their

---

31 Magnusson A (2006) *The Quarriers Story*. Birlinn Ltd, Edinburgh. p. 112.

condition. Residents could be self-funded, and those with no financial means were taken in if they were willing to undertake menial work there. Alexander wrote a textbook entitled *The Treatment of Epilepsy*, and because of his background in surgery he developed an interest in surgical treatments for the condition. The need for residential care for epilepsy gradually diminished as treatments improved, and in 1987 the Maghull centre became a residential care home for the elderly.

In the rest of Europe, epilepsy centres were well established by the mid-nineteenth century. The world's first nursing home for people with epilepsy, largely from affluent families, was opened in 1855 in an isolated rural area near Görlitz in the Prussian province of Silesia. The first European centre to offer specialized support and care for those with epilepsy was La Teppe in Tain-l'Hermitage, France. Founded in 1856 and originally privately run, it was subsequently taken over by a religious charity known as The Company of the Daughters of Charity. It offered a cure based on the medicinal properties of the plant *Galium album* (lady's bedstraw), which was harvested from the local hillsides and mixed into a remedy using a secret formula that was passed down through generations of the same family. Such was the reputation of La Teppe that patients were referred there from all over France. Today it continues to function as a centre that provides multidisciplinary care for patients with complex drug-resistant epilepsy.

Records of the Epilepsy Centre Bethel in Bielefeld, Germany, date back to 1865, when a resolution was passed at a conference on providing 'Care for Epileptics', as there were very few asylum places available for epileptic patients. The centre was established initially for young male patients, and the main emphasis was on education. However, many of the residents had severe mental or physical impairments and so were unable to receive formal education. In 1874 a carpentry workshop was established, which together with opportunities for farm work enabled residents to gain employment and achieve some degree of independent living. The history of the Bethel Centre was reviewed recently by a current staff member, Philip Grewe, and his colleagues.[32]

By the early twentieth century, multiple centres across Europe were providing residential care and training for people with epilepsy. In 1892 the Kork Epilepsy Centre had opened in Kehl-Kork, Germany. In 1905 a centre opened in Oslo, Norway, and in 1919 a monastery was founded to provide care for men with epilepsy at Kempenhaeghe, in the Netherlands.

In the USA, too, treatment approaches for people with epilepsy had gradually advanced from housing them with deviants and the insane to the establishment of specialized institutions for the care of epileptic patients.[33] In 1867 the Epileptic and Paralytic Hospitals

---

32 Grewe P, Siedersleben C and Bien CG (2017) Epilepsy Center Bethel, Bielefeld, Germany. *Epilepsy & Behavior* 76 (Suppl.), S17–S20.

33 Rothman DJ (1971) *The Discovery of the Asylum: Social Order and Disorder in the New Republic.* Little, Brown &

were established on Blackwell's Island, New York. The Blackwell's Island Asylum was the first lunatic asylum for the city of New York. Now called Roosevelt Island (best known for its remaining central octagonal tower, and a popular location for film makers), in its heyday it was known locally as 'Welfare Island', as it provided long-term care for those with epilepsy, smallpox, or paralysis who had either been rejected by society or were too ill to return to it.

In 1893 the first North American institution to be established specifically for the care of people with epilepsy, known as the Asylum for Epileptics and Epileptic Insane, was opened in Gallipolis, Ohio. It was one of the first publicly funded epilepsy centres in the world. Up until then, those with epilepsy were housed in the state poorhouses, prisons, and asylums. Much bureaucracy and state legislation had to be cleared, and the project was 30 years in the planning. It seems likely that the success of the project was down to Governor William McKinley (who went on to become the 25th US President), whose wife Ida had epilepsy. The centre was based on the German model at the Epilepsy Centre Bethel, with provision for over 400 men and women who were transferred from 'insane' secure wards to independent cottages. Governor McKinley appointed fellow Republican Henry Rutter as the first medical superintendent; a pathology laboratory was founded for the study of causes of epilepsy; and various treatments, including bromide, hot and cold baths, and diet, were evaluated. The early achievements of the centre, and also its opposition to the Eugenical Sterilization Law (1914), which aimed to authorize the sterilization of those deemed to be 'socially inadequate', have been described in detail in a historical review.[34] Sadly, the Marriage Law, which prevented the 'habitual drunkard, epileptic, imbecile, or insane' from obtaining a marriage license, was enacted by Ohio State and by the hospital in 1904.

Given that William McKinley was so instrumental in establishing the Ohio hospital, some background information about his wife's epilepsy is relevant. Ida Saxton McKinley was a vivacious socialite from an affluent family, but her life changed at the age of 26, following childbirth and bereavement. The family medical records were kept secret, but the picture that emerged from eye-witness accounts was that of a worsening seizure disorder with both major and minor attacks. John DeToledo and his colleagues have pointed out that the word 'epilepsy' was taboo and that, on hearing that her aunt had epilepsy, one of the First Lady's nieces said that the Democrats would 'stoop so low as to invent lies about McKinley's wife'.[35]

DeToledo and his colleagues also listed the strategies that the President used to conceal what was happening when his wife had an attack in public. She once had a seizure on the

---

Company, Boston, MA.
34 Kissiov D, Dewall T and Hermann B (2013) The Ohio Hospital for Epileptics—the first 'epilepsy colony' in America. *Epilepsia* 54, 1524–1534.
35 DeToledo JC, DeToledo BB and Lowe M (2000) The epilepsy of First Lady Ida Saxton McKinley. *Southern Medical Journal* 93, 267–271.

night of the Inaugural Ball, and thereafter at functions she was placed where she could be removed at a moment's notice, and she was prevented from carrying out the usual White House duties. She died 6 years after her husband's assassination in 1901. Her physicians consistently downplayed her illness, leaving no description of her attacks in their records, although a mild form of epilepsy was acknowledged. It is clear that the McKinleys and their physicians concealed her medical condition due to fear of the public reaction, although McKinley himself did much, through the Ohio hospital, to improve the lot of 'epileptics'. Had he lived until 1904 he would have been dismayed to find out that, by enacting the Marriage Law, his home state of Ohio had all but nullified his own happy marriage.

In 1886 the Pennsylvania Epileptic Hospital and Colony Farm opened on the outskirts of Philadelphia at Westtown. A total of 140 acres of land was set aside for those with epilepsy to farm. A brother and sister, Eckley and Rebecca Cox, donated the first few acres, and further donations of land soon followed. By 1898 there were 30 residents, a medical superintendent, a matron, two nurses, various farm assistants, and laundry and domestic staff. Women were often admitted after having a single seizure and, regardless of diagnostic accuracy, were consigned to spend the rest of their lives there. The Church was central to the whole operation, and there were many generous donations from benefactors. However, despite this, the public clearly did not want people with epilepsy living in the community with them, and in the same year as the Pennsylvania colony opened, the State of Connecticut introduced laws to prevent anyone who was epileptic, an imbecile, or feeble-minded from marrying. The opening of special institutions for those with epilepsy served to banish the condition from public view and to reinforce the idea that it was incurable. The Commission for the Control of Epilepsy and its Consequences calculated that across the USA half a million people with epilepsy were still living in special institutions or psychiatric facilities well into the 1950s.[36] Through the 'colony movement' it was now believed that fits could be reduced by improving the overall health and welfare of the epileptic individual. Against this backdrop of pastoral care emerged the first Victorian clinicians to study epilepsy in analytical detail and to provide the knowledge that would lead to scientifically based treatments. The first part of the nineteenth century had seen the gradual accumulation of the pathological and clinical studies of epilepsy tainted with medical nihilism with regard to whether an effective treatment or even a cure could ever be found. At the same time, many theories were proposed as to the nature of the physiological process that culminated in a seizure.

At this point, let us consider the then current controversy of mapping the brain. According to one school of thought the brain was organized in such a manner that discrete

---

36 Commission for the Control of Epilepsy and its Consequences (1978) *Plan for Nationwide Action on Epilepsy. Volume 1.* US Department of Health, Education, and Welfare, Public Health Service, National Institutes of Health, Bethesda, MD.

regions or areas were responsible for specific functions. The other school of thought claimed that functions were spread uniformly throughout the brain and that no one area could be regarded as having the role of executing or perceiving a particular act. In other words, there was no particular zone tasked with moving a limb, perceiving a sensation such as touch or smell, or creating and understanding language. Isolated case reports had shown loss of a specific function in relation to a discrete brain injury. The most famous of these was the observation by the French surgeon Paul Broca (1824–1880) of loss of language with right-sided paralysis in a 51-year-old man with damage to the left frontal lobe.[37] However, the experimentalists were seeking more than the occasional case report, and in particular they required laboratory evidence.

At this point in time two protagonists, namely the Scottish physiologist **David Ferrier** (1843–1928) and the German physiologist **Friedrich Golzt** (1834–1902), enter the story, and the game-changing Seventh International Medical Congress, which took place in London in 1881.[38] This conference was attended by thousands of scientists and physicians from all over the world, and one of its highlights was the debate on whether brain function could be mapped. Ferrier and Golzt held opposing views about the organization and functioning of the brain. Both of them conducted vivisection experiments that involved removing different parts of the brain from living animals and then observing the effect of this on function. Goltz was unable to induce paralysis or other deficits in dogs by removing various parts of the brain without knowledge of their function. However, Ferrier was able to consistently produce paralysis, blindness, and loss of hearing in monkeys by removing specific areas of the brain that he had chosen based on his previous research findings. After all of the experimental animals had been examined independently, Ferrier was judged the winner of the debate, and the theory that specific functions were located in discrete areas of the brain was accepted by the scientific community. This would subsequently have a huge impact on the understanding of seizures and the localization of their origins within the brain.

Ferrier's triumph was short-lived, as in 1881 he was taken to court by the anti-vivisectionists. The *British Medical Journal* came to his aid, claiming the importance of his work in providing maps of the brain that would now allow surgeons to operate with confidence on the basis of symptoms alone, and he was therefore acquitted.[39] Ferrier's experimental work was published in the *Medical Reports* of the West Riding Lunatic Asylum, one of the most important centres of scientific research between 1866 and 1876, where he undertook much of his early work before moving to London. He was knighted for his research in 1912.

---

37 Broca PP (1861) Loss of speech, chronic softening and partial destruction of the anterior left lobe of the brain. *Bulletin de la Societé Anthropologique* 2, 235–238.
38 Finger S (2000) *Minds Behind the Brain*. Oxford University Press, Oxford.
39 French RD (1975) *Antivivisection and Medical Science in Victorian Society*. Princeton University Press, Princeton, NJ.

Ferrier's career overlapped with that of **John Hughlings Jackson** (1835–1911), an English physician who made a significant contribution to our modern understanding of epilepsy. His research was mainly conducted at the National Hospital for the Paralysed and Epileptic between 1862 and 1906. Hughlings Jackson was born in the village of Green Hammerton in Yorkshire, the youngest of five children of a prosperous local brewer and farmer. His early medical training was by apprenticeship to a physician in York, and then at York Medical School. He started his London career in 1859 as a journalist on the *Medical Times and Gazette*, but later that year took up freelance appointments as a practical physician at several London hospitals as well as giving physiology lectures to medical students. He went on to obtain an MD from the University of St Andrews, and then studied at Cambridge University and at the Martin Luther University of Halle-Wittenberg in Germany.

His first published article on epilepsy, entitled 'Cases of epilepsy associated with syphilis' (1861),[40] contained a mixture of his personally observed cases and those reported by others. In it he commented that 'the convulsions were limited to one side (of the body) and in one of them the fit was not complete, there being no loss of consciousness.' He was describing unilateral or one-sided seizures that do not always progress to generalized (bilateral) seizures with unconsciousness, and he observed that these cases were associated with abnormal tissue on the brain's surface. In the Victorian era, seizures were commonly encountered in people with syphilis, a sexually transmitted disease that was rife at that time.

Over the next two years, Hughlings Jackson observed seizures in the minutest detail in further studies, correlating the symptoms with the anatomy of the brain and the areas of specific function as set out by Ferrier. He noted from post-mortem studies of patients who had died of syphilis that the cause was an obvious organic disease process 'on the side of the brain opposite to the side of the body convulsed.' His paper on this subject, entitled 'Convulsive spasms of the right hand and arm preceding epileptic seizures' was published in the *Medical Times and Gazette* in 1863. It was to be followed by a series of case reports describing a plethora of seizure-related symptoms, such as temporary loss of speech, distortion of the sense of smell, temporary paralysis, eye deviation, and the relationship between seizures and chronic ear infections (the temporal lobe lies adjacent to the inner part of the ear).

The University of St Andrews had gained an unfortunate reputation for awarding the degree of Doctor of Medicine (MD) on the basis of references alone. Hughlings Jackson had been among the many (including Edward Jenner, the pioneer of smallpox vaccine, and Jean-Paul Marat, physician and famous French revolutionary) to benefit from what was seen by other institutions as an unregulated qualification provided for a fee. In order to assert its academic credibility, the university established a journal entitled *Transactions of the St*

---

40 Jackson JH (1861) Cases of epilepsy associated with syphilis. *The Medical Times and Gazette* 2, 648–652.

Andrews Medical Graduates Association. It was in this publication in 1873 that Hughlings Jackson published his landmark paper, 'A Study of Convulsions', which would transform the study of epilepsy.[41] He suggested that epilepsy was a symptom of a range of different possible causes, such as syphilis, stroke, or head injury. He attributed the seizure to 'an excessive and disorderly discharge of nerve tissue on muscle'. He recognized two types of seizure, namely those that affected both sides of the body and which occurred without warning symptoms or an aura, and those that involved only one side and were usually associated with premonitory symptoms or an aura. He believed that the seizure was caused by the instability of the grey matter of the brain, and he attempted to identify the seizure origin or 'focus' in the various areas from which he believed the features of the attack originated. Hughlings Jackson's landmark paper focused on the unilateral attacks with localizable symptoms. He speculated that several steps led to the occurrence of a convulsion: first, a lesion in the grey matter of the brain with destruction or instability of nerve tissue; second, an excessive or disorderly discharge from within that tissue; and finally, a circumstance or set of circumstances that provoked such a discharge into erupting.

When considering what these circumstances might be, he listed (among others) emotional excitement, but also speculated how a change in the blood supply to the lesion might influence its excitability. He was adamant that it was not the abnormal brain tissue (due to whatever cause) that produced the discharge, but rather the normal tissue lying adjacent to it. He eventually settled upon a scientific definition that holds to this day, when he described epilepsy as 'occasional sudden excessive rapid and local discharges of grey matter'.[42] Based on this definition, he added that 'a sneeze is a sort of healthy epilepsy'.

Hughlings Jackson brought a scientific rationale to the understanding of epilepsy in recognizing that a focal lesion within a particular area of the brain would produce its own unique symptoms depending on which region or lobe of the brain was affected. He suggested that epilepsy was the outward visible manifestation of occasional, sudden discharge within the brain, and that the location of this defined the characteristics of the attack. The 'Jacksonian march' that is named after him refers to the 'march' of symptoms in the focal motor seizures that arise in the frontal lobe or motor cortex of the brain. These so-called 'Jacksonian seizures' typically take the form of a twitch of the thumb or face that then spreads to involve the whole of one side of the body. Hughlings Jackson also suggested that the so-called 'dreamy state' of a seizure arose from the temporal lobe.

His papers on the various types of epilepsy have seldom been improved upon either in their descriptive detail or in the analysis of their relationship to specific areas of the brain.

---

41 Jackson JH (1870) A study of convulsions. *Transactions of the St Andrews Medical Graduates Association* 3, 162–204.
42 Jackson JH (1873) *On the Anatomical, Physiological, and Pathological Investigation of Epilepsies.* Spottiswoode & Co., London.

He also re-introduced the term 'automatism' to describe the twilight state following a seizure when the individual is on 'automatic pilot' although they can perform basic tasks. Hughlings Jackson's definition leads to the conclusion that epilepsy is not a single disease, but rather that there are many different types of epilepsy with a variety of causes, outcomes, and treatments.

Hughlings Jackson had married his cousin Elizabeth Dade Jackson in 1865. She died after a sudden illness in 1876, apparently as a result of a cerebral thrombosis or stroke followed by Jacksonian seizures. Her tragic demise seems a poignant postscript to her husband's observation that epilepsy is not a single disease but a symptom of many conditions.

Sir William Gowers (1845–1915) was working at the National Hospital for the Paralysed and Epileptic in London at the same time as Hughlings Jackson. Gowers, a shoemaker's son, encountered a family with muscular dystrophy after he became apprenticed to a local physician and surgeon, and this fuelled his desire to specialize in conditions of the nervous system. In 1881 his first monograph, *Epilepsy and Other Chronic Convulsive Diseases*, based on over 1000 personally observed cases, was published. He elaborated on the concept of electrical overactivity within the brain to explain why seizures occurred, and he commented that 'epilepsy is thus a disease of grey matter, and has not any uniform seat. It is a disease of tissue, not of structure.' Here Gowers was attempting to explain seizures in cases where a structural cause, such as a tumour or head injury, could not be found. He proposed a situation in which a combination of electrical overactivity and inhibition resulted in brain instability and seizures. He went on to suggest that overactivity would in turn inhibit other areas of the brain, resulting in loss of consciousness during the seizure, as well as temporary loss of function such as memory on recovery. Gowers recognized epilepsy and hysteria as two different categories of convulsion, and attempted to provide criteria for distinguishing between them, highlighting the coordinated purposeful movements of 'hystero-epilepsy' in contrast to the involuntary movements of 'genuine epilepsy'.

In 1907, Gowers published his second monograph, *The Border-land of Epilepsy*. In it he discussed those conditions that lay 'in the border-land of epilepsy – near it, but not of it', introducing the reader to disorders such as fainting, migraine, dizziness, and sleepwalking, among others, and setting out the basis for distinguishing them from seizures. Gowers was the first to suggest that epilepsy and hysteria could coexist in the same individual, but that they were separate conditions. Up until the nineteenth century the possibility of misdiagnosis of epilepsy had not really been considered. Hysteria had been regarded as a variety of epilepsy, with the terms 'uterine epilepsy' and 'hystero-epilepsy' commonly used to describe it. Although hysteria in men was recognized, it was generally accepted that it was predominantly a disorder of women, who were considered to be predisposed to it because of their 'greater sensitivity'.

The French physician **Jean-Martin Charcot** (1825–1893), known as the 'father of neurology' (and also renowned for his theatrical teaching style), worked, conducted research and taught at the Salpêtrière Hospital for 33 years. He began to study hysteria by creating a special ward for non-insane female patients with a condition that he termed 'hystero-epilepsy'. Charcot believed that epilepsy and hysteria were different conditions, and he described the features that could be used to distinguish an attack of hysteria from one of epilepsy. Like Gowers, he insisted on a complete separation of the two conditions, but unlike him he did not believe that they could coexist in the same individual. He noted that tongue biting could occur in either condition, and that in hysteria movements were more like contortions than jerking movements, and that body arching was common. He came to the conclusion that many of his patients were suffering from a form of hysteria that had been induced by their emotional response to a traumatic incident or accident in their past. For Charcot, research was based on making observations and, as he put it, being able to see things that others might overlook. Sigmund Freud was briefly his student and was greatly impressed by Charcot's reasoning and treatment approaches, to the extent that he experimented with some of them on returning to Vienna. Since Charcot's time a number of different terms have been used to describe what are believed to be psychologically based episodes that resemble seizures. These include non-epileptic attack disorder (NEAD), psychogenic non-epileptic seizures, psychogenic seizures, pseudo-seizures, and functional seizures.

As the scientific explanation for epilepsy became better understood, its depiction in the arts became more positive. Public attitudes towards people with epilepsy were beginning to be influenced by the written word, both through the popular press and in fiction. Not all Victorian literature provided a compassionate depiction of those with epilepsy, although significantly enlightened attitudes were introduced. Charles Dickens (1812–1870) made frequent visits to prisons and workhouses, where he would have encountered a disproportionate number of people with disabilities, including epilepsy. In his novels he portrayed numerous characters with the condition, including some compassionate and insightful depictions. The Russian writer Fyodor Dostoevsky (1821–1881) suffered from epilepsy himself, so had a unique insight into the condition, and he included characters with epilepsy in many of his novels. (For a detailed discussion of the contribution of Dickens and Dostoevsky to the positive portrayal of epilepsy, see Chapter 4.)

Drug treatments

Early nineteenth-century treatments had been based on purging or bloodletting. However, by 1857 potassium bromide had been introduced as the first anti-epileptic drug (AED), mainly on account of its sedative properties. Its discovery was pure serendipity. **Sir Edward**

Sieveking (1816–1904), an Edinburgh-trained physician, published a book about the classification of epilepsy, entitled *On Epilepsy and Epileptiform Seizures* (1858). At the time a third of the patients who were admitted to the London hospital where he worked had epilepsy, for which no effective treatment was then available. In 1857 he was approached by **Sir Charles Locock** (1799–1875), Queen Victoria's obstetrician, who mentioned to Sieveking that he had heard that potassium bromide suppressed libido in men and so might be a logical candidate for controlling uterine epilepsy (which he believed to be caused by sexual arousal) in women.

In an article published in the *Medical Times and Gazette* in 1857,[43] Locock reported that he had tried potassium bromide with benefit in 14 out of 15 women, although he never published these data himself. Despite initial scepticism, where it was available bromide soon became the treatment of choice for epilepsy. Indeed at the National Hospital at Queen Square, which opened in 1860 and was the first specialist neurological hospital, Sieveking and his colleagues used two and a half tons of the drug each year. However, no drug trials were conducted, and until the late nineteenth century all reports of the beneficial or adverse effects of potassium bromide were anecdotal. Several studies of the efficacy of bromide therapy for controlling epilepsy were then published, one of which showed that potassium bromide was ineffective in nearly 50 per cent of patients who took it, although in a third of patients, control of their epilepsy had been achieved for up to two years.[44]

Apart from bromide, other drugs that were used in patients with epilepsy included chloral hydrate (a sedative and hypnotic) and Borax (a compound used in detergents), but these had little effect. Zinc salts, opium, and even strychnine had their advocates, but bromide remained the drug of choice, despite its side effects.

Surgical treatments

The suggestion that brain surgery might benefit certain patients with epilepsy assumes that the cause of the problem lies within the skull. The earliest surgical treatments were designed to release the cause from the head by drilling a hole in the skull. This procedure was called trepanning or alternatively trephining (from the Greek noun *trypanon*, meaning 'to bore'). Trepanation is probably the oldest surgical procedure for which there is archaeological evidence, from skulls excavated from burial sites dating back to 6500 bce in Europe, Siberia, China, and the Americas. In the ancient world the main superstitious reason cited for trepanning was to release harmful vapours or even demons from the brain. It is unclear exactly when this procedure first started to be used as a treatment for epilepsy. The Greeks

---

43 Locock C (1857) Discussion of paper by Dr Sieveking: analysis of fifty-two cases of epilepsy observed by the author. *Medical Times and Gazette* 1, 524–526.
44 Turner WA (1907) *Epilepsy: A Study Of The Idiopathic Disease*. Macmillan, London.

certainly practised it, and written evidence of its use for this purpose can be found in the thirteenth-century medieval surgical text, *Quattuor Magistri (The Four Masters)*, in which it was recommended for 'melancholics, epileptics and others'. Owsei Temkin's comprehensive account of the history of epilepsy describes how a French nobleman with epilepsy was robbed and beaten, as a result of which he sustained a severe wound to the head. He was treated by a surgeon and lost a large amount of his skull bone, but became free of seizures thereafter.[45] Temkin also cites a fifteenth-century text, *The Compleat Practice of Physick*, which states that when all else has failed 'the last remedy is to open the fore part of the skull – that the evil air may breathe out. By this means many desperate epilepsies can be safely cured.'

By the eighteenth century the notion that trephining allowed the release of harmful vapours or devils had been largely dismissed, but the technique continued to be used for patients with epilepsy right up until the early twentieth century, and not just in countries where superstitious beliefs persisted. In 1838 an account of successful trephining performed at the Massachusetts General Hospital was published in the *Boston Medical and Surgical Journal*. The individual concerned had a 12-year history of seizures, which had started after the healing of a scalp ulcer. The author attributed the seizures to a build-up of pressure within the head that was relieved by trephining. The account described how the patient progressed from having several seizures a week to only one every couple of months. In 1889 a report published in the *British Medical Journal* described the case of a man who had sustained a head injury while drunk, and then went on to experience 16 seizures a day, which responded to trephining. However, such anecdotal reports are difficult to verify, as detailed background information about the patient's epilepsy in these cases is not available.

In fact, the development of pioneering epilepsy surgery was just around the corner, the key players being the English surgeon **Sir Rickman Godlee** (1849–1925) and the Scottish surgeon **Sir William Macewen** (1848–1924). Macewen's contributions to surgery were immense, and he had benefited from working at the Glasgow Royal Infirmary at the same time as Joseph Lister, who introduced techniques that minimized the risk of post-surgical infection. This transformed surgery, allowing new and more ambitious operations to be considered. Macewen contributed to many fields of surgery, and could be described as the world's first neurosurgeon. The twelfth son of a marine engineer, he studied medicine at Glasgow University. He followed with interest the research of David Ferrier (described earlier in this chapter), and soon, like him, concluded that the causes of the neurological symptoms displayed by patients were located in specific areas of the brain. In 1876 he localized an abscess to the language centre of the brain in an 11-year-old child who had briefly lost the

---

45 Temkin O (1971) *The Falling Sickness: A History of Epilepsy from the Greeks to the Beginnings of Modern Neurology*, 2nd edition. Johns Hopkins University Press, Baltimore, MD. p. 235.

power of speech after a seizure. The family declined Macewen's offer of surgery, and after the child's death the post-mortem examination showed that the abscess was located exactly where Macewen had predicted it would be, which he said gave 'poignancy to the regret that the operation had not been permitted during life.'[46] The following year a teenage girl came to see him with seizures involving the right side of her face and arm. Macewen assumed that the cause of the seizures was located on the left side of the brain in what Ferrier had earlier mapped as being the motor cortex. Using antiseptic techniques, he removed a tumour from the lining of the brain from the very area where he had suspected it was located, and the young girl survived. By the end of 1883, Macewen had performed seven operations on the relevant part of the brain and spinal cord, guided solely by the individual patient's symptoms and signs.

Several years after Macewen's pioneering surgery, Rickman Godlee gained even greater acclaim, in 1884, for the first reported operation on a brain tumour that had been the cause of a patient's epilepsy. The patient was a young farmer called Henderson from Dumfries, Scotland, who for two years had suffered from seizures that affected the left side of his face, after which he would lose consciousness. The twitching of his face would often spread into his hand and then into his leg. Much of Godlee's success was in fact due to the guidance he received from the neurologist **Alexander Hughes Bennett** (1848–1901), who believed that the cause of the epilepsy must be on the right side of the brain in what the neurologist David Ferrier had defined as the motor cortex (the part of the brain from which movement on the opposite side of the body is initiated). Henderson's condition worsened and urgent surgery was performed under chloroform anaesthesia in a hastily assembled operating theatre at the National Hospital for Paralysis and Epilepsy in London. When Godlee probed just beneath the surface of the brain, a walnut-sized tumour was located in the precise area where it had been predicted to be, and was removed. Despite the use of a carbolic spray machine to try to prevent infection, Henderson died four weeks later from meningitis. Nevertheless, that operation marked the start of surgery within the brain to treat epilepsy that could be localized on the basis of clinical symptoms. Godlee, dismayed by his patient's death, abandoned brain surgery two weeks after his landmark operation.[47]

The year after Godlee's landmark surgery, the renowned physician **Sir William Osler** (1849–1919), then based in Montreal, published an account of a colleague's child who had a 12-year history of seizures. These attacks again took the form of uncontrollable twitching of one side of the body (so-called Jacksonian seizures), and culminated in the child's death. At post-mortem a small tumour in the leg centre of the brain was found. Osler said that this

---

46 Macewen W (1888) An address on the surgery of the brain and spinal cord. *British Medical Journal* 2, 302–309.
47 Rose FC (2011) Neurosurgery. In: *History of British Neurology*. Imperial College Press, London. pp. 213–227.

was 'an instance in which operation would have been justifiable and possibly have been the means of saving life'.[48]

The next major contributor to the development of epilepsy surgery was **Sir Victor Horsley** (1857–1916), an English surgeon who also had links with the Brown Animal Sanitory Institution, a London-based veterinary institute that had animal research facilities, where he conducted his experimental research on epilepsy. As had been the case with Ferrier, his vivisection techniques attracted strong criticism and protests. To some extent building on Ferrier's earlier work, he used electrical stimulation of the animal brain to study the limb responses and to map areas of the brain that had specific functions. He realized that any pathology that caused irritation of the brain in these regions would produce predictable symptoms that would indicate the site of irritation, allowing the possibility of removing the cause and thereby achieving a cure. In 1886, Horsley operated on a 22-year-old man who during childhood had been run over by a horse-drawn cab in Edinburgh. This accident had resulted in severe epilepsy that was manifested as twitching of the leg, spreading to the arm and face, followed by complete loss of consciousness with twitching of all four limbs.

Operating under chloroform anaesthesia, Horsley enlarged the hole in the patient's skull that had resulted from the childhood injury, and located a scar lying in the leg area of the brain. The surgery, which resulted in a cure for the patient, had been based on the use of skull defects to guide Horsley to the correct site. In subsequent operations, with no such landmarks, he began to operate using the nature of the seizure alone as a guide, and had similar success. Realizing that locating the motor strip in the brain was not a straightforward matter, due to the lack of anatomical landmarks, he went on to electrically stimulate the brain in human patients during surgery. This enabled him to produce increasingly accurate maps of brain function.[49] The *Lancet* reported on a famous address given by Horsley to the British Medical Association in 1886 on 'the technique of operations on the central nervous system'.[50] He described three patients with epilepsy (caused by head injury in two cases and a brain tumour in the third) for whom surgery had proved successful. Horsley emphasized that without Ferrier's earlier animal experiments, those operations would have been impossible. His admiring audience included the acclaimed neurologists Jean Martin Charcot from Paris and John Hughlings Jackson.

In the early nineteenth century there was a growing interest in the use of maps to guide diagnosis and surgery. **Fedor Krause** (1857–1937), a German neurosurgeon who

---

48 Osler W (1885) A contribution to Jacksonian epilepsy and the situation of the leg centre. *American Journal of the Medical Sciences* 89, 31–37.
49 Horsley V (1909) The Linacre Lecture on the function of the so-called motor area of the brain. *British Medical Journal* 2, 121–132.
50 Horsley V (1906) Address in Surgery on the technique of operations on the central nervous system. *Lancet* 2, 484–490.

had originally studied music at the Berlin Conservatoire before he embarked on a career in medicine, was responsible for the introduction of epilepsy surgery into German hospitals. By 1912 he had performed 96 operations in which he used brain stimulation to map out the most excitable areas, which he assumed were the source of the patient's seizures. His maps of the motor cortex indicated to surgeons which areas of the brain could be removed without language loss or paralysis. He studied the specimens removed during his operations and observed that the causes of epilepsy ranged from small tumours to areas of scarring from previous injuries or infections. He noted that the area of the brain that was more excitable and thus the origin of the seizure was often a short distance from the scar or tumour that was irritating it, rather than the lesion itself being the 'epileptic focus'. This led him to suggest that removal not only of the lesion but also of the epileptic focus was necessary if optimum results were to be achieved.[51] It is important to bear in mind that this pioneering work was carried out without any of the sophisticated imaging and electrical tests that are available today, and that nearly all of Krause's patients had the Jacksonian form of twitching epilepsy that could be clinically localized to the motor cortex. Krause's map, which was annotated in German, showed how he was able to use electrical stimulation to map the movement of limbs at their joints to discrete regions of the motor cortex. Unlike most surgeons of his day, Krause followed up his patients by letter. Of the 29 patients whom he contacted, four had died, eleven were no better, three were worse, eight were considerably better, and three were completely cured.

The twentieth century

Drug treatments

In the early twentieth century a major contributor to advances in drug treatment for epilepsy was **William Aldren Turner** (1864–1945), a leading British neurologist based at the Chalfont Epileptic Colony near Chalfont St Peter in Buckinghamshire, and at the National Hospital for the Paralysed and Epileptic in London. He studied medicine at Edinburgh University, and through his research into the prognosis and treatment of epilepsy, and the value of institutional care for the condition, went on to become a major figure in the field of epileptology. He published a landmark textbook entitled *Epilepsy: a Study of the Idiopathic Disease* (1907), and he provided written accounts of around 45 different bromide salt preparations that were available for the treatment of epilepsy, as well as documenting

---

51 Feindel W, Leblanc R and de Almeida AN (2009) Epilepsy surgery: historical highlights 1909-2009. *Epilepsia* 50 (Suppl. 3), 131–151.

their severe side effects. Prolonged use of bromides resulted in 'bromism', the symptoms of which included impaired concentration and memory, lethargy, tremor, unsteadiness, nausea, flatulence, slowing of the heart, poor circulation, and loss of libido. Turner also described cosmetic changes (such as coarsening of facial features), personality changes, and impaired vision. Bromides could be bought over the counter and their use was widespread; they accounted for 1 in 5 prescriptions in the USA.[52] By that time it was possible to measure blood levels of bromide. This enabled physicians to monitor whether the drug was being taken regularly, and thus gave them a sense of greater control over the use of the drug.

The next effective AED did not become available until some years later. The sedative effect of barbituric acid and its derivatives (barbiturates) suggested the possibility that these compounds might be effective in the treatment of epilepsy. (Several explanations have been offered for the coining of the term 'barbiturates'. One possibility is that the German chemist Adolf von Baeyer, who discovered the compounds in 1864, celebrated this breakthrough in a local tavern on St Barbara's day, and that barbiturates are named after this patron saint. An alternative explanation is that he named them after a young woman called Barbara whom he had recently befriended.)

Evidence for the effectiveness of the barbiturate phenobarbitone in the treatment of epilepsy was provided by **Alfred Hauptmann** (1881–1948), a German neurologist, who first used it in 1912, when it was marketed by the drug company Bayer as Luminal.[53] Accounts of Hauptmann's discovery of the drug's effects describe how when he was a junior doctor in Freiburg he slept in a room above the epilepsy ward. After having been kept awake for many nights by his patients, he prescribed the hypnotic drug phenobarbitone for them with the sole intention of himself getting a good night's sleep. To his surprise he found that their seizures became less frequent. He went on to select patients who had proved resistant to potassium bromide, and he gradually worked out the most effective dose for them.[54] Hauptmann used the medical records in the clinic at the University of Freiberg to compare the patients' seizure frequency the previous year, when they were taking potassium bromide, with their current seizure frequency while on phenobarbitone. He noted that their seizures were now not only less frequent, but also less severe.

In 1922 a study by Dr C Brook, resident medical officer at the Chalfont Epileptic Colony in England, reported that phenobarbitone was not only effective for the treatment of epilepsy in patients under his care, but was also superior to bromides. His successor, Dr F Haward, reported the effects of the drug on 124 patients who were treated for a period

---

52 Friedlander WJ (2000) The rise and fall of bromide therapy in epilepsy. *Archives of Neurology* 57, 1782–1785.
53 Scott DF (1992) The discovery of anti-epileptic drugs. *Journal of the History of the Neurosciences* 1, 111–118.
54 Magiorkinis E, Diamantis A, Sidiropoulou K et al. (2014) Highlights in the history of epilepsy: the last 200 years. *Epilepsy Research and Treatment* 2014, 582039. doi: 10.1155/2014/582039.

of more than six months.[55] One-third of them showed a dramatic reduction in the number of attacks they experienced. Among the remaining two thirds, in only 25 per cent of cases did the drug have no effect at all. Thus phenobarbitone was established as the first truly effective AED. In 1928, Haward produced guidelines stating that every newly admitted patient would be started on potassium bromide, and that if no improvement was observed they would be switched to phenobarbitone. If there was still no improvement the two drugs would be combined.[56]

Phenobarbitone (now known as phenobarbital) remained the most widely used treatment for epilepsy well into the 1970s, and is still included in the World Health Organization's list of essential drugs. It is a highly effective but inexpensive medication, although it has significant side effects. Its low cost has resulted in it being widely used in developing countries whose healthcare systems cannot afford the newer, more expensive drugs.

The success of phenobarbitone led to the investigation and development of other AEDs related to the barbiturates in terms of their chemical structure. The first of these was phenytoin, the structure of which is characterized by a five-membered barbiturate ring. It was first produced in 1908, and was initially used as a sedative or hypnotic. Separation of the sedative effect (excessive sleepiness) from the anti-epileptic effect (reduction in the frequency and severity of seizures) was to become the 'holy grail' of anti-epileptic drug development. Phenytoin was considered to have a less sedative effect than phenobarbitone. Between 1919 and 1931 around 30 people with epilepsy had been treated with a form of phenytoin that was quite toxic. However, despite its side effects, the drug reduced the frequency of seizures.

In 1929, **Stanley Cobb** (1887–1968), a leading neurologist and pathologist working at the Boston City Hospital in America, was asked by an eminent lawyer whether there was anything more effective than a starvation diet for controlling his son's epilepsy. Cobb had tried various treatments, including diet and dehydration, to control seizures. His interest in the role of glucose in preventing attacks had resulted in the use of the ketogenic diet (also known as the starvation diet, discussed in more detail later in this chapter), which had met with some success. The lawyer's question triggered a programme of research and the formation of the Harvard Epilepsy Commission. During the Depression it was difficult to obtain funding for medical research, especially in the field of epileptology. However, the Rockefeller Foundation came to the rescue, aiding the search for better treatments.[57] **Tracy Jackson Putnam** (1894–1975) and **Hiram Houston Merritt Jr** (1902–1979), both of whom were leading neurologists at the Boston City Hospital, drew up a list of possible anti-

---

55 Haward F (1928) *Report of the Medical Officer*. The National Society of Epilepsy, Chalfont.
56 Shorvon SD (2009) Drug treatment of epilepsy in the century of the ILEA: the first fifty years,1909–1958. *Epilepsia* 50 (Suppl. 3), 69–92.
57 Friedlander WJ (1986) Putnam, Merritt, and the discovery of Dilantin. *Epilepsia* 27 (Suppl. 3), S1–S21.

epilepsy drugs, and developed an animal model of epilepsy with which to test them. This involved comparing the effectiveness of different potential anti-epilepsy drugs in cats in order to determine the best candidate for testing in humans. The experimental animals were given an electric shock that resulted in a convulsion, and for each drug the minimum intensity of shock necessary to cause a seizure (known as the seizure threshold) was measured. The more effective the drug, the higher the seizure threshold would be.

Phenytoin was found to be the most effective of the many drugs tested, and Putnam and Merritt conducted several clinical trials in human patients with epilepsy between 1938 and 1940, the final trial involving 267 patients.[58] These researchers not only developed a model that enabled drugs to be tested, but they also refined the methods for evaluating their effectiveness and side effects in large clinical trials. Phenytoin became the mainstay of epilepsy treatment for the next 50 years. Many drugs were added to the list of anti-epileptic medications during the twentieth century, the most notable ones being carbamazepine, sodium valproate, gabapentin, and lamotrigine, names that will be familiar to many readers of this book.

The search for new drug treatments with fewer side effects continued, and as the biological basis of epilepsy became better understood, an increasing number of candidate drugs emerged. The basic mechanism underlying all anti-epileptic drug treatments is a reduction in excitability or excessive electrical activity within the brain. The early drugs were discovered by chance or as a result of using animal models, without understanding the precise mechanism of drug action, while trying to achieve a balance between achieving seizure reduction and avoiding excessive sedation. We now know that substances called neurotransmitters pass information from one nerve cell to the next, and therefore must play a role when those cells become overexcited. Neurotransmitters influence the excitability of cells by acting on 'receptor sites' on the cell wall, thereby altering the flow of chemicals in and out of them.

To summarize a very complex process, these receptors are the targets for drugs that might control epilepsy better while at the same time having more tolerable or even negligible side effects. Modern AEDs act by a number of different mechanisms. For example, they may modulate sodium, calcium, and potassium ion channels, increase gamma-aminobutyric acid (GABA)-mediated inhibition, or block glutamate receptors. Drugs that have been identified as acting via such mechanisms then undergo toxicity studies to ensure that they are not harmful, followed by studies in healthy human volunteers, and small studies in patients with epilepsy. Finally they are tested in randomized controlled trials (RCTs), in which human

---

58 Merritt HH and Putnam TJ (1938) Sodium diphenyl hydantoinate in the treatment of convulsive disorders. *Journal of the American Medical Society* 111, 1068–1073.

subjects are randomized to receive either the new drug, an existing drug, or a placebo (a treatment that has no therapeutic effect). RCTs are usually conducted at several independent epilepsy centres across several different countries. They are independent of the drug company that developed the drug, they involve large numbers of subjects, and the results must be interpreted by individuals who have not been informed of which patients are taking which treatment. Finally, regulatory approval is sought with a view to gaining a license for the drug.

The process of drug evaluation outlined above is expensive, and this will in turn determine the cost of the drug and hence its affordability. The older anti-epileptic drugs are much less expensive than the most recently developed ones, and for this reason many healthcare systems across the world still use the older drugs, such as phenobarbitone and phenytoin. At the time of writing there were 25 approved AEDs (marketed under 35 different brand names). Despite this promising situation, many people with epilepsy continue to be 'drug resistant', deriving little or no benefit from their treatment. Approximately one-third of epilepsy patients continue to have seizures despite taking their drugs regularly. If two different drugs have been tried without success, the probability of a third drug being effective is less than 1 in 20.

The selection of a suitable AED for a particular individual is now based on the type of seizure, the epilepsy syndrome, and individual factors such as age, gender, coexisting medical conditions, and the relative acceptability of different potential side effects. Treatment is initiated with a single AED, and the dose is then gradually increased until either seizure control is achieved or toxicity (unacceptable severity of side effects) occurs. If the use of a single drug proves to be inadequate for seizure control, a second drug is introduced. There is some controversy in the medical community as to whether the second drug should be added to the first, or whether the first drug should be withdrawn. In fact this is a risk/benefit issue that needs to be approached on an individual basis. If the second AED is effective, withdrawal of the first drug should be considered. If two or three AEDS have failed to achieve seizure control, the epilepsy should be considered medically refractory and referred for further evaluation and consideration of additional non-drug treatments, such as surgery (see below) or a technique known as vagal nerve stimulation.

Surgical treatments

During the early years of the twentieth century, a growing number of surgeons were mapping the brain by electrical stimulation, the most famous of whom was the American neurosurgeon **Harvey Cushing** (1869–1939) at the Johns Hopkins Hospital in Baltimore. Using local anaesthetic with the patient awake, and a newly designed electric stimulator probe, he was able to map out the parietal lobe (the part of the brain that is responsible for understanding spatial relationships and identifying objects).

However, it was not until the 1930s, in Montreal, Canada, that surgery for epilepsy began to develop into its present-day form. The American-Canadian **Wilder Penfield** (1891–1976) studied medicine at Princeton University, and after training in Oxford, Spain, Germany, and New York he became the first neurosurgeon in Montreal. His vision was to establish in that city an institute of surgeons, physicians, physiologists and research scientists who could jointly bring about advances in the understanding and care of neurological disorders, including epilepsy. The Montreal Neurological Institute opened in 1934 and soon became a model for similar establishments throughout the world. From his days in Oxford, Penfield had developed an interest in electrical brain stimulation and mapping, in Germany he had come into contact with the eminent neurologist and neurosurgeon Otfrid Foerster, and in Spain he had studied pathology. All of this experience equipped him well for his future research.

Using local anaesthetic and electrical stimulation, Penfield moved beyond mapping the motor and sensory areas of the brain to mapping those regions responsible for language, vision, and, most crucially of all, memory. His refinements of the mapping of the motor cortex resulted in the 'homunculus' (miniature human being) – that is, a cartoon of the size and order of the representation of movement overlying the cortex itself. This concept is perhaps easier to illustrate than to describe (see Figure 2). For instance, because hand movement is so much more intricate than movement of the hip, the hand area of the human cortex, and thus the number of cells or neurons involved, will be larger than the hip area. The same applies to the sensory cortex, where the sensation of, for example, the hand or lips is so much greater than that of the chest or stomach. With regard to mapping of other functions, it is in relation to memory that Penfield's studies are most relevant to epilepsy. We have already mentioned the aura (or 'breeze') that occurs before a seizure (see Chapter 1). This can often take the form of a memory from the past, which may or may not be real (*déjà vu* or *jamais vu*). Through electrical stimulation, Penfield was able to show that memory was a function of the temporal lobe. He found that when he stimulated the lower part of the brain on either side (the temporal lobes) he could elicit memories of events, sounds, and even colours. If he repeatedly stimulated the same area in the same individual he reproduced the same memory, which might be as sophisticated as a song learned in childhood. He had not only located the physical site of memory, but had also shown that the temporal lobe was the origin of the aura that is experienced by many people with epilepsy. The temporal lobe was now the new target for epilepsy surgery, and there were many more patients with temporal lobe epilepsy than there were with the twitching epilepsy of Jacksonian seizures.

In 1937, **Herbert Jasper** (1906–1999) came to work with Penfield, pioneering the use of a relatively new technique that had been devised by Hans Berger (see Chapter 3), namely the electroencephalogram (EEG), to investigate the electrical activity of the brain. This investigation and its subsequent refinements were used to classify epilepsy more scientifically, and specifically to confirm those cases in which epilepsy was of temporal lobe origin. The main focus of interest was now the deepest part of the temporal lobe, where scarring was believed to be responsible for the development of this type of epilepsy. The main problem with removing this part of the brain was that no one was quite sure what damage it might cause to the memory. As a result, operations focused on removing those parts of the temporal lobe that were least likely to harm memory, namely the front end and the surface. Penfield's initial series of operations had a 50 per cent success rate, and this only improved when deeper structures were also removed.

Over the last 50 years, epilepsy surgery has developed further. It is now being offered more widely, and has better outcomes in terms of seizure control and retention of memory function. Temporal lobe surgery has focused increasingly on the deep structures where the causal scarring can be found. The nature of the scarring and its causes has been investigated, and the use of magnetic resonance imaging (MRI) and computerized tomography (CT) as imaging techniques has greatly improved surgical accuracy. In addition, the use of the EEG to record measurements at the brain surface or deep within it during surgery has enabled surgical benefit to be achieved in areas of the brain that were hitherto 'no go' areas.

Non-pharmaceutical treatments

At the same time that drug treatments were being explored there was also an ongoing search for non-pharmaceutical therapies. Initially these took the form of diets, in particular the ketogenic diet (also known as the starvation diet). This high-fat, low-carbohydrate diet is termed 'ketogenic' because it results in the liver producing ketones to be used as an alternative energy source. The resulting high levels of ketones in the blood are believed to have an anticonvulsant effect. Despite the fact that it is still being used after nearly a century, the exact mechanisms underlying the clinical efficacy of the ketogenic diet remain unknown. Interestingly, fasting diets designed to 'starve' epilepsy date back to the time of Hippocrates. Stanley Cobb's interest in the ketogenic diet was mentioned earlier in this chapter, but it was **Hugh William Conklin** (1877–undated), an American osteopath, who re-introduced fasting as an epilepsy treatment in the early twentieth century. He believed that seizures were caused by toxins released from the gut, and that 18 to 25 days of fasting would allow this toxin to disperse and disappear. He claimed to have treated hundreds of epilepsy patients with his 'water diet', and boasted of cure rates of 90 per cent in children and 50 per cent in adults.[59] The ketogenic diet is one that is high in fat and low in carbohydrate, with a moderate

---

59 Wheless JW (2004) History and origin of the ketogenic diet. In: Stafstrom CE and Rho JM (eds.) *Epilepsy and the Ketogenic Diet*. Humana Press Inc., Totowa, NJ.

but adequate protein content. It was introduced in the 1920s, became very popular in the 1930s, and is still used by some, especially for the control of childhood epilepsy. In recent times it has been used in cases of intractable epilepsy, and it has also become established as a first-line therapy for a few specific epilepsy syndromes that have a metabolic cause related to glucose metabolism.

Some authors believe that the avoidance of specific foods can help to control epilepsy. For example, some food additives, such as monosodium glutamate (MSG), have been reported to trigger seizures in those who have the condition. This observation is perhaps not surprising, in view of the known effects that additives can have on behaviour, especially in children, but gathering the evidence to link cause and effect unequivocally is difficult. Similarly, there are many reports of the use of distraction strategies to halt a seizure at an early stage when an epilepsy aura or warning has occurred. People with epilepsy have reported that performing a mental task, such as mental arithmetic, at the onset of a warning can abort or reduce the severity of a seizure. Again this evidence is anecdotal and would be difficult to test scientifically, but once more it is not surprising and should not be discounted.

Other non-pharmacological treatments include yoga, meditation, and Ayurveda, all of which have their champions. The term 'Ayurveda' is derived from the Sanskrit words *ayur* (meaning 'life') and *veda* (meaning 'science' or 'knowledge'), and is one of the oldest systems of medicine in the world. Ayurvedic practices pre-date written records and were handed down from one generation to the next by word of mouth. Eventually they were recorded as written Sanskrit texts more than 2000 years ago. Ayurvedic physicians prescribe individualized treatments, including compounds of herbs or proprietary ingredients, as well as making diet, exercise, and lifestyle recommendations. The majority of the population of the Indian subcontinent and many people in South-East Asia use this form of medicine in combination with conventional modern drug treatments. The effect of Ayurveda on seizure control is not known, but again should not be dismissed.

Other unproven but widely used non-pharmacological treatments include biofeedback, aerobic exercise, music therapy, acupuncture, and traditional Chinese herbal remedies. Music therapy is of particular interest in relation to epilepsy. Several studies have shown that it can be effective in reducing the number of seizures, providing a useful alternative treatment option for people with epilepsy, although the underlying mechanism involved is unclear. A study conducted in Toronto in Canada found a link between music, specifically listening to Mozart's Sonata for Two Pianos in D major (K. 448), and a very significant reduction in epileptiform discharges as measured by an electroencephalogram (EEG) in patients with poorly controlled epilepsy.[60] The growing interest in the effects of music on the

---

60 Hughes JR, Daaboul Y, Fino JJ et al. (1998) The "Mozart effect" on epileptiform activity. *Clinical Electroencephalography*

brain has led to the development of a new specialty known as neuromusicology. Listening to music increases the level of the neurotransmitter dopamine in the brain. Indeed, professional musicians have some more highly developed cognitive skills than the general population. The relationship between music and epilepsy is discussed in more detail in Chapter 6.

Conclusion

The nineteenth century saw epilepsy at last emerging from the shadows. Not only was it more openly spoken about, but also an increasing number of medical books, scientific papers, and conferences were devoted to the subject. People with chronic epilepsy were no longer housed in prisons but in asylums, and then, as understanding of the condition improved, in designated wards and colonies. Much improved care was provided by specialist staff in these specialized centres, and data could now be collected on the incidence of the condition, and the outcome and social circumstances of those affected by it. This led to a growing understanding of the social implications of having epilepsy. During the Victorian period, despite the stigma that was resurfacing, writers such as Dickens and Dostoevsky finally gave a voice to those with epilepsy.

Meanwhile, a scientifically based understanding of the causes of epilepsy had replaced the early medical theories about vapours and contagion. Rational effective treatments had yet to be developed, but it was now widely accepted that epilepsy and hysteria were completely separate conditions. Many of the early drug treatments for epilepsy were discovered serendipitously. Although the use of animal models to test potential new drug and surgical treatments would be considered unacceptable today, at the time few alternatives were available. If these pioneering but controversial methods had not been used by the early researchers, it would have taken much longer to develop many of the effective pharmaceutical and surgical treatments for epilepsy, thus withholding therapeutic benefit from large numbers of patients. Thankfully, advances in the identification of potential anti-epilepsy drugs and the development of functional brain imaging techniques have now made animal studies largely redundant.

The last 120 years have seen huge advances in the treatment of epilepsy, from diagnostic tests to management based on a genetic understanding of the condition. Nevertheless, attitudes to the condition among the general public have continued to lag behind medical progress, and epilepsy is still widely perceived as a stigmatized disease.

CHAPTER 3

The investigation, classification, and causes of epilepsy

The development of techniques for investigating epilepsy has had five main aims: (1) to improve understanding of the condition; (2) to aid its diagnosis; (3) to investigate its causes; (4) to identify and classify the different types of epilepsy; and (5) to enable targeted treatments to be developed. In much the same way as headaches can be caused by a large number of conditions, ranging from poor eyesight to a brain tumour, epilepsy is not in itself a disease, but rather it is a symptom of myriad conditions.

There are now a number of different approaches that can be used to investigate epilepsy. The most important of these involve measuring the electrical activity within the brain during or between seizures, and the use of brain scanning to image the cause of the epilepsy and to identify chemical changes within the brain. For many years, however, a recording of the changes in electrical activity in the brain was the only test available for confirming whether or not epilepsy was a cause of seizures, 'funny turns', and blackouts, and for identifying the type of epilepsy present.

The electroencephalogram (EEG)

Electrical activity within the brain consists of 'brainwaves' that are produced when brain cells or neurons communicate with each other by means of synchronized electrical impulses; they are the basis of all of our thoughts and emotions. Once scientists had established that such electrical activity was present and could be measured, they went on to determine how it was affected by physical diseases of the brain and by mental disorders.

In 1875, **Richard Caton** (1842–1926), an English physician and physiologist, published his observations that electrical currents could be detected in the brains of rabbits.[61] Several other researchers based in Russia and Poland confirmed these findings, but the exact location in the brain from which these currents arose remained unclear. Caton demonstrated the suppressing effect of the anaesthetic chloroform on the wave forms, which supported his view that they had a biological basis and arose from the brain cells. However, it would be around another 50 years before the possible application of brainwave measurements to the diagnosis of epilepsy would be considered.

The nineteenth-century studies by Caton and others of the electrical activity of the cerebral cortex in a range of laboratory animals, including dogs and primates, laid the foundations for the clinical application of the electroencephalogram (EEG). By the 1920s, **Hans Berger** (1873–1941), a German neuropsychiatrist working at the University of Jena, had started recording these electrical potentials from the scalps of patients who had skull defects resulting from head injuries or surgery. Berger coined the term 'electroencephalogram', and made his first recording in a human subject in 1924, during a neurosurgical operation on a 17-year-old boy. He next reported on that same case in 1929, using the terms 'alpha wave' and 'beta wave' to describe the two different wave forms that he observed in the brain. The alpha waves that he had noted disappeared when the subject closed their eyes, and returned when they opened them again. A few years later, using more sensitive equipment, Berger was able to obtain recordings through the intact skulls of human subjects, without the need for a hole or defect.

Berger noted that the brainwaves of adults were different from those of children, and with the advent of improved amplification and ink-writing technology developed by the German company Siemens, he was able to produce paper recordings as permanent documentation of his findings. He published over 20 papers on his 'electroencephalogram', and recorded the first motor or Jacksonian seizure in 1930. He also noted that in patients with epilepsy there could be an unusual pattern of brain activity between seizures, which he termed 'inter-ictal activity'. Because he published his research findings in psychiatric journals rather than in physiological ones, his pioneering scientific work would not become internationally recognized until nearly a decade later.

Outside his scientific work, Berger had some controversial views. He had been motivated to study brainwaves by his belief in telepathy and psychic phenomena. It was formerly

---

61   Caton R (1875) The electrical currents of the brain. *British Medical Journal* 2, 278.

believed that it was Berger's ambivalence towards the Nazi party that compelled him to take early retirement, and led him to commit suicide in 1941. However, recent evidence has shown that he was in fact a willing participant in the Nazi courts that reviewed appeals for forced sterilization of neuropsychiatric patients, thus maintaining his professional standing by becoming complicit with policies of oppression.[62]

The American neurologist **William Lennox** (1884–1960) was responsible, along with several of his fellow neurologists at Harvard Medical School, for a major scientific breakthrough that established the EEG as a valuable tool for the investigation of epilepsy. Lennox had first become interested in the condition when he encountered cases while working as a medical missionary in China. After returning to the USA he estimated that nearly half a million of his fellow citizens were suffering from epilepsy, but that little was being done to diagnose the condition, let alone treat it. He commented that 'To the epileptic writhing on the road of medicine, the investigator has perhaps given a cup of cold water, but then has passed by to succour those with illnesses which seemed more likely to reward his efforts. From the humanitarian point of view, epileptics are peculiarly in need of help.'[63]

In 1934, Lennox and his colleagues recorded brainwaves during petit mal attacks (or 'absences') in children, and found that all of these patients showed a similar pattern of brain electrical activity while they were experiencing the seizure. The researchers reported that a 'spike and wave' burst of activity occurred three times per second for the duration of the attack. These children were easier to study as they were motionless rather than convulsing during the attack. Convulsive seizures would have disturbed the recording electrodes that had been pasted to the hair of the scalp. Using a larger number of more robustly attached electrodes, the researchers went on to study grand mal attacks and temporal lobe epilepsy, as well as observe the brain electrical activity between attacks. Lennox later damaged his reputation by becoming involved in the eugenics movement, by joining the advisory council of the Euthanasia Society of America, and by recommending the 'mercy killing' of children with severe brain diseases.[64] He also advocated social engineering by limiting the ability of certain races to have children.

By the late 1930s the EEG was established as a method of diagnosing epilepsy. As the technology improved so did the reliability of the EEG, and its value in enabling an international classification of the different types of seizure. Before imaging techniques became available, the EEG was the central investigation in epilepsy neurosurgery programmes, and for 30 years it was the only diagnostic tool available to the epilepsy specialist. However,

---

62 Zeidman LA, Stone J and Kondziella D (2014) New revelations about Hans Berger, father of the electroencephalogram (EEG), and his ties to the Third Reich. *Journal of Child Neurology* 29, 1002–1010.
63 Goodkin HP (2007) The founding of the American Epilepsy Society: 1936–1971. *Epilepsia* 48, 15–22.
64 Lennox WG (1938) Should they live? Certain economic aspects of medicine. *The American Scholar* 7, 454–466.

subsequent technological advances have seen the development of sleep studies, the use of prolonged recordings combined with visual capturing of the seizure, the introduction of wireless technology, and the use of intra-operative recording either deep within or on the surface of the surgically exposed brain.

Early techniques for visualizing the brain

Before the techniques of computerized tomography (CT) and magnetic resonance imaging (MRI) were developed, visualization of the brain in health and illness was complex. In 1918 the American neurosurgeon **Walter Dandy** (1886–1946) perfected the technique of X-raying injected air in order to define the brain and outline the various ventricles (cavities) within it. Initially this required the drilling of a hole in the skull, through which the air could be injected. However, as Dandy knew that air inside the body rises, he suggested that the air should be administered by lumbar puncture, thus avoiding the need to operate on the patient. In recognition of this work he was nominated for the Nobel Prize for Medicine. Air was injected in the lumbar region (lower back) into the fluid-bathed space that surrounds the spinal cord and brain. Then, by manoeuvring the patient, the air could be made to spread around the surface of the brain and through the ventricles within it. Any distortion or asymmetry of the normal configuration of the ventricles would indicate either swelling or loss of brain tissue. This investigation enabled assessment of the shape of the temporal lobes of the brain in patients with epilepsy, and allowed the outline of the presence of a tumour or the shrinkage from damage to be seen. This investigation, known as the lumbar air encephalogram (LAEG) or pneumoencephalography, was often complicated by severe headaches that lasted for several days. However, it remained the most accurate method of locating brain lesions until the technique of computerized tomography (CT) scanning was introduced in the 1970s.

In the early 1920s, **Egas Moniz** (1874–1955), a Portuguese neurologist and the founder of psychosurgery, sought a method of visualizing the blood vessels of the brain. Since the days of Thomas Willis the anatomy of the blood supply to the brain had been well established, but it could only be examined post-mortem. Moniz believed that if the blood vessels could be visualized in living patients, the anatomy of the brain that was supplied by the vessels could be inferred. For instance, a mass within the brain would displace the blood vessels, and this displacement would become evident when one side of the brain was compared with the other. To this end, Moniz developed the technique of cerebral angiography. He used bromide (as he believed that this would show up in the lumen or interior of arteries on X-ray film), which he administered to human subjects prior to taking X-rays of the head. The bromides caused headaches, and the X-rays revealed nothing. After further experiments continued to yield poor results, Moniz turned his attention from bromide to iodide. After eventual success in 1927, he went on to publish over 60 papers on this new technique for studying brain anatomy, and iodide became the 'contrast agent' of choice in radiology for many years thereafter.[65]

The era of brain scans

Sir Godfrey Hounsfield (1919–2004) was an English electrical engineer who developed the computerized tomography (CT) scanner, allowing the production of images of the brain within the skull without the need for injections of air or iodide. During the 1960s, Hounsfield, by applying the work of the South African theoretical mathematician **Alan Cormack** (1924–1998), with whom he shared the Nobel Prize for Medicine and Physiology in 1979, developed a system in which clusters of X-rays were passed at multiple angles through the human body. By means of sophisticated computer calculations based on the measurement data, images of different cross sections of the body could then be created, allowing three-dimensional images of internal organs to be obtained.

Up until that time the approach to investigation of epilepsy had varied from one part of the world to another, depending on the availability of resources. In resource-rich countries the diagnosis of adult-onset epilepsy required the exclusion of a brain tumour, despite the general acceptance that brain tumours are rare and epilepsy is common. Exclusion of such a tumour would require EEG studies followed by an angiogram and a lumbar air encephalogram. These would necessitate hospital admission for a period of one to two weeks, and thus demand considerable resources, despite the probability (given the relative incidences of brain tumour and epilepsy) that the test results would be normal. The availability of CT scans would become the game changer, requiring far fewer resources as all of the necessary information was provided during a brief outpatient visit, with no risk of harm to the patient.

Hounsfield considered that the brain would be the most suitable organ (given that its detailed anatomy was known and that it was enclosed within the rigid boundaries of the skull) for testing whether his CT images were interpretable and of diagnostic value. He tested a prototype head scanner first on the brain of a cow from a local butcher's shop, and then on himself. Despite the relatively poor resolution of the early images compared with those from future generations of scanners, his machine entered clinical practice in 1971. Now that the contents of the brain could be visualized and analysed in living subjects, epilepsy was near the front of the queue of common disorders awaiting investigation.

---

65 Doby T (1992) Cerebral angiography and Egas Moniz. *American Journal of Radiology* 159, 364.

CT scanning can be used to identify a number of possible causes of epilepsy, including tumours, knots of blood vessels and strokes, head injury, and some infections. However, the early scanners could not show the subtle brain scars that caused epilepsy in many cases, and the majority of scanned patients with the condition were described as 'CT negative'. An important group of infectious conditions that cause epilepsy and which are visible on CT scanning are those caused by tapeworms, which are common parasites of pigs, dogs, and cats that can spread to humans. The condition of neurocysticercosis is caused by the pork tapeworm (*Taenia solium*), and can affect up to 25 per cent of people living in some parts of Asia and sub-Saharan Africa. When the brain becomes infected, multiple cysts around 5–20 mm in diameter can be seen on CT (see Figure 3). In developing countries, neurocysticercosis is the cause of nearly a third of all cases of epilepsy.

The most recently developed CT scanners have excellent spatial resolution, with an ability to detect abnormalities with a diameter of 0.5 mm. This is in fact superior to the resolution achieved by magnetic resonance imaging (MRI) (see below), which typically only identifies abnormalities with a diameter of 1–2 mm or larger. However, CT does not have a high enough sensitivity and specificity to show the subtle changes in brain tissue that occur in many patients with epilepsy.

Magnetic resonance imaging (MRI)

The next major advance in brain imaging was the development of magnetic resonance imaging (MRI). In **1882**, **Nikola Tesla** (1856–1943), a Serbian-American inventor and engineer, discovered the rotating magnetic field – a fundamental discovery in physics. The tesla, which is the unit of magnetic field intensity in the SI system of physical units, was named after him. To this day, MRI scanners are characterized according to their 'field strength' and thus their resolution in tesla units.

It was not until the 1970s that the potential clinical applications of MRI, which had so far been used solely for chemical and physical analysis, were recognized. **Raymond Damadian** (1936–), a New York physician, observed that tumour cells contained more water than normal cells and thus had a different hydrogen signal. He believed that MRI might be able to detect this, and he obtained a patent allowing MRI to be applied to the study of tumour tissue. In 1971 he performed the first full body MRI scan of a human subject, which allowed the detection and thus diagnosis of cancer.[66] He then went on to study healthy human controls as well as those with cancer, using an MRI scanning machine that he himself had invented.

---

66   Damadian RV (1971) Tumor detection by nuclear magnetic resonance. *Science* 171, 1151–1153.

Sir Peter Mansfield (1933–2017), an English physicist, developed scanning programmes that enabled images to be built up within seconds, and by the beginning of the twenty-first century, *brain, heart and whole body MRI* was well established, along with *functional MRI (fMRI)*, which, by measuring small changes in blood flow, was able to show brain activity – that is, the actual functioning of the brain. By 2010 approximately 30 million MRI examinations were being performed annually worldwide.[67] The more powerful the field strength in tesla units, the shorter the scan time and the higher the quality of images obtained. A detailed scan of the brain currently takes between 10 and 30 minutes.

The MRI scanner consists of powerful circular magnets surrounding a large tube containing a moveable bed on which the patient can be moved in and out of the scanner. When the patient is lying under the magnets, a small number, approximately three in a million, of the hydrogen ions in the body tissues line up in the same direction at any given time. Images can be generated from the rate at which those hydrogen ions settle back into their previous position. Radio waves are directed at certain parts of the body, knocking the hydrogen ions out of alignment. After the radio waves have been switched off the hydrogen ions realign themselves, and as they do so they send out radio waves that are detected by the scanner, and used to build up a detailed image of the part of the body that is being scanned. Normal and abnormal tissue with different hydrogen ion concentrations can then be displayed as a simple image or photograph. Bone has the lowest concentration of hydrogen ions and appears dark on the image, fat has the highest concentration and appears white, and all other tissues are of intermediate shades.

We shall now compare the information that CT and MRI scanning can provide about patients with epilepsy. CT depends on X-ray technology, so is very useful for examining the bones of the body (e.g. for arthritis and fractures), although it can also be used to visualize soft tissues such as the brain and spinal cord. However, MRI will give a clearer picture of abnormal function in these soft tissues, because it builds up images based upon the relative differences in water content between tissues. For this reason, CT is often used as a screening test for soft tissue conditions such as tumours, with a normal CT scan rendering MRI unnecessary, whereas an abnormal CT scan will usually result in an MRI scan being performed to provide clarification. When investigating epilepsy we are often trying to detect very subtle brain changes, and a negative CT scan will often lead on to a more probing MRI examination if this is warranted by the nature and type of seizure. In the case of brain tumour, MRI is now used in addition to CT to provide better definition of the extent of the tumour and its relationship to surrounding, often critical, structures, in order to enable the safest possible surgery to be planned (see Figure 4).

---

67 European Magnetic Resonance Forum (2014) MR imaging: facts and figures. *Magnetic Resonance: A Peer-Reviewed Critical Introduction.* www.magnetic-resonance.org/ch/21-01.html

In recent times it has become increasingly apparent that epilepsy is in many cases caused by macroscopic changes in the brain. At one end of the spectrum this might be a tumour, while at the other end it might be an area of scarring with loss of brain tissue, or a variation from normal brain anatomy and development. MRI does not indicate whether a person has epilepsy, as many of the subtle findings that are observed in individuals who have seizures can also occur in those without seizures.

Specialized scan sequences can be used to examine the grey matter both on the surface of the brain and deep within it, as well as areas of brain tissue scarring and loss. These more sophisticated scans are generally reserved for patients who have failed to improve on drug treatment, and for whom the option of surgery is being considered. One of the possible causes of epilepsy in this patient group is *mesial temporal sclerosis (MTS)*. Deep in the temporal lobe of the brain this is manifested as a loss of brain cells or neurons associated with shrinkage and scarring (see Figure 5). As a result of this process the surrounding brain cells have become more excitable, resulting in seizures of temporal lobe origin. There seems to be an association between such brain changes and childhood seizures due to a high temperature (febrile convulsions) or a complicated delivery or pregnancy. Thus this part of the brain appears to be particularly vulnerable during fetal development and early infancy. As the brain develops normally during pregnancy, the grey matter (the brain cells) migrates from deep within the brain to the surface, resulting in the development of the cerebral cortex. The white matter contains all of the fibres that extend from the grey matter or neurons, sending signals to other areas of the brain or spinal cord, rather like a large number of telephone wires connecting telephone exchanges to each other. The white appearance is due to the presence of myelin, an insulating layer of fatty material around the nerves that helps to speed up the rate at which messages pass down the 'telephone wires'.

Epilepsy cannot arise in white matter, as the latter does not normally contain any neurons. However, sometimes the process of migration of grey matter to the surface of the brain during development is incomplete, and a small area of grey matter becomes arrested deep within the brain in the white matter. This is termed *focal cortical dysplasia (FCD)*, and the isolated grey matter becomes electrically over-excitable or unstable, and acts as the source of seizure onset. On MRI, using a scanning sequence known as a FLAIR (Fluid-attenuated inversion recovery) image, these are seen as areas of higher intensity, often lying deep in one of the valleys of the grey matter of the brain that give it its typical 'walnut' appearance (see Figure 6). Sometimes cortical dysplasia is more widespread and appears as a blurred ribbon, whereas normally the grey and white matter areas are sharply demarcated. Cortical dysplasia often coexists with MTS, which suggests that they have similar developmental causes. Other patterns of abnormal brain development associated with seizures include shrunken regions (microgyria) and enlarged regions of grey matter, unusual childhood tumours, and features of specific inherited conditions that can affect the brain, such as tuberous sclerosis. The latter is an inherited condition caused by one of two gene mutations that result in the development of non-cancerous growths or tubers in the skin, brain, kidney, and other organs. On brain MRI scans the tubers are visible, as are islands of arrested grey matter deep within the white matter.

In summary, imaging has had a major impact on our knowledge and treatment of epilepsy. CT has shown us the more visible causes of the condition, such as head injury, stroke, and tumours, whereas MRI has provided new information about the hitherto unknown seizure-related consequences of abnormal brain development. Imaging has added a new dimension to our understanding of what causes epilepsy, and of why it is often (although not always) associated with other problems, such as learning disability. It has also enabled the option of surgical treatment for many patients with drug-resistant epilepsy. Finally, imaging has led to a more logical classification of epilepsy into many different seizure types, and has allowed a larger number of causes of the condition to be identified.

The classification of seizures

Why should we attempt to classify seizures and the disparate disordered processes that cause them? The basis of all medical and life sciences is the need to bring order to knowledge. In 1893 the first international classification of diseases was adopted by the International Statistical Institute, based on the Bertillon Classification of Causes of Death developed by the French statistician **Jacques Bertillon** (1851–1922). With regard to human illness, it is only by recognizing that there are many subtly different subtypes of the same condition that we can understand how each of them might behave individually, how they respond to the treatments that are given, and how to narrow down the possible underlying causes. The drawback of systems of classification is that if they become overly obsessive and detailed, as perhaps in psychiatry, there is a risk that the extremes of the normal range may be regarded and classified as abnormal.[68] However, such 'medicalization' of behaviours does not cause problems where epilepsy is concerned, and systems of classification of this condition have been of great benefit.

The first attempts to classify the different types of seizure were made in the late nineteenth century, when John Hughlings Jackson formulated his definition of epilepsy. The development of the technique of electroencephalography (EEG) provided a scientific basis

---

68   Anon. (2016) Medicalization and its discontents (editorial). *Lancet Psychiatry* 3, 591.

for distinguishing between seizures with a localized onset, which were described as 'focal' (see Figure 7), and those with immediate involvement of both sides of the brain, which were termed 'generalized' (see Figure 8). For decades the terms that were most commonly (and somewhat loosely) used to describe seizures were 'grand mal' and 'petit mal', resulting in a simplistic and imprecise system of classification. The present-day classification of seizures is based on three key features: (1) the seizure's site of origin in the brain; (2) whether consciousness or awareness is lost; and (3) the presence of any specific additional features. When seizures arise from a network of cells in a specific location on one side of the brain they are described as *focal*. When they arise simultaneously from both sides of the brain they are described as *generalized*.

Seizures that start focally and then rapidly involve both sides are referred to as *focal seizures with secondary generalization*. The level of consciousness is more pertinent to the categorization of focal seizures. When awareness is present throughout a focal seizure – for example, when a person with twitching of a hand or leg is able to converse throughout and is fully aware of the attack – this is referred to as a *simple focal seizure*. This is the type of attack that Hughlings Jackson described, formerly known as Jacksonian epilepsy, and which was operated upon, as its focal origin could be carefully pinpointed. When there is confusion or impaired awareness, this is referred to as a *complex focal seizure*. In the past, as these symptoms most commonly originated in the temporal lobe, this was termed *temporal lobe epilepsy*. However, it is not always easy to establish whether or not awareness has been retained, especially if the patient lives alone or has seizures during sleep.

Generalized seizures originate across wide areas of the brain, and affect both of its sides from the very beginning. They include the *tonic–clonic seizure* (also known as grand mal) as well as the *absence attack* (also known as petit mal). Generalized seizures can also manifest as *drop attacks*, where the individual simply drops to the ground (*atonic*), or as episodes of jerking (*myoclonic*). There are still a large number of cases that do not fit within a precise classification of seizures. What is clear, however, is that when a person has epilepsy, their attacks tend to be very similar on each occasion. The repeated stereotypic form of attacks in an individual is a characteristic feature of the condition, to the extent that if variability is observed, the diagnosis of epilepsy should be questioned. Much useful information can be found in the revised classification of seizure types published by the International League Against Epilepsy (ILAE) in 2017 (see Table 1).

It may seem curious that a classification of a medical condition does not address its causes. There is a logical reason for this. Identifying that an individual has epilepsy is the first stage in investigation and treatment. Once the type of epilepsy (focal or generalized) has been ascertained, the appropriate investigations and treatments can be selected. Focal epilepsy requires a search for a lesion within the appropriate area of the brain, whereas generalized epilepsy is likely to have a non-structural cause (for example, no scars, tumours, or other localized brain conditions). Focal epilepsy that does not respond to drug treatment may benefit from surgery, whereas generalized epilepsy is less likely to do so.

We have now discussed two of the three key features of the present-day classification of seizures, namely the site of origin of the seizure, and the maintenance or loss of consciousness or awareness. With regard to the third, namely the presence of any specific additional features, the situation becomes more complicated, reflected by the fact that there are over 50 different recognizable types of epilepsy. Indeed, given the complexity of the human brain it could be argued that, just as no two snowflakes are the same, each individual's epilepsy has its own unique characteristics. If focal epilepsy can originate from any location within the human cortex, it could have myriad initial manifestations before spread to adjacent areas of the brain produces a more standardized picture.

This can be explained by considering some examples. Seizure onset in the area of the brain that perceives smell might give the affected individual a false sensation of the smell of burning rubber, and as the attack becomes more widespread there would then be a loss of awareness associated with a vacant expression. Similarly, there could be an unpleasant taste in the mouth, a feeling of unfamiliarity (jamais vu) or familiarity (déjà vu), or a host of other subjective sensations before the more general form of the attack ensues. The list of such initial sensations or 'auras' is almost endless, although because certain areas of the brain are more susceptible to epilepsy, some sensations are more common than others. The nature of the initial symptom identifies a specific area of the brain as the source or focus of the attack. Generalized epilepsy does not have this kind of 'pinpointing' onset. Both sides of the brain are affected simultaneously, so there is no aura or warning, and the attack causes loss of awareness from the onset, usually with shaking, stiffening, or jerking movements of all four limbs.

The causes of epilepsy

Anyone can develop epilepsy, irrespective of age, gender, or ethnic origin. Surprisingly, in about 50 per cent of individuals with the condition no definite cause can be identified. To aid the reader, a simple although not exhaustive guide to the various causes of epilepsy is provided in Table 2. In individuals for whom there is a demonstrable cause, the condition can be attributed to an acquired or developmental disorder of the brain. Acquired causes include head injury, stroke, infections, and degenerative diseases. Infections can include encephalitis (inflammation of the brain), meningitis (infection of the membranes surrounding the brain), and focal infection (cysts or abscesses within the brain). Degenerative diseases are those in which the brain ages prematurely, such as Alzheimer's disease. A brain injury sustained just before birth or around the time of delivery is also regarded as an acquired injury, as the nervous system had developed normally up until that point. At this stage the baby's brain is more susceptible to damage caused by factors such as maternal infection, poor nutrition, drug or alcohol misuse, and lack of oxygen. Brain damage caused by any of these factors can result in epilepsy and associated problems such as learning disability or cerebral palsy. Developmental disorders are the result of impairment of the normal process of fetal brain development and maturation during pregnancy, and are very distinct from those in which a normally developed nervous system has been subject to any of the external insults mentioned above. These disorders are often manifested as complex syndromes in which epilepsy is only one of the symptoms present. Common examples of developmental disorders include autism and focal cortical dysplasia (FCD).

Many of the hitherto unexplained forms of epilepsy can be attributed to genetic factors, as it has been known since ancient times that the condition can run in families. The first scientifically based link between heredity and epilepsy was established over 100 years ago in relation to a form of generalized epilepsy that is now known as *progressive myoclonic epilepsy*. In 1936, based on the perceived importance of inheritance, the report of the American Neurological Association Committee for the Investigation of Eugenical Sterilization recommended voluntary sterilization for people with epilepsy. Researchers have linked some types of epilepsy to specific genes, but in most cases genes are only one factor in causation, in that they may make an individual more sensitive to environmental factors that trigger seizures, such as head injury. In 1990 a link between a specific chromosome and epilepsy was demonstrated, and this has since become an expanding area of research that may eventually explain why people with no other demonstrable cause of their seizures are prone to the condition.

The interaction between genes and environmental factors is evident in relation to febrile convulsions. Only a minority of individuals who have a single seizure with a high temperature go on to develop recurrent epilepsy with scarring in the temporal lobe visible on MRI scans. Those who do so often have either a prolonged febrile seizure or a family history of epilepsy, highlighting the fact that it is an inherited genetic factor that determines the long-term outcome. It is to be hoped that the growing research-based evidence for the link between specific genes and different types of epilepsy may lead to better diagnosis and more targeted drug treatment.

The origins of the epilepsy societies

This chapter would not be complete without a brief discussion of the development of the 'epilepsy movement', which has been responsible for spearheading understanding of, support for and research into the condition. It has been and continues to be led by people with epilepsy and those who care for them, who have advocated for a greater understanding of the condition and for the upholding of the human rights of the individual and their family.

The first national association for patients with epilepsy was founded in America in 1898 by **William Letchworth** (1823–1910), a businessman and philanthropist. He was from a Quaker family, and had made his money in the iron industry. He spent several years travelling around Europe and the USA, at his own expense, during which time he studied the treatment of epilepsy. His book entitled *The Care and Treatment of Epileptics*[69] was based on this research. In 1896 he established Craig Colony, a state institution for patients with epilepsy, in New York. He served as President of the National Association for the Study of Epilepsy and the Care and Treatment of Epileptics, and edited the proceedings of its first annual meeting.[70] Membership was offered to 'any person interested in the scientific study of epilepsy, or in the study of ways and means to improve the condition of epileptics, or in sociological subjects generally'. The first meeting was held in May 1901 in Washington, DC. Letchworth served on the New York State Board of Charities, and the development of epilepsy centres and the New York fostering system can be directly attributed to him.

The American Epilepsy Society was established to promote research, and it joined the **International League Against Epilepsy (ILAE)** when this was established in 1909 in Budapest, Hungary. The ILAE's stated purpose was 'the study of the pathology, therapy and social legal aspects of epilepsy'. During the last two decades it has published classifications of the different types of epilepsies, outlined diagnostic criteria, and provided guidelines on standards of care. The International Bureau for Epilepsy (IBE), which was established in 1961, has enabled national epilepsy organizations to network globally for the benefit of those with epilepsy. During the last 60 years many countries have produced guidelines on epilepsy care to ensure a standardized approach to diagnosis, investigation, and treatment.

In 1997 the World Health Organization (WHO), in combination with the ILAE and the IBE, launched a global campaign to 'bring epilepsy out of the shadows and further improve diagnosis, treatment, prevention and social acceptability'. It is significant that social acceptability was the last of their listed aims, whereas for people living with the condition it would be the first priority. The national and local epilepsy charities that have emerged from

---

69 Letchworth WP (1900) *The Care and Treatment of Epileptics*. G. P. Putnam's Sons, New York.
70 Fine EJ, Fine DL, Sentz L et al. (1993) William P. Letchworth: philanthropist and pioneer epileptologist. *Archives of Neurology* 50, 313–316.

the 'epilepsy movement' provide information and support, including websites and helplines, as well as campaigning on policy matters, providing training, and raising awareness. Pressure exerted by the charities on healthcare providers has led to improvements in the services available for those with epilepsy, such as the introduction of the epilepsy specialist nurse to improve accessibility to care and advice. Although the epilepsy charities have improved the public's awareness of epilepsy, there is still much work to be done in changing long-held negative attitudes.

Conclusion

The last 100 years have seen the development of surgical treatment for epilepsy, the emergence of anti-epileptic drugs, and a growing understanding of the molecular processes and genetic factors that underlie seizures. A much wider range of investigations is now available, and they have made a huge contribution to establishing the diagnosis, causes, and classification of epilepsy. Given the global nature of the condition, we can no longer ignore the glaring inequalities in the availability of the benefits of these advances, most notably access to good-quality medical care for epilepsy. Moreover, social understanding and acceptance of epilepsy lags far behind the major scientific advances that have been made. The challenge now is to educate the wider public, as only a better understanding of epilepsy can overcome long-held attitudes and prejudice.

PART II

Epilepsy in the arts

CHAPTER 4
Epilepsy in literature and in authors

It has been claimed that a significant number of writers, including Gustave Flaubert, Charles Dickens, Edgar Allan Poe, Fyodor Dostoevsky, Lord Byron, Dante Alighieri, Sir Walter Scott, Edward Lear, and Jonathan Swift, were affected by epilepsy. However, with the exception of Flaubert, Dostoevsky, and Lear, there is little evidence to support these claims. For example, it has been suggested that Edgar Allan Poe's 'difficult' personality was due to his being an 'epileptic', whereas in fact he experienced blackouts caused by binge drinking, but there is very little evidence that he suffered from epilepsy. It seems likely that Dickens had severe renal colic that caused him to collapse occasionally. Speculation that Byron had epilepsy is based on the single line stating that he 'fell prey to violent convulsions' when, at the age of 16 years, he heard that a woman he loved was thinking of getting married.

The appearance of characters with epilepsy in fiction and drama can be traced back through history. Seizures have been used for dramatic effect as well as for plot and character development. As early as the sixth century bce, the Greek playwright Euripides had linked epilepsy to madness and violence.

William Shakespeare (1564–1616)

We have already referred in Chapter 1 to William Shakespeare's *Julius Caesar* (Act 1, Scene 2), where the 'falling sickness' makes its first appearance in classic literature. Here epilepsy is being used as a metaphor for Caesar's vulnerability. In *King Lear*, Shakespeare uses the word 'epileptic' in a derogatory manner in the insult 'a plague upon your epileptic visage'. Epilepsy plays a significant role in *Othello* (Act 4, Scene 4). When Iago tells Othello that Cassio has confessed to having an affair with Desdemona, this proves too much for Othello, who has a seizure, with the stage direction stating that he 'falls in a trance'. Enter Cassio.

Cassio: What's the matter?
Iago: My lord is fall'n into an epilepsy. This is his second fit. He had one yesterday.
Cassio: Rub him about the temples.
Iago: No, forbear. The lethargy must have his quiet course. If not, he foams at mouth and by and by breaks out to savage madness. Look, he stirs. Do you withdraw yourself a little while.

This perceptive dialogue tells us, as all modern first aiders know, that one should never disturb someone who is having a seizure, except to ensure that they are in the recovery position. The shame and stigma attached to seizures are implied in the advice to withdraw. Finally, when Othello recovers, Iago asks him if he has struck his head, Othello being unaware of the fact that he had fallen. The play centres on Othello's obsessive jealousy and his stigmatization on account of the colour of his skin, his emotional vulnerability, and his epilepsy, which is portrayed as possession by demons. The description of his seizures suggests focal epilepsy with secondary generalization, and the tendency to speak nonsensically on recovery suggests that the dominant (probably left) side of the brain is affected. Later in the play Othello murders his wife in a jealous rage. The links between seizures, rage, violence, murder, and demonic possession have been well and truly made. John Emery in *The Psychoanalytic Review*[71] writes briefly about the trigger for Othello's seizure, namely the mental image of Desdemona and Cassio's adultery, and elaborates on how sexual arousal might provoke seizures. It should be noted that all of this is speculative, being based on opinion rather than fact, with the author quoting Democritus of Abdera (born *c.* 460 bce), who claimed that 'coition is a slight attack of epilepsy'.

How did Shakespeare know about epilepsy? Walter Friedlander[72] mentions that Shakespeare's son-in law, John Hall, was a physician. However, Friedlander also quotes a study of the medical references, metaphors, and similes used by Shakespeare, which found that the frequency with which these occurred did not change after his son-in-law's arrival on the scene.[73] Friedlander also suggests the possibility that Shakespeare's granddaughter

---

71 Emery JP (1959) Othello's epilepsy. *Psychoanalytic Review* 46D, 30–32.
72 Friedlander WJ (1963) Shakespeare on epilepsy. *Boston Medical Quarterly* 14, 113–120.
73 Simpson RR (1959) *Shakespeare and Medicine*. E. & S. Livingstone, Edinburgh.

Elizabeth (John Hall's daughter) had convulsions, as documented in the physician's own observations. Throughout Shakespeare's plays there are frequent dramatic blackouts, both genuine and feigned. Lady Macbeth's contrived loss of consciousness when she learns that Duncan's murder has been discovered is perhaps the best known example of the latter. The term 'fit' is often ambiguous, and may be used by Shakespeare to imply rage or madness. In *Hamlet* (Act 5, Scene 1) his mother says 'This is mere madness: and thus awhile the fit will work on him', and reference is made to 'his fits, his frenzy, and his bitterness'. Shakespeare certainly used fits and faints for dramatic effect throughout his writings, and there is a danger of reading too much epilepsy into a host of blackouts, feigned or otherwise. These blackouts were invariably linked to physical or emotional events such as drunkenness, fatigue, surprise, anger, fear, or hearing bad news. Most experts accept that in *Othello* and *Julius Caesar* the unconsciousness was due to epilepsy, and in both circumstances Shakespeare showed a clear knowledge of the condition and an awareness of the prejudices of his time. His knowledge and dramatic use of medical conditions has been the subject of a major review.[74]

William Makepeace Thackeray (1811–1863) was a British writer who specialized in satirical works that criticized the greed and corruption of English society. His most famous work was *Vanity Fair* (1848), which is seen as satirizing the greed and corruption of the aristocracy and the middle classes. In it he describes a minor character, Lord Castletoddy, as 'an epileptic and simple-minded nobleman'. In Chapter 46 he writes 'Dear Rhoda Macmull will disengage the whole of the Castletoddy property as soon as poor dear Lord Castletoddy dies, who is quite epileptic.' The novel follows the lives of Becky Sharp, Emmy Sedley, and their friends and families during and after the Napoleonic Wars. In the characterization of Lord Castletoddy, an association between epilepsy, feeble-mindedness, and ridicule is made, and the general uselessness of people with epilepsy is also implied. Castletoddy's seizures are triggered by his emotions, in particular his upset at his daughter's fanatical outbursts on religion: 'The physicians declared his fits always occurred after one of her Ladyship's sermons.'

Alfred Lord Tennyson (1808–1892) was Poet Laureate during the reign of Queen Victoria and is still one of the most popular British poets. He is perhaps best remembered for his epic poem 'The Charge of the Light Brigade'. His upbringing was harsh, and was dogged by the possibility of epilepsy. He was one of 12 children born to George Clayton, an unfulfilled pedestrian clergyman, and his long-suffering wife Elizabeth. One of his brothers was committed permanently to an asylum, and another intermittently. The family had a history not only of alcoholism, drug abuse, and mental instability, but also of the 'black blood' of epilepsy – this at a time when epilepsy was commonly attributed to sexual excess

---

74 Simpson RR (1959) *Shakespeare and Medicine*. E. & S. Livingstone, Edinburgh.

and shrouded in shame. For most of the first half of his life, Tennyson laboured under the belief that he had inherited the condition from his father, and found it hard to endure the thought that the clergyman had indulged in carnal excesses. It is known that the poet was prone to 'trances', and when he was hospitalized in 1848 a doctor attributed the trances not to epilepsy but, somewhat surprisingly, to gout. Tennyson readily accepted this explanation, which gave him the confidence to consider marriage and parenthood without fear of passing on the 'black blood' to his offspring. The long and popular narrative poem 'The Princess' was published in 1847, and was then revised by the author over the next four years. Tennyson wrote the poem, after discussing the outline with his future wife, Emily Selwood, in response to those critics who had accused him of avoiding serious subject matter. The main theme is a feminist one, in that a betrothed princess enters a women's university where men are forbidden. Her future husband, himself a prince, and his two friends disguise themselves as women students in order to follow her. They are found out, flee, are attacked and wounded, and eventually everyone is reconciled. Although the poem is about emancipation and gender role reversal, ultimately the reconciliation is dependent upon the men and women resuming their more traditional roles. In later revisions of the poem, Tennyson introduces the prince's 'weird seizures' that he has inherited from his family, and from which he can only be released by the love of Princess Ida. The seizures are attributed to an ancestor who was also burnt as a sorcerer. During the seizures, which occur at times of stress, the princess becomes like a shadow to the prince. Barbara Wright suggests that the seizures are epileptic in nature, and the description of derealization and depersonalization associated with them implies a focal temporal lobe origin.[75] The account of the brevity of the trance and his ability to continue his activities during them provides further support for their epileptic nature. The inherited background and the causal sorcerer's curse mirror both Tennyson's personal experiences and the perceptions of the time. The happy ending here is that true love banishes the curse of epilepsy. Tennyson's trances also feature in three further works, namely 'In Memoriam', 'Maud', and 'Idylls of the King'. In these poems the trances are seen in a more transcendental light as something to enjoy rather than fear. We shall never know for sure whether Tennyson himself had epilepsy. After his death his wife and son burnt his personal letters, and there is little evidence of the nature of his own trances (which, incidentally, his son did not inherit).

No discussion of Tennyson can ignore **Edgar Allan Poe** (1809–1849). These two writers admired each other's work. Poe was a critic and editor, but is best known for his poems (especially 'The Raven'), for his macabre short stories, and for blazing a trail for science fiction and the detective novel. His life was short but confrontational, and his literary output was relatively small. His own history of blackouts or memory loss can be attributed to his binge

---

75 Wright BH (1987) Tennyson, the weird seizures in *The Princess*, and epilepsy. *Literature and Medicine* 6, 61–76.

drinking rather than to epilepsy. However, as alcohol abuse can lead to the development of seizures, and conversely people with epilepsy may resort to the use of alcohol, the distinction between the two conditions is by no means clear, and will be discussed later (see p. 00). Poe's complex life has been the subject of several biographies.[76]

His Gothic short story 'Berenice' (published in the *Southern Literary Messenger* in 1835) features two conditions – epilepsy and cataplexy – that merge and become difficult to distinguish from each other. It relates the tale of Egaeus, a studious young man, who shares a dark mansion with his beautiful but doomed cousin Berenice. Both appear to experience trances, with Berenice being described as having 'a species of epilepsy not infrequently terminating in trance itself'. Egaeus himself has daydreams in which he appears separate from the world around him. The two become engaged, but Berenice's beauty begins to fade, and she also starts to experience episodes in which she stands motionless and unable to communicate. Egaeus then becomes obsessed with Berenice's white teeth, which increasingly figure in his daydreams. After one of her seizures Berenice is found dead, and she is subsequently buried. Egaeus falls in and out of a trance state and has a vague recollection of a shameful deed associated with shrill screaming. He then hears that Berenice's grave has been desecrated and that it seems as if she was buried while still alive. He notes beside him a spade as well as a box containing a dental instrument, 'thirty-two small, white and ivory-looking substances', and a poem he has about visiting his beloved's grave. The reader is left to assume that Egaeus, while in his trance state, has opened Berenice's grave, killed her, and removed the teeth that had obsessed him – all of this while he was in a post-seizure or 'fugue' state. A fugue state is characterized by reversible memory loss for events and personal identity. Although linked to stress or traumatic events, it can occur after a seizure, especially a focal one of temporal lobe origin. Based on the circumstances in which it arises in this short story, epilepsy seems the most likely cause. Poe is showing us that in the twilight state following a seizure, a person with epilepsy can carry out the most vile and unimaginable acts of evil. Clearly this is not a good advert for epilepsy. Poe was not unaccustomed to long periods of memory loss, which were usually alcohol related, and ironically such memory loss surrounds the mystery of his own death. Cataplexy is a state characterized by a sudden and passing episode of muscle weakness accompanied by full conscious awareness, typically triggered by emotions such as laughing, crying, or terror. Although the individual with cataplexy is awake, they cannot move. This condition features in two other stories by Poe, 'The Fall of the House of Usher' and 'The Premature Burial', and reflects both Poe's personal fear and the universal human fear of being buried alive. This led to all sorts of devices being fitted to coffins to act as an

---

76 For example: Barnes N (2009) *A Dream Within a Dream: The Life of Edgar Allan Poe*. Peter Owen Publishers, London; Silverman K (1991) *Edgar A. Poe: Mournful and Never-Ending Remembrance*. HarperCollins Publishers, New York.

alarm in the event of anyone being buried prematurely. Whereas Berenice may have had cataplexy, which resulted in her burial while she was still alive, the evidence from the story suggests that Egaeus had epilepsy.

For writers who did not have a personal knowledge of epilepsy, one possible source of information about the condition would be John Quincy's *Lexicon Medicum*. First published in 1717 (the first London edition was not published until 1805), this dictionary of medical terms and conditions was created by an apothecary with little knowledge of the practice of medicine, despite having a medical qualification (earned for a dissertation) from the University of Edinburgh. Authors would refer to this book for information on diseases, and on the basis of descriptive similarities it appears to have been consulted by the English writer **George Eliot** when she was creating the character of Silas Marner. George Eliot was the nom de plume of the author Mary Ann Evans (1819–1880). The daughter of a mill owner, and having received little formal education, Evans adopted a male name in order that her writing might be taken more seriously, and to escape the female stereotype of being an author of trite romances. She wrote seven novels, of which *Silas Marner* (1861) was the third. Because of her 25-year-long relationship with a married man, George Lewes, and her disdain for Christian worship, she was denied a burial at Westminster Abbey, and was instead buried at Highgate Cemetery alongside Karl Marx.

Silas Marner is an impoverished linen weaver who resides in the fictitious town of Lantern Yard. He is known to have 'fits' that last from a few minutes to an hour, and during these episodes he becomes motionless, is unresponsive, and has an empty look about him. Afterwards he has no memory of the attack. These features all strongly suggest a focal seizure arising in the temporal lobe. His fellow townsfolk, who represent an unspecified religious sect, interpret his attacks as some form of divine visitation that marks him out as a chosen person. All goes wrong when a bag of gold disappears during Marner's watch over a dying man. This theft during a death wake leads to his fall from grace, and despite his explanation that the gold was stolen during a trance he is found guilty of the deed and is exiled to a foreign land. His seizures are no longer considered saintly, but are now perceived as demonic. Marner has become an outsider, and is exiled for many years. During this time, due to his frugal lifestyle he amasses some wealth, which ironically is then stolen from him. When those who had previously banished him learn of this new misfortune, they take pity on him and invite him back into the community. After another 'trance' he wakes to find an orphan girl in his humble hut, and he raises her as his adopted child, at last finding contentment. His lost money is also recovered, so all ends happily. Here epilepsy is used to bring attention to the injustice of being accused of theft and then being unable to refute the accusation on account of loss of memory. It also highlights the ambivalence of the townsfolk as to whether Marner's 'trances' are a sign of divinity or of demonic possession. Epilepsy serves as the vehicle for the themes of Marner's misfortune, vulnerability, and dependence on the goodwill and perceptions of others.

The French writer **Gustave Flaubert** (1821–1880) is best known for his debut novel *Madame Bovary* (1857). Flaubert suffered from chronic syphilis, and died from a brain haemorrhage in his late fifties. It is unclear whether he had epileptic seizures or whether his 'nerve sickness' was caused by neurosis or hysteria. Whatever the explanation, his illness led him to isolate himself from others, and had a very destructive effect on his life. Flaubert was treated with regular bleedings, mercury massages, and the anti-epileptic drug bromide, which may well have had an impact on his cognitive function and writing skills. If Flaubert did have epilepsy, he chose not to give any of his fictional characters the condition, although there is a suggestion of it in *Madame Bovary*. There were also hints that vivid visual and psychic auras were to feature in his planned novel *La Spirale*, but the latter was never completed. There are several lines of evidence that Flaubert had epilepsy. The first event occurred when he was 23 years old,[77] and it was documented by his friend Maxime Du Camp: 'Gustave was thrown down and fell. His brother bled him right there on the spot hoping and believing that he had witnessed an isolated event. Other episodes followed, and he went on to have four seizures over the next three weeks.'[78] Flaubert's father and brother were both doctors, with the former working at the Hôtel-Dieu hospital in Rouen. The bleeding treatment administered by Flaubert's brother was at the time considered an effective way to treat epilepsy. Soon after this initial attack, Flaubert resigned from the Faculty of Law in Paris, where he had been a student. In a subsequent attack, he sustained burns to his hand from scalding water applied by his brother to purge the episodes. When describing his condition, Flaubert commented that 'no one else ever had the slightest idea [of it]'. Some authors have attributed certain personality changes to his epilepsy.[79] These authors outline in Flaubert features of the 'epileptic personality' or 'interictal dysphoric disorder' that had been described by others, namely aggressiveness, irritability, depression, and hyposexuality. The latter observation was based on a reduction in Flaubert's sexual activity with prostitutes (which had been the cause of his chronic syphilis) as he grew older and his epilepsy progressed. Further evidence to support the view that epilepsy was the cause of Flaubert's nervous disease comes from the analysis of his handwriting. Two American neurologists had noted rapid writing in patients with epilepsy, including diminishing spaces, much underlining and repetition, and the generally

---

77 Jallon P and Jallon H (2005) Gustave Flaubert's hidden sickness. In: Bogousslavsky J and Boller F (eds.) Neurological Disorders in Famous Artists. *Frontiers of Neurology and Neuroscience* 19, 46–56.
78 Du Camp M (2002) *Souvenirs Littéraires: Flaubert, Fromentin, Gautier, Musset, Nerval, Sand*. Hachette, Paris.
79 Arnold LM, Baumann CR and Siegel AM (2007) Gustav Flaubert's "nervous disease": an autobiographic and epileptological approach. *Epilepsy & Behavior* 11, 212–217.

frenetic nature of the handwriting.[80] This is clearly evident in Flaubert's manuscripts, with the author himself commenting that he was 'progressively, painfully, spoiling considerable quantities of paper'.[81]

His friend Maxime Du Camp, in his *Souvenirs Littéraires*, gives a most compelling account of the seizures: 'Abruptly without reason Gustave would raise his head and become very pale: that was when he was feeling his aura, this mysterious sensation that he would have in his face as though a ghost had just walked through him. ... He would walk to his bed quickly and lie down, dejected.' Du Camp goes on to describe Flaubert shouting out and moaning, and he also mentions visual hallucinations that Flaubert likened to fireworks with exploding colours. It appears from the letters that he wrote to friends that the seizures, which would occasionally progress to convulsions, would now be termed focal seizures with or without secondary generalization. During his nine-year relationship with the married poet Louise Colet, she documented his seizures in her diary, and wrote that 'he begs me not to call for help; his convulsions, the noises in his throat, the foam coming out of his mouth, the marks his nails left in my arm. He came round after about ten minutes, vomiting.'

After the breakdown of his relationship with Colet, he wrote his masterpiece, *Madame Bovary*, which led to his prosecution for obscenity, on grounds of being offensive to public morality, but he was acquitted. Thereafter, perhaps as a consequence of his attacks, he rarely travelled away from home, but instead lived quietly with his mother, niece, and maid. His last few years were spent in solitude and financial hardship. The term 'epilepsy' was rarely mentioned; Flaubert referred to his attacks as 'nervous hallucinations' or 'nervous sickness'. Just before his death, according to Du Camp he had 'a nervous attack which he tried to ward off with ether' followed by a 'golden vision' and a 'convulsive movement', after which he died. He was 58, and whether he died of a seizure or a stroke, possibly syphilis related, is uncertain.

The philosopher Jean-Paul Sartre considered Flaubert's seizures to be due to neurosis or hysteria rather than epilepsy, and attributed this to Flaubert's unreconciled hatred of his medical father and brother.[82] This seems to be an unduly judgmental view, as the documentation of Maxime Du Camp and Louise Colet would seem to confirm the diagnosis of epilepsy. Flaubert's condition, which he describes as a 'dark illness', prevented him from studying law and led him to adopt a sheltered and withdrawn life. He never considered writing about the condition (except in the planned but never completed *La Spirale*, as mentioned earlier). His own letters offer a revealing picture of his life and the limitations and advantages that it gave him: 'My illness has benefited me in that I am able to spend my

---

80   Waxman SG and Geschwind N (2005) Hypergraphia in temporal lobe epilepsy. *Epilepsy & Behavior* 6, 282–291.
81   Wall G (2001) *Flaubert: A Life*. Faber and Faber, London.
82   Sartre JP (1971) *L'Idiot de la Famille*. Gallimard, Paris. pp. 1771–2136.

time as I like.' The solitary life that Flaubert was forced to lead due to his epilepsy ultimately resulted in a major literary legacy for future generations. Nevertheless, his biographer and friend Maxime du Camp wrote that 'this illness has destroyed his life; it forced him to isolate himself and has rendered him almost savage' and that 'if it were not for the nervous ailment that plagues him he would have been a man of genius'.

In his relative youth, Flaubert became a close friend of the author **George Sand** (1804–1876). George Sand was the nom de plume of Amantine Lucile Aurore Dupin, who had love affairs with a number of the artistic luminaries of her time, including the composer Frederic Chopin, and was believed to have had lesbian relationships, too. She corresponded extensively with Gustave Flaubert, and despite their differences they became close friends. What did she know of his epilepsy, and did this influence her novel *La Mare au Diable* (*The Devil's Pool*) (1845), in which epilepsy plays a prominent part? That book is one of four pastoral novels that drew upon her childhood experiences. It depicts a congenial gravedigger with epilepsy who is the organizer, not to mention the heart and soul, of village life. His epilepsy is seen as a positive affirmation of his life by those who know about it. However, his own personal feelings of shame about his condition are the cause of his eventual downfall. In an attempt to conceal his epilepsy from relatives, as he senses that a seizure is imminent, he climbs up to the solitude of the hayloft, only to fall to his death. Sand understands the stigma and the need to conceal, as well as the worthiness of the individual. Did she learn this from Flaubert?

Despite their 17-year age difference they corresponded intimately for over 12 years. Sand referred to Flaubert as 'my Old Troubadour' and he called her 'My Master'. Although he never identifies it specifically, Flaubert frequently alludes to his nervous condition in this correspondence.[83] In October 1869 he wrote 'I have wanted for several days to write you a long letter in which I should tell you all that I have felt for a month. It is funny. I have passed through different and strange states. But I have neither the time nor the repose of mind to gather myself together enough.' In March 1870, Flaubert wrote to Sand, saying 'I am very tired in mine (my brain) or rather it is very low for the moment! However hard I work, it doesn't go! Everything irritates me and hurts me; and since I restrain myself before people, I give way from time to time to floods of tears when it seems to me as if I should burst.' The level of their shared intimacies about health is demonstrated by Sand's suggestion that Flaubert should see her doctor. In April 1870, Flaubert commented upon the consultation, writing 'I have seen your physician, M. Favre, who seemed to me very strange and a little mad, between ourselves. He ought to like me for I let him talk all the

---

83 Sand G and Flaubert G (McKenzie AL trans., 1921) *The George Sand-Gustave Flaubert Letters*. Norilana Books, Los Angeles, CA.

time. There are high lights in his talk, things which sparkle for a moment, then one sees not a ray.' Finally, in July 1873, he wrote 'I am exhausted, and I am now sleeping ten hours a night, not to mention two hours a day. That is resting my poor brain.' Their shared correspondence dwells mainly on literary, political, and social issues, but the fragility of Flaubert's health and the recurring theme of his nervous condition are always apparent. If it is accepted that Flaubert indeed had epilepsy, there can be little doubt that Sand was aware of the nuances of that condition.

Peter Wolf, a Danish neurologist, has studied how epilepsy is used by writers to symbolize vulnerability and weakness, religiosity, mental instability, and sexuality. He has also reviewed the epileptic aura as described in literature, and has commented that some written observations are more insightful than descriptions in medical textbooks.[84] The contribution of Dickens and Dostoevsky to the positive portrayal of epilepsy has already been mentioned. However, in early fiction, individuals with epilepsy were generally perceived as being possessed and a threat to others, although occasionally, particularly when female, they were viewed as being touched by God, holy and gifted.

Fyodor Dostoevsky (1821–1881) is generally the first name that springs to mind when epilepsy and literature are discussed. He is regarded as a great writer who chronicled the social conditions of nineteenth-century Russia. Like Flaubert, his father was a medical practitioner, and he was prone to what were described as nervous breakdowns. Dostoevsky trained as a naval engineer in St Petersburg and, after a period in which he focused on gambling, embarked upon a literary career. In 1846, at the age of 25 years, he experienced a seizure while attending a funeral. Voskuil describes an episode at a party when Dostoevsky's face 'changed queerly and a frightened look came into his eyes. A few minutes passed and in a hollow voice he asked "Where am I?"' After this he left the company and was later found convulsing.[85] Thereafter minor attacks and more severe generalized attacks with a preceding 'visage of terror' are described. By this stage he had become involved in the revolutionary movement, and this resulted in his capture, trial, and death sentence, which was commuted to deportation to Siberia. Throughout this period frequent seizures are described, with foaming at the mouth and twitching, followed by exhaustion. Seven years later, at the end of his prison sentence, Dostoevsky married, and subsequently experienced further seizures while on his honeymoon, which were attributed to sleep deprivation, excitement, and alcohol consumption. A diagnosis of epilepsy was eventually made. In 1863 he went abroad to seek expert advice from Moritz H. Romberg (in Germany) and Armand Trousseau (in France), two of the leading neurologists of the time.

---

84 Wolf P (2016) Epilepsy and metaphors in literature. *Epilepsy & Behavior* 57, 243–246.
85 Voskuil PH (1983) The epilepsy of Fyodor Mikhailovitch Dostoevsky (1821–1881). *Epilepsia* 24, 658–667.

Epilepsy features in seven of Dostoevsky's eleven novels. This strongly suggests that, unlike Flaubert, he wished to bring his own personal experiences of epilepsy to the fore. It is in *The Idiot* (1868–1869) that he develops this theme most fully. Prince Myshkin, the hero, is sent to a Swiss sanatorium to receive treatment for his epilepsy. At the age of 26 he is considered to be fully recovered, and returns to St Petersburg to claim his inheritance. While travelling back to St Petersburg by train he meets Rogozhin and tells him of his epilepsy, of being fostered after the death of his parents, and of his sizeable inheritance. Due to his innocent nature he is regarded by many as an idiot, whereas in fact he has exceptional intelligence and wisdom. Dostoevsky, drawing upon his own first-hand knowledge, describes the build-up to the Prince's grand mal seizure at an evening reception, culminating in the breaking of an extremely valuable Chinese vase. Myshkin is epilepsy's first and possibly only superhero, and Dostoevsky depicts him as 'the positively good and beautiful man'. The novel examines the consequences of placing such an individual in the world of conflict, vested interest, and egoism; the Prince rises above all of these. When his adversary and former friend Rogozhin is about to stab him, a seizure saves the Prince's life. After several attempts to deprive him of his inheritance, and after his betrothed, Nastasya, has run off with Rogozhin on their wedding day, he returns to St Petersburg to hear that she has died. Heartbroken, he goes to view Nastasya's body and is then found by the police in a catatonic state. This results in his return to the Swiss clinic, where his condition is pronounced incurable.

In *Crime and Punishment* (1866), Svidrigailov expresses his love of Raskolnikov's sister by stating 'I truly thought I was getting the falling sickness.' Dostoevsky's writings are peppered with references to epilepsy, most notably in the case of the character Smerdyakov in *The Brothers Karamazov* (1879–1880), who fakes a seizure as an alibi for his father's death and then, as a possible punishment, develops life-threatening epilepsy. In all of these novels except for *The Idiot*, death, suicide, or murder appear inextricably linked to epilepsy. This is a deeply pessimistic view and must be regarded as Dostoevsky's perception of the unfair treatment that could be expected if one had the condition. In *The Possessed* (1872), one of the main characters, Kirillov, experiences frequent auras and is informed that these will eventually become full-blown seizures. He is told that this is the way epilepsy starts and that it always becomes more severe as time passes. In one of Dostoevsky's earlier works, *The Lodging Woman* (1847), he describes the pro-convulsant effects of alcohol and the resultant ecstatic feelings, which were so similar to those he experienced during his own attacks. In *The Insulted and Injured* (1861) he describes the gentle character Nelly's experiences of generalized seizures, and her post-seizure feelings.

What do we know about the cause of Dostoevsky's epilepsy? Some have suggested that it was the consequence of syphilis contracted a year or two before his first seizure. Although he may well have had syphilis, any link between this and his epilepsy is purely speculative and runs the risk of equating epilepsy with sexual excess. It seems likely that his seizures were of temporal lobe origin, and were probably unrelated to any intercurrent venereal disease. His friends described the attacks as occurring on a monthly basis, and being heralded by a strange long scream followed by a fall to the floor with twitching of the body and foaming from the mouth. Dostoevsky himself referred to his 'ecstatic aura', in which he would feel in harmony with the world and have visions of paradise before collapsing.

Two of his characters, Prince Myshkin in *The Idiot* and Kirillov in *The Possessed*, experienced such feelings as well as a sense of celestial peace during their seizures. Dostoevsky's own account of his aura or warning best describes the ecstatic state: 'I experience a happiness that is impossible in an ordinary state and of which other people have no concept. I feel in full harmony in myself and in the whole world, and the feeling is so strong and sweet that for a few seconds of such one could give up ten years of life, perhaps all life, before an attack.'[86] He also noticed the effect that stress had on the frequency of his seizures.[87] The rising hollow feeling at onset and the ecstatic aura suggest that Dostoevsky probably had temporal lobe epilepsy with occasional generalized seizures.

In 1881, a year after completing *The Brothers Karamazov*, Dostoevsky died, most likely from tuberculosis. He had survived a lifetime of epilepsy, and this condition had helped to shape his work as a great writer and social commentator. Dostoevsky's case illustrates how a remarkable writer integrated his suffering into his art, and turned a disadvantage into an artistic advantage. He showed that his characters with epilepsy should be judged by their personality and not by their condition. Dostoevsky's epileptics were generally pure, noble, and principled. He championed the condition from which he suffered, and never attempted to conceal it from anyone. Gastaut commented on his 'extraordinary defence in favour of the countless persons who have been subjected to the unacceptable prejudice that they are destined to intellectual decline because of the repetition of their seizures, and those exceptional epileptic persons whose genius has erroneously been considered as a byproduct of their disease'.[88]

Wilkie Collins (1824–1889), an English author, was a friend and contemporary of Charles Dickens, with whom he collaborated on short stories such as 'The Perils of Certain English Prisoners' (1857). His book *The Moonstone* (1868) is considered to be the first modern English detective novel. He developed an addiction to opium, having originally taken it for gout, and this may have significantly reduced his literary output. In his novel *Poor Miss*

---

86 Morgan H (1990) Dostoevsky's epilepsy: a case report and comparison. *Surgical Neurology* 33, 413–416.
87 Voskuil PH (1983) The epilepsy of Fyodor Mikhailovich Dostoevsky (1821–1881). *Epilepsia* 24, 658–667.
88 Gastaut H (1978) Fyodor Mikhailovich Dostoevsky's involuntary contribution to the symptomatology and prognosis of epilepsy. *Epilepsia* 19, 186–201.

Finch (1872), epilepsy is the cornerstone of the plot. Lucilla, who is blind, is being pursued by Oscar, who has a ruthless twin brother called Nugent. Oscar has been disfigured by silver nitrate that was used to treat his epilepsy. Nugent hopes that if Lucilla's vision can be restored by an eye specialist, she will see Oscar's disfigurement and prefer him instead. Oscar supports Lucilla in her pursuit of the operation, and once she can see she prefers Oscar, despite his blemishes, to Nugent. This is a study in psychology, with disability ultimately triumphing over the conniving Nugent. Collins makes Oscar's epilepsy 'respectable' by providing the back story that it was acquired from a head injury that he sustained while preventing a robbery. This 'sanitizing' of epilepsy by attributing it to a head injury received while carrying out an honourable deed is a theme that we shall encounter again, especially in the depiction of epilepsy in the movies (see Chapter 6).

Charles Dickens (1812–1870) is without doubt the greatest social commentator, observer, and chronicler of Victorian Britain. He accurately described seizures in five characters, namely Edward Leeford (also known as Monks), who is Oliver Twist's villainous half-brother in *Oliver Twist* (1838); Bradley Headstone, who is Charley Hexam's schoolmaster in *Our Mutual Friend* (1865); Guster (Augusta), a housemaid in *Bleak House* (1852–1853); John Jasper, the choirmaster in *The Mystery of Edwin Drood* (unfinished at the time of Dickens' death in 1870); and Walter Wilding in *No Thoroughfare* (1867) (a stage play and novel written with Wilkie Collins). Before we consider Dickens' razor-sharp observations on epilepsy, we first need to explore how he acquired such knowledge. He had been a court reporter, and had witnessed the disenfranchised at first hand. He was also a frequent visitor to prisons and workhouses. In addition, he witnessed Dr John Elliotson's magnetic treatment of the epileptic Elizabeth O'Key in 1838, and had read the writings of Gabriel Andral (1797–1876), a distinguished French pathologist and professor at the University of Paris, on epilepsy in the *Lancet*.[89] Dickens was in fact a regular reader of the *Lancet* and a friend of the founding editor, and after his own death was honoured by an obituary in that journal as well as in the *British Medical Journal*. He probably based his realistic descriptions of epilepsy on a number of sources. His son Charlie was described as having 'a strange fading [that] comes over him', and his sister Letitia was 'a delicate child subject to fits'. His work as a court reporter and frequent prison and poorhouse visitor might also have given him a special insight into the condition. In both prison and poorhouse settings he would have encountered a disproportionate number of people with disabilities, including epilepsy. The possibility that Dickens himself had epilepsy can be discounted. He certainly had mental health problems and was prone to severe kidney pain, and eventually died from a stroke, but there is no evidence to support the frequently cited view that he had epilepsy.

---

89 Eysell J (2005) *A Medical Companion to Dickens's Fiction*. Peter Lang, Frankfurt.

In *Oliver Twist,* Monks is physically unattractive, with a scar on the left side of his jaw, and he also has a cowardly nature, as well as suffering from severe epileptic fits. His seizures are triggered when he experiences feelings of anger: '[Monks] shook his fist, and gnashed his teeth … and advancing towards Oliver as if with the intention of aiming a blow at him, fell violently on the ground, writhing and foaming, in a fit.' His seizures can also be induced by the weather: 'These fits come on me triggered by thunder.' A young woman called Nancy describes his injuries, noting that 'his lips are often discoloured and disfigured with the marks of teeth; for he has desperate fits, and sometimes even bites his hands'. He had a broad burn or scald on his neck, probably from the same cause. Monks' fate is also attributed to his epilepsy in that 'he sunk under an attack of his old disorder and died in a prison cell.' Dickens typically uses disfigurement and disability in adults as a metaphor for negative or criminal traits. In Monks, epilepsy adds to the generally unsavoury nature of the character.

Bradley Headstone, Charley Hexam's schoolmaster in *Our Mutual Friend,* fares little better. He falls in love with Lizzie Hexam and pursues her in a passionate, relentless, and violent manner. His personality swings between respectability and wild jealousy, and his propensity for violence is constantly present in the background. His seizures are an integral part of his unattractive persona. When describing Headstone's seizures, Dickens states that he is 'accustomed to be seized with giddiness', 'to pull at his neck cloth as though he were trying to tear it off', and 'biting and knocking about him furiously'. This sounds like a description of a focal seizure with secondary generalization. The fear that his attacks engendered, and the tendency for them to occur one after another, is made clear: 'This horrible condition brought on other fits. He could not have said how many, or when: but he saw in the faces of his pupils that they had seen him in that state, and that they were possessed by a dread of his relapsing.'

Whereas Dickens demonized his male characters through their disability, in the case of children and women he used illness as a metaphor for vulnerability and pitifulness. Guster (Augusta), the Snagsbys' housemaid in *Bleak House,* is a clear example of his patronizing approach to young female characters. Guster is a clumsy, emaciated young woman, fresh from the workhouse and fearful of being returned there. Her seizures are triggered by excitement and fear. She plays only a minor role in the novel, but Dickens draws upon her vulnerability as part of the storyline. When she enters the novel it is stated that she 'goes cheap with this unaccountable drawback of fits; and is so apprehensive of being returned on the hands of her patron Saint [to the workhouse] that except when she is found with her head in the pail, or the sink, or the copper, or the dinner, or anything else that happens to be near her at the time of her seizure, she is always at work'. Dickens conveys the impression that Guster has to work as hard as she can, in the face of her epilepsy, in order to remain employed by the Snagsbys. There is also an account of prolonged fits or *status epilepticus*: 'Guster murders sleep by going ... out of one fit into twenty' and '[she] fell into a fit of unusual duration, which she only came out of to go into another, and so on through a chain of fits, with short intervals between.' Mr Snagsby comments that she was 'timid and has fits, and ... [taking fright at a foreigner's looks and way of speaking] gave way to it [epilepsy], instead of bearing up against it, and tumbled down the kitchen stairs out of one into another'. It is noted that 'Guster falls into a staring and vacant state' frequently. Finally, Mr Bucket, a detective, tells Dr Woodcourt that 'the girl's subject to fits, and has 'em bad upon her tonight'. He then makes the following request: 'I understand you are a medical man. Would you look to this girl and see if anything can be done to bring her round?' Dickens' portrayal of this minor character is full of sympathetic understanding of the problems that she faces, and is in stark contrast with his unsympathetic treatment of the characters of Monks and Headstone.[90] Finally, Dickens was aware that seizures could be caused by many different illnesses. Little Nell, in *The Old Curiosity Shop* (1840–1841), describes her grandfather as having been 'taken very ill – found in a fit on the floor' with a fever and a weakened mind. In *David Copperfield* (1849–1850), David Copperfield's father-in-law falls out of a horse-drawn, doorless carriage, or phaeton, and is found 'lying partly on the roadside, and partly on the path, upon his face'. It is suggested that he either took a fit which led to his fall, or that the seizure was a consequence of falling. He dies soon afterwards, and a head injury or stroke are the most strongly suspected causes. Dickens also realized that excessive alcohol consumption could cause a seizure. Joe Gargery in *Great Expectations* (1861) describes his father as given to drink, and states that he died as a result of a 'purple leptic fit'. Finally, in *Martin Chuzzlewit* (1842–1844), the protagonist gives the following advice: 'Don't you drink too much of that sour wine, or you'll have a fit of some sort.'

In Peter Levi's lengthy biography[91] of **Edward Lear** (1812–1888), the English illustrator, musician, and poet, epilepsy does not feature significantly – indeed the word itself does not appear in the index. Lear would have endorsed this reticence, because of the shame he felt and the lengths to which he went to conceal his condition. He was the youngest of 21 children born to a wealthy London stockbroker and his wife, and is best remembered now for his nonsense poems for children, such as 'The Owl and the Pussycat', published in *A Book of Nonsense* (1846). He was also an accomplished artist (he illustrated Tennyson's poems), and could play the accordion, flute, and piano, as well as compose (he set Tennyson's poems to music).

His seizures started at the age of five, occurred up to four times a week, and no one outside his close family knew about them. He once stated: 'It is wonderful that these fits

---

90 Cosnett JE (1994) Charles Dickens and epilepsy. *Epilepsia* 35, 903–905.
91 Levi P (1995) *Edward Lear: A Biography*. Macmillan, London.

have never been discovered.' Levi describes Lear as brooding over his epilepsy when he went to school, and fearing it 'every morning in the little study when learning my lessons, all day long, and always in the evenings and at night. The strong will of sister Harriet put a short pause to the misery, but very short.' Jane, another sister, also had epilepsy, and Harriet, presumably based upon what she had witnessed, helped Edward to control his attacks to such an extent that they could pass unnoticed. As he grew older his seizures became more severe but less frequent. In his diary he would place an 'X' next to the dates when he had seizures, and a score of 1 to 10 as a measure of their severity. While he was staying in Corfu, a typical diary entry read as follows: 'January 5th. Worked irregularly and suddenly came to awful grief X:3.' He learned when he became aware of the warning symptoms to go to another room that gave him complete privacy, and lie down. Lear had witnessed his older sister Jane having frequent seizures while dying in adolescence, and was convinced that his own epilepsy would eventually lead to a loss of his mental faculties, and ultimately death. He referred to his epilepsy as 'the Demon', as though it had its own persona, and when looking back over his life reflected that the Demon's presence 'would have prevented happiness under any sort of circumstances. It is a most merciful blessing that I have kept up as I have, and have not gone utterly to the bad mad sad.' Lear lived a sad, melancholic life that is belied by the humour of his limericks. He had difficulty forming relationships, may have had unresolved issues with regard to his sexuality, and eventually died alone in St Remo on the Mediterranean coast, with few people attending his funeral. There can be no doubt that his life was significantly affected by his 'Demon' and the shame that he felt as a result of it.

Lorna Doone is the only novel for which the English writer **R.D. Blackmore** (1825–1900) is now remembered. Born into the middle-class comfort of an Oxfordshire rectory, he had a privileged upbringing until his mother died of typhus, his father remarried, and he was sent to Blundell's boarding school in Devon (his father's former school). There he was treated harshly and bullied. In Victorian boarding schools, physical and mental punishment was acceptable and indeed expected, and it was here that Blackmore fell foul of a senior student named Frederick Temple, the future Archbishop of Canterbury, who struck him on the head with a brass-headed hammer. It is possible that it was this injury that brought on his epilepsy and altered the course of his life. After leaving school he attended Oxford University, where his seizures spoiled his chances of obtaining a First Class degree. His subsequent career as a barrister ended because of his fear of having seizures in the courtroom. In correspondence with a friend he wrote that 'ill health drove me from chamber practice [as a barrister]; my once excellent health has become impaired. My medical advisor said I would have to give up my profession, seek an outdoor employment or die young.' He became a schoolteacher, and took a great deal of physical exercise in the form of walking. It was during his early days of teaching that he started to write poems and novels. An inheritance from his uncle subsequently allowed him to stop teaching, an occupation that he did not enjoy, and become a full-time writer and horticulturalist in the Teddington area of London.[92] He pursued a career in market gardening for the next 40 years.

In addition to *Lorna Doone*, Blackmore published 12 other novels, as well as poems, translations, and short stories. *Lorna Doone* was initially unsuccessful, with only 300 copies being sold, and it was Blackmore's inheritance and market gardening that supported him and his wife, Lucy. They had no children, and after Lucy's death he was cared for by his two nieces. The extent to which epilepsy dominated his life is uncertain. The same fear that made him abandon a career in law due to fear of a courtroom seizure also prevented him, later in life, from making speeches to literary gatherings. We also know from his years as a barrister that the pressure of work and worry had the effect of worsening his seizures. By now his life had become a lonely and solitary one, and he rarely ventured from his home. With increasing age he developed other health problems, such as arthritis and stroke, and his epilepsy lessened. He died in early 1900 at the age of 75, a couple of years after completing his last novel, *Dariel* (1897). He was buried next to his wife, and a memorial to him in Exeter Cathedral was established through the efforts of several of his fellow authors, including Thomas Hardy, Rudyard Kipling, and James Barrie. Although his epilepsy, and especially the stigma attached to the condition at that time, determined both the course of his life and the manner in which he lived it, that illness also resulted in his legacy, the novel *Lorna Doone*.

Sadness and isolation in a person's life often suggest the existence of an underlying physical or mental health problem. The recent film *A Quiet Passion* (2016), directed by Terence Davies, poetically conveys the reclusive life of the American poet **Emily Dickinson** (1830–1886). Dickinson was ill for most of her life, although her medical notes do not provide a definitive explanation for her poor health. She published only ten poems in her lifetime, but left hundreds of letters and poems, which were to be fought over by generations of heirs. Her biographer Lyndall Gordon notes that epilepsy is at the centre of a number of Dickinson's poems.[93] In the early 1850s, Dickinson regularly took glycerine, which has antiepileptic properties, and then for the rest of her life took chloral hydrate, which has similar effects. Gordon also describes a family history of epilepsy, which suggests that Dickinson had the genetically inherited form of the condition. Born into one of Massachusetts' most distinguished families, she lived the privileged but restricted life of an unmarried woman of that time. She spent much of her life in reclusive isolation, withdrawing increasingly from the outside world. During her lifetime a physician diagnosed her as having 'nervous

---

92 Matthew HCG and Harrison B (eds.) (2004) *Oxford Dictionary of National Biography. Volume 6*. Oxford University Press, Oxford.
93 Gordon L (2010) *Lives like Loaded Guns: Emily Dickinson and Her Family's Feud*. Viking, New York.

prostration'. One can only speculate as to whether this was a euphemism for epilepsy. Dickinson's increasingly bizarre behaviour – for example, always wearing white clothing, rarely going out, and only speaking to visitors through a closed door – adds support to the view that there was an underlying problem. Her poems reflect a lifelong fascination with illness, dying, and death. As in the case of Edward Lear, it has been suggested that her sexuality might be a possible explanation for her withdrawal from life. However, if epilepsy was present, as Gordon suggests, then the stigma attached to the condition might explain her reclusiveness, and the fear of passing it on to the next generation might account for the fact that she never married.

In 1926, the English writer **Graham Greene** (1904–1991), author of *Our Man in Havana* (1958) and *Brighton Rock* (1938), among many other novels, was told by his doctor that he had a condition that should make him 'consider carefully before marriage'. After this diagnosis was made during his childhood, his parents insisted to the family doctor that Greene 'ought not to be told what the matter is in any terms that included the word epilepsy'. He attended a private school where his father was headmaster, and he soon displayed a rebellious streak and unwillingness to conform. Greene's troubled childhood and adolescence led to him seeing a psychoanalyst in early adulthood. The psychoanalyst, with whom he lived for six months, suggested that Greene should see a specialist about his blackouts. It was at a Harley Street appointment with an eminent neurologist that Greene, without any investigations having been undertaken, was told for the first time that he had epilepsy. In the first volume of his autobiography, *A Sort of Life* (1971), Greene recalls that even though his physician optimistically held out hope that the seizures could be controlled by taking long walks and Kepler's malt extract, he was distraught as he had just planned to get married. In Britain at that time a diagnosis of epilepsy was sufficient legal grounds for annulment, and Greene had been informed that his condition could be inherited by his offspring. The failure of his neurologist to offer treatment with phenobarbitone (now known as phenobarbital) is surprising, and suggests that the doctor himself did not have any particular interest in epilepsy.

The day after Greene was given this news, he described himself 'standing on an Underground platform and trying to summon the will and the courage to jump. It was not my new Catholicism which restrained me. ... I was simply tired out by the thought of starting a completely different future than the one I had planned. But suicide requires greater courage than Russian roulette, the trains came and went, and soon I took the moving staircase to the upper world.' Greene was fortunate in that he experienced no further seizures in adulthood, and did not have to live the 'completely different future' that he had imagined and feared. At the time when he considered ending his life he had published only one book,

The Man Within (1929). He went on to write a further 25 novels, including *The Power and the Glory* (1940), *Our Man in Havana* (1958), *Travels with my Aunt* (1969), *The Third Man* (1949), and *The Quiet American* (1956), many of which have been made into classic films. Interestingly, he turned to a priest for solace when he was diagnosed but, like his fictional characters who consulted a priest in their hour of need, he derived no comfort as a result. According to Greene's biographer, Norman Sherry,[94] his seizures did not persist. Moreover, Greene's brother, who was a doctor and the medical correspondent of *The Times*, and who had witnessed an attack, was sceptical about the diagnosis. Greene married and had two children, neither of whom subsequently developed epilepsy. Greene never wrote about epilepsy in his novels, but was profoundly affected by the diagnosis that he had been given. He was quoted as saying that epilepsy, leprosy, and cancer were the conditions that, through ignorance, caused the greatest public fear. In 1971 he was asked whether he felt that the diagnosis he had been given 45 years previously had been correct. He responded that 'With the hindsight of forty years free of any recurrence, I do not believe it, but I believed it then.' The lesson here is that in 1926 the diagnosis of epilepsy, whether or not it was correct, could have a life-changing effect on a 22-year-old with their whole life ahead of them. It is not known how the diagnosis affected Greene after he had contemplated suicide.

Only a few writers have drawn from their own personal experience of having epilepsy. One such author is **Margiad Evans** (1909–1958), also known as Peggy Williams or Whistler. Born Peggy Whistler, she married a Welshman, George Williams. She took her pen name from her mother's maiden name, which was Evans. Her fifth book, *A Ray of Darkness* (1952), was an autobiographical account that followed her diagnosis of epilepsy. She experienced her first generalized or tonic–clonic seizure eight years before she died from the brain tumour that had caused her epilepsy. She incorporated her own experiences of the first convulsive seizure into the narrative of the book, setting out every detail of the events that occurred up to and including her epilepsy. She was known to have experienced auras from early childhood, and she described the aura that preceded an attack as 'like a tiny wheel – the wheel, say, of a watch, whirring at blurring speed, quite soundlessly, in my head while I went on with whatever I was doing, guided by the consciousness left over rather than the consciousness of the moment.' She gave the following description of her first generalized seizure, which occurred at night while she was alone, writing poetry, in her cottage: 'I made the tea, looked up at the clock – a strange chance – saw that it was ten minutes past eleven. The next thing I was still looking up at the clock and the hands stood at five and twenty minutes past midnight. ... I discovered I was lying on the floor on my back, my head against the rungs of a rocking-chair and my body, full length, crowded between the steel fender and

---

94 Sherry N (1989) *The Life of Graham Greene, Volume 1: 1904–1939*. Jonathan Cape, London.

the little table at which I had been writing.' She goes on to express her surprise that she had not been seriously injured, given the fact that she was alone, the cottage had a stone floor, and a fire was burning in the open fireplace: 'My sleeve was charred by an ember, but that was all.' This observation touches upon the relative infrequency of severe seizure-related injuries as though, at a subconscious level, the instinct for self-preservation is still functional. Evans refers to the humiliation caused by the seizure, describing how she 'felt a cold dampness and it came upon me stunningly, terrifyingly, that my clothes were wet. My urine had escaped me then.' Andrew Larner, in an article about her epilepsy in *Clinical Medicine*, describes how she was frustrated and annoyed by 'inexpert opinion, disbelief and the wrong sort of kind advice' that was offered by well-meaning relatives and friends.[95]

Evans found that her drug treatment with phenobarbitone (phenobarbital) affected her ability to write, and commented that 'the drugs I have to take ... make me apathetic, have faded and dulled and dimmed the powers of imagination and concentration'. Larner comments that while on drug treatment she had a successful pregnancy, which was complicated only by a post-delivery seizure and being denied the opportunity to breastfeed. Evans' outspoken 'warts and all' descriptions of what it was like to live with epilepsy were criticized as being too negative and self-indulgent by the British Epilepsy Association, a charity that provides support for those with epilepsy. Undeterred, before her death Evans made a broadcast on the national radio about her epilepsy and the need for better understanding of the condition. Sadly, few writers since have been willing to describe their epilepsy with such candour.

Laurence 'Laurie' Lee (1914–1997) was an English novelist and poet who is best known for his autobiographical trilogy *Cider with Rosie* (1969), *As I Walked Out One Midsummer Morning* (1969), and *A Moment of War* (1991). The latter describes how he travelled to Spain in the 1930s to join the Republican International Brigades, where his services were declined on the grounds that he had epilepsy. In her biography of Lee,[96] Valerie Grove mentions the Spanish Civil War incident but provides very little information about his epilepsy. In *Cider with Rosie*, Lee describes a biking accident that occurred when he was 10 years old, which he thought might have triggered his epilepsy: 'That blow in the night – put a stain of darkness on my brow and opened a sinister door in my brain.' Later on there is a description of Lee going rigid and falling on the floor while listening to Handel's *Largo*. Grove refers to the fact that people knew about Lee's epilepsy in the 1950s, but little detail is provided. She subsequently quotes from a letter written by a friend of Lee in 1973, which stated that 'epilepsy allied to a simple mind is difficult enough, but in conjunction with such sharpness of focus as Laurie has it is more difficult. It's not even a cure that Laurie needs as such, but

---

95 Larner AJ (2009) 'A ray of darkness': Margiad Evans's account of her epilepsy (1952). *Clinical Medicine* 9, 193–194.
96 Grove V (1999) *Laurie Lee: The Well-Loved Stranger*. Viking, London.

a man with deep understanding and insight, with sympathy and humility.' Lee's doctor and confidant was a general practitioner called Jim Hoyland, who himself had epilepsy and adopted an idiosyncratic approach to treatment. Grove quotes him as saying 'All epileptics are shy about epilepsy. There is a stigma; people are afraid that you might pass out and start frothing at the mouth.' Lee confided to a friend that he was 'pursued by caravanserais of demons' and was terrified of having an attack in a public place. His daughter Jessy stated in an interview with *Cotswold Life* magazine long after her father's death that 'it was very difficult being his daughter, as he did suffer from epilepsy',[97] and in subsequent articles she mentions how difficult he was to live with, as well as his need for long-term medication. Valerie Grove describes Lee as 'a person of concealment' despite 'his entire opus consisting of fragments of autobiography'. Herein lies the clue, in that the vanity of Lee was to appear to open himself up to his readers while at the same time concealing any information, such as the fact that he had epilepsy, which might diminish him in their eyes.

The International Brigades were set up by Communist International to oppose the attempt by the Nationalists, under General Francisco Franco, to take over Spain. To suppress fascism the Brigades attracted working-class socialists and intellectuals from all over Europe. Of the 35,000 members who served in the Brigades, nearly a third died in combat. Those who fought included literary luminaries such as George Orwell, Ernest Hemingway, Stephen Spender, W.H. Auden, and Arthur Koestler, and it was with this brotherhood and cause that Lee wished to align himself.

According to Valerie Grove, Lee was one of 912 volunteers who slipped into Spain in December 1937. Wilma Gregory, who was Lee's mentor at the time, seemed to sense that he might not be medically fit to fight, and wrote to the Spanish Minister of Defence, stating that 'I understand so well how irresponsible an epileptic is – volatile as the Victorians would say.' While he was waiting to be pronounced fit to serve, Lee had two seizures in Figueres, which he latter attributed to the shock of exploding shells and the increased excitement of being in Spain. His International Brigades file states that 'it seems clear that generally speaking he is physically weak, he will not be any use at the front. He agrees that the added excitement would be too much for him.' Thereafter, according to Grove, he appeared to be non-combatant and was continuing to have seizures. It seems that he was deeply ashamed about eventually being sent back to England because he was deemed not medically fit to serve. In his own account of the Spanish Civil War, *A Moment of War*, which was not published until nearly 50 years later, there is very little mention of his epilepsy, but instead a bravado account of imprisonment and a narrow escape from death by firing squad. This contentious book has been described as 'fantastical' by those who fought in Spain, despite the fact that it

---

97 *Cotswold Life* (2013) March issue, pp. 116–120.

entered the pantheon of literary classics about war. By concealing his epilepsy and justifying his return to England, Lee placed himself alongside George Orwell (*Homage to Catalonia*, 1938) and Ernest Hemingway (*For Whom the Bell Tolls*, 1940) as having written one of the three classic eye-witness accounts of the Spanish Civil War.

Lee's complex personality, his difficulties with relationships, his mood swings, and his secrecy are evident, but how much of this relates to his epilepsy is speculative. That he concealed much of his condition from the documents that he left his most hailed biographer is beyond doubt. We shall never know the nature of his epilepsy, the treatment that he was prescribed, and the extent of his feelings of shame. The fact that he wished to conceal the condition and leave no trail behind speaks for itself. Both his personal flaws and his literary achievements should now be viewed in the light of the disabling condition from which he clearly suffered.

The American writer **Thomas Pynchon** (1937–) has remained silent about any personal experience of the condition, but epilepsy is a recurring theme in several of his novels. For example, in *Gravity's Rainbow* (1973) an aura is described as 'an odour, one he knows but can't quite name, an aura that threatens to go epileptic any second'. Such specific detail can only come from a close personal knowledge of epilepsy. In his short story 'Lowlands' an epileptic aura also features, and in his first novel, *The Crying of Lot 49* (1966), he introduces one character, a poet, by stating that he 'had the misfortune to be both homosexual and epileptic'. The author's private life remains a mystery. He has had virtually no contact with the media over a 40-year period, the only available photographs of him date back to his school and college days, and even his whereabouts are unknown. One can only speculate about this, but perhaps he is another Flaubert or Lear, in terms of the reason for his chosen lifestyle.

There are many other twentieth-century English-language novels in which epilepsy makes a fleeting appearance, a selection of which will be briefly discussed here.

In her novel *Owls Do Cry* (1957) the New Zealand author **Janet Frame** (1924–2004) draws upon her own experiences of poverty, illness, and tragedy. Her older brother was severely epileptic and was routinely beaten by their father, and Frame herself was frequently admitted to psychiatric hospitals, narrowly avoided having to undergo a lobotomy, and was considered to be on the autistic spectrum. She gives a powerful description of the seizures experienced by Toby, one of the main characters in the novel: 'a dark hood would be thrown over his head by Jesus or God, and he would struggle inside the hood, pushing at the velvet folds, waving his arms and legs in the air till the sun took pity.'

In *The Apprenticeship of Duddy Kravitz* (1957), **Mordecai Richler** (1931–2001) describes the dangers of epilepsy and driving, when one of the characters, Virgil Roseboro, becomes paraplegic as a result of a seizure-related car accident indirectly caused by his friend, Duddy. Subsequently Duddy takes advantage of Virgil when he requires some financial assistance, highlighting the vulnerability of the 'epileptic'.

In *The Bachelors* (1960) by **Muriel Spark** (1918–2006), two of the main characters are Matthew, a barrister, and Ronald, his flatmate. Ronald has epilepsy, which he believes has ruled him out of the priesthood and, if he was not to become a priest, marriage. Ronald's epilepsy is sympathetically portrayed and is linked to his spiritualism. The Edinburgh-based author stated that she was inspired to include epilepsy in the storyline in an empathetic manner after she witnessed a seizure for the first time, in the street.

In his novel *One Flew over the Cuckoo's Nest* (1962), **Ken Kesey** (1935–2001) exposes the harsh treatment that can be experienced by people with mental health problems and epilepsy, at the hands of the very people who are employed to care for them. Set in a psychiatric hospital in Oregon, it follows the lives of some of the inmates, including Sefelt and Frederickson, both of whom have epilepsy. Nurse Ratched (also known as Big Nurse) is the cold-hearted tyrannical head nurse, who feels that she is superior to those for whom she is meant to provide care. Sefelt has a seizure while he is standing in line for his lunch. Nurse Ratched and her orderlies attend to him, and as he recovers she mocks him for saying that he thought he had no need for medication. Frederickson takes sides against Nurse Ratched, and tells her that she is crucifying his friend. Sefelt pretends to take his medication (phenytoin), but often passes it on to Frederickson, who believes that his own epilepsy is being undertreated by the staff and that he requires a higher dose. Frederickson becomes infuriated by the way that his friend is being treated, and when someone asks why Sefelt is reluctant to take his phenytoin, he opens his mouth to show the gum rot that has been caused by the drug. Kelsey gives an accurate portrayal of the dilemma that many people with epilepsy face, and the choices that they have to make. Sefelt would rather take his chances than develop gum rot, whereas Frederickson would rather develop gum rot than risk having a seizure. Rather than attempting to understand this, Nurse Ratched ridicules Sefelt for the choice that he has made. The novel also describes a practice that would today be regarded as extremely dangerous, namely putting a wallet in the mouth of a person who is having a seizure, in order to prevent tongue biting. The film adaptation of the book (released in 1975) won five Academy Awards.

Epilepsy features prominently in the novel *Lamb* (1980), by **Bernard MacLaverty** (1942–). Owen Kane is a 10-year-old resident in a care home in rural Ireland that takes in boys with behavioural problems. Owen runs away to London with a former priest, Michael Lamb, who has been left a small inheritance. The boy has major seizures that are preceded by an aura, and is dependent on medication. Michael becomes Owen's father figure, and the history of the boy's seizures and criminal activities is revealed in flashbacks. In London, after a series of misfortunes, including drug use and a sexual encounter with another man, as well as lack of money, Michael decides to save Owen from being returned to the care home by killing him. He drowns him in the sea during a seizure, and then tries unsuccessfully to drown himself. Clearly Owen's epilepsy adds to his overall vulnerability, which, together with his behavioural problems, makes his future appear bleak enough for Michael to decide to offer 'salvation'.

In her book *The Shell Seekers* (1987), **Rosamunde Pilcher** (1924–2019) paints a depressing but truthful picture of the social consequences of being a young man concerned about the possible diagnosis of epilepsy. Danus is a mysterious gardener who, because of his personal problems, has become reclusive, has stopped driving and drinking alcohol, and ceased studying to be a lawyer. He regards marriage as out of the question, and believes that gardening is the only employment that he can safely undertake. These anxieties help to explain this complex although somewhat peripheral character, and will be recognized as very familiar concerns by any reader with epilepsy. However, the novel is misleading in its depiction of how epilepsy is diagnosed, as it implies that this is based solely on tests such as CT scans and electroencephalograms.

In *The Satanic Verses* (1988), **Salman Rushdie** (1947–) mentions the doomed false prophet Ayesha who has the falling sickness and is 'possessed by the demon of epilepsy', which brings us back to the ancient prejudices that surround the condition.

The most powerful of the recent novels in which epilepsy features is undoubtedly *Electricity* (2006), by **Ray Robinson** (1971–). We do not know the source of the author's knowledge of epilepsy, but it is sufficient for him to have produced a compelling and award-winning account. This book has been adapted for the silver screen, and the film and its impact will be discussed in Chapter 6. The main character, Lily O'Connor, who is also the narrator, has had epilepsy ever since her mother hurled her down the stairs when she was a small child. An early pronouncement by Lily sets the scene: 'If epilepsy does have a face, it looks something like mine: a bit lopsided, scars on the eyebrow and forehead and chin. Leftovers of bruises and black eyes. ... Teeth missing, gums cut.' Lily was taken into care as a child, and the novel centres around her search for a long-lost brother. Her attitude to her fits is summarized as 'thrash, get up, and get on with it'. This doggedness alongside her vulnerability moulds her personality, which is characterized by defiance, lack of self-pity, and a refusal to be defined by her illness. The dangers of having a bath or simply being alone in a locked flat are emphasized, and to many non-epileptic readers the hazards of such everyday activities will come as a surprise. Life is punctuated by the need to take pills ('six a day, two in the morning, two in the afternoon, and two at night'), as well as to avoid injury, exploitation, and theft, and to continue her search. She leaves notes around her flat so that she can re-orientate herself during the aftermath of an attack, and she has run-ins with the doctors who try to change her trusted drug treatment. She has to accept that if she goes on a night out, at some point she is likely to 'be down there lying in a puddle of piss and sweat'. *Electricity* is an uncompromisingly candid account of a 30-year-old who is on a mission while simultaneously coping with the effects of epilepsy on her life. Its subject matter may not be palatable to all, and the ending is somewhat saccharine, but as a contemporary account of what it is like to live with epilepsy it is unparalleled.

Colin Grant (1961–) is a UK writer, historian, playwright, and radio producer with a Jamaican background. In *A Smell of Burning* (2016)[98] he provides an account of his younger brother Christopher's epilepsy – a journey that ended in sudden unexplained death in epilepsy (SUDEP) in 2008. The book explores family relationships, the meaning of living with epilepsy, interactions with the doctors, and the impact of stigma and prejudice. It is a highly personal account interspersed with vignettes on the history of epilepsy and famous people who have had the condition. The text describes Colin's attempts to share with his brother what it means to have epilepsy and the transcendental meaning of seizures. Having developed epilepsy at the age of 15, Christopher's life from that point on is described as a war of attrition, as with each seizure 'a bit more of him was chipped away'. The title of the book, *A Smell of Burning*, refers to the hallucinatory aura that he experienced as the onset or aura of each attack. Grant, a former medical student, owns up to his early prejudice by admitting to a sense of revulsion when he witnessed a seizure for the first time in the hospital wards. He paints a depressing picture of the family's early denial of Christopher's epilepsy, and comments on how the condition (temporal lobe epilepsy) had ruined his brother's life, which would now 'never be perfect – far from it'. This biography of illness is an articulate and compassionate account of the resultant loss and grief. Its negativity might be too much for some readers, although I suspect that many with epilepsy will readily identify with most of the sentiments expressed. In a review published in *The Guardian*,[99] the critic Gavin Francis wrote that *A Smell Of Burning* was a very individual account of epilepsy, rather than being the full story, and that the newly diagnosed person who wanted to understand more about their condition might be well advised to look elsewhere. This is a harsh assessment of the book, and it is a pity that many of the book's detractors focus unduly on the frequent use of the word 'epileptic', rather than appreciating the work as an honest and informative eulogy to a much loved brother.

---

98 Grant C (2016) *A Smell of Burning: A Memoir of Epilepsy.* Jonathan Cape, London.
99 Francis G (2016) *A Smell of Burning* by Colin Grant review – how people with epilepsy have been persecuted. *The Guardian*, 19 August 2016.

The crime novel and epilepsy

It is in crime fiction that many of the myths and misconceptions about epilepsy are most likely to be found. **Raymond Chandler** (1888–1959) in *The Big Sleep* (1939) created the character Carmen Sternwood, who kills her sister's husband while in a twilight state that is attributed to her epilepsy. Chandler's private detective, Philip Marlowe, takes on the assignment to investigate blackmail against Carmen, the beautiful but half-witted 'wild child' daughter of oil millionaire General Guy Sternwood. Marlowe describes how 'the hissing noise came tearing out of her mouth as if she had nothing to do with it. There was something behind her eyes, blank as they were, that I had never seen in a woman's eyes.' This can be assumed to be a description of her seizures. Ultimately Marlowe takes Carmen to a deserted field, where she tries to kill him, but the gun is filled with blanks, and when he laughs at her the shock causes Carmen to have an epileptic seizure. The story ends with her being sent to an institution for the insane. Through the character of Carmen the book associates epilepsy with promiscuity, insanity, instability, and murder. Interestingly, the film version, in order to avoid censorship, did not end with Carmen's incarceration in an asylum. Chandler was influenced by the theories of the Italian criminologist and physician Cesare Lombroso (1835–1909), who believed that criminal degenerates were 'born criminal', and that this state was manifested by certain physical characteristics and conditions, one of which was epilepsy. We shall consider Lombroso and his legacy in more detail later in this book.

The novel *Perchance to Dream* (1991) by **Robert B. Parker** (1932–2010) is a homage to Chandler, in which Carmen Sternwood reappears. It is set some time after *The Big Sleep*, and Carmen has been staying in a luxury psychiatric hospital from which she has recently disappeared. Phillip Marlowe is hired to find her. The novel has rather unkindly been called 'The Big Snooze', and Carmen's epilepsy is mentioned only in passing. Indeed we don't know whether she is still having seizures or whether she received treatment for them while in the sanatorium, although there is an evil psychiatrist thrown in for good measure.

The British crime writer **Agatha Christie** (1890–1976) was born into a wealthy upper-middle-class West Country family, and this upbringing is certainly reflected in the upper-class-based plots of her novels. Before marrying and moving to London she worked in a Devon hospital, where she helped to care for troops returning from the trenches during the First World War, and she would certainly have acquired considerable medical knowledge from this work. One can speculate that she would have been likely to have witnessed seizures in those who had sustained head injuries, and epilepsy does play an important role in two of her novels.

In *The Murder on the Links* (1923), the Belgian detective Hercule Poirot (who appears in 33 novels and 54 short stories by Christie) and Captain Hastings (his 'Dr Watson') are called to France to investigate blackmail by an individual called Paul Renaud. On their arrival they are informed that Renaud has been found dead beside a golf course, stabbed in the back with a letter opener, and that his face is disfigured almost beyond recognition. A lead pipe has been buried alongside him. His wife claims that he was abducted from their home the previous night by intruders, while she was bound and gagged. She collapses in grief on identifying her husband's body. Another body is then found, stabbed through the heart with the same letter opener, and with roughened hands like those of a tramp. In the denouement it transpires that Reynaud had encountered a tramp having an epileptic seizure, from which he died. Renaud, who was trying to build a new life for himself and his wife, saw this as an opportunity to fake his own murder, so he stabbed the dead body and planned to bury it in a newly dug grave. He disfigured the face of the tramp sufficiently to ensure that his wife, who was in on the scheme, could give a false identification but others would not realize that it was not his body. It transpired that a neighbour, Marthe Daumbreuil, had been blackmailing Renaud and had much to lose financially if he disappeared, but would benefit from his death. She had overheard Renaud and his wife discussing the plan, followed him to the golf course and stabbed him there before he could bury the tramp. We do not know whether the tramp died as a result of inhaling vomit, choking, or experiencing SUDEP, which can occur in relation to a seizure. In this novel, epilepsy in a homeless tramp has provided Renaud unexpectedly with the dead body that he needed in order to feign his own murder. The homeless epileptic is viewed as expendable, and his loss goes unmourned.

In *The ABC Murders* (1936), a person with epilepsy is the victim, and the detective Hercule Poirot is his saviour. The falsely accused is a travelling salesman. He is epileptic, having fought in the war and received a blow to the head, which has made him prone to blackouts. Following one such a blackout on leaving a cinema he is found to have a murder weapon in his pocket and blood on his sleeve. By a process of deduction, the detective proves that the accused is innocent, saves him from hanging, and the real murderer is apprehended. This novel is sympathetic to the character with epilepsy, showing the vulnerability caused by loss of memory and being unable to give an account of one's whereabouts and actions. However, the epilepsy is made more 'respectable' by the fact that it was acquired as a result of a head injury sustained while the accused was defending his country, this being a stereotype of public acceptability. It is possible that the war injury and resultant epilepsy were based on Christie's wartime nursing experiences. Epilepsy is briefly mentioned in the novel *Nemesis* (1971), when the discovery of a dead body in the house raises the question 'An epileptic fit?' The fact that those with epilepsy need special care and support is also mentioned – in other words, the novel presents a sympathetic view.

The Belgian crime writer **Georges Simenon** (1903–1989) wrote over 500 novels and short stories. With such a huge output it is not surprising that epilepsy features in at least one of his works. He used 17 different pen names and lived a colourful life, rubbing shoulders with the criminal population about whom he wrote. In *The High Evil* (1977), Jean Naillier, a young farmer with epilepsy, is pushed to his death through a hatch in a barn by his mother-in law. The term 'high evil' refers to Jean's epilepsy. Madame Pontreau, the mother-in-law, camouflages the crime as an accident caused by Jean's seizures. Her accomplice in the murder, which was committed in order to obtain ownership of the farm, is a young farmworker who eventually denounces her. We know little of Jean's epilepsy other than that it is falsely used to explain his fall to his death and thus cover up his murder. The title of the book would appear to reflect Simenon's negative perception of epilepsy.

Tony Fennelly (1945–) was a New Orleans barmaid before she began to write crime fiction, and was subsequently nominated for the Edgar Allan Poe Award by the Mystery Writers of America. Her novels *The Closet Hanging* (1987) and *Kiss Yourself Goodbye* (2003) feature the gay lawyer and antique dealer Matt Sinclair. Matt has epilepsy as a result of a riding accident, and the seizures are used to explain why he was not drafted into the US armed services (if a man did not have an honourable military record, he had to provide good reasons for this). The author draws from a family history of epilepsy, as a result of which she had a knowledge of seizures and their treatment with Dilantin (phenytoin) and phenobarbitone (phenobarbital). Despite the fact that Matt Sinclair has epilepsy, this does not feature in the storyline of all the books in which he appears. In *The Closet Hanging*, a drug addict changes Matt's drug treatment for placebo. Having been seizure-free he now suffers a relapse, and as a result he ends up being suspected of murder. In *Kiss Yourself Goodbye*, an attempt is made on Matt's life by administering an electric shock while he is gagged, in an attempt to trigger a seizure that will lead to suffocation. After removal of the gag he would then appear to have died naturally as a result of a seizure. Fennelly deals with her hero's epilepsy without attaching any stigma to it. The condition is part of the character, like the colour of his hair. It is not used to make him vulnerable, or to evoke pity or distrust, but simply to develop the plot, and does not in any way hinder him.

Epilepsy also appears in some science fiction novels. In *The Terminal Man* (1972), the writer **Michael Crichton** (1942–2008), who was also a qualified doctor although he never practised medicine, links explosive violence with epilepsy. The main character, Harry Benson, is a computer scientist in his thirties, who is described as suffering from psychomotor epilepsy following a car crash. He has seizures that are followed by memory blackouts, after which he has no knowledge of what he might have done. During a recent seizure he violently attacked two people and was arrested whilst assaulting a third. He is now regarded as a prime candidate for an experimental operation that involves implanting a 'brain pacemaker' or stimulator in the area of the brain that is responsible for rage. Two surgeons plan to perform the operation, but two psychiatrists, Dr Ross and Dr Manon, question the wisdom of the procedure, pointing out that Benson is psychotic and has strong views about machines controlling human beings. The surgeons respond by explaining that the pacemaker will only 'kick in' when a seizure is about to occur, and then, by preventing it, will abort the associated violence. The operation goes ahead, a total of 40 electrodes are implanted in Benson's 'rage centre', and he is provided with a plutonium-powered backpack that will drive the stimulator. He is tagged on leaving hospital, and is told to contact the surgeons in the event of any mishap, as the backpack is radioactive. Benson continues to exhibit delusional thoughts about machines and computers taking over the world, and this, together with concerns that he might become addicted to the pleasure of stimulating his own brain, results in all the doctors having second thoughts about the wisdom of performing the procedure. The technicians who operate the pacemaker have found that stimulating different electrodes produces different effects, particularly sexual pleasure. By now, equipped with his pacemaker and the knowledge of how to turn it on and off, Benson has escaped from the hospital and is planning to attack its mainframe computer. The search is on to find him, both at his workplace and at the 'strip clubs' that he has begun to frequent. Benson turns up at the house of his psychiatrist, Dr Ross, has a seizure and attacks her. Just before she lapses into unconsciousness she turns on her microwave oven, the radiation from which damages the plutonium in his backpack. The surgeon, Dr Morris, then traces Benson to an airport hotel, where he in turn is assaulted with a metal pipe that destroys the lower half of his face. Benson next turns up at the hospital and goes down to the basement to locate the mainframe computer in order to destroy it. There is a chase through a maze of underground corridors, followed by a struggle that culminates in the psychiatrist, Dr Ross, accidently shooting Benson fatally. In a postscript (and probably in response to criticism) the author did concede that any kind of violent behaviour in epileptic patients is extremely rare, but nonetheless the seed of the idea had been sown and the concept was central to the plot. A film adaptation of the story was released in 1974.

In some respects the author of this novel was well informed. The concept of neurostimulation was just around the corner in relation to conditions such as Parkinson's disease (the actor Michael J. Fox, who starred in the film *Back to the Future* (1985), was an early recipient of such treatment for that condition). Furthermore, the area of Benson's brain in which the electrodes were inserted, the amygdala, is indeed the centre for rage. However, neurostimulation has never been used as a treatment for epilepsy, and the association between epilepsy, rage, and acts of violence is disingenuous at best. Michael Crichton's book and subsequent film did a disservice to people with epilepsy by perpetuating the stereotype that individuals with epilepsy are potentially violent. We shall consider this in more detail in Chapter 11.

Young adult fiction

We should not forget the potential value of the literature, including eBooks, available for children and young adults, as it is through informing this age group that their attitudes in adulthood can be appropriately influenced. I was able to find around 30 books in this genre where epilepsy featured, although it was usually peripheral to the plot. Two bestselling young adult novels, *Conversion* (2014) by Katherine Howe (1977–) and *Shiver* (2009) by Maggie Stiefvater (1981–), mention epileptic seizures merely in passing, and in a derogatory way. It is disappointing that this powerful tool for change has not been used in a more positive manner.

An example of a positive, informative, and attitude-changing work is **David B's** *Epileptic* (2005), which is the English translation of the *L'Ascension du Haut-Mal* series. David B is a comic artist, and he produced this six-volume graphic work about growing up with his older 'epileptic' brother. His family lived in Orléans in France, and he describes his childhood being disrupted when his brother, Jean-Christophe, developed epilepsy at the age of 11. He outlines the family search for a 'cure' from an assortment of conventional medical practitioners and alternative therapists, the latter comprising mediums, acupuncturists, dietitians, and magnetotherapists. Each avenue would generate false hope, followed by eventual disappointment. Jean-Christophe would experience brief periods of remission, which would play into the hands of the alternative therapists, but overall his condition continued to worsen. Illustrated with striking black-on-white drawings, the book is an astonishing and intimate account of the way that epilepsy strikes at the whole family.

Talia Jager's *Teagan's Story: Her Battle With Epilepsy* (2011) follows the experiences of a 16-year-old girl who has lost both her parents in a car crash and is struggling to cope with this, the resultant life changes, and her epilepsy. It deals with epilepsy in a sensitive and informed manner. Teagan's battle is not just with the seizures, but also with the reactions of others, both informed and uninformed. The book is targeted at 8th Grade readers in the USA, equivalent to Year 9 in UK schools. It provides an excellent example of how, in the hands of an empathetic author, books on health issues aimed at a young readership can influence attitudes and opinions.

Conclusion

This account of epilepsy in literature is selective and by no means inclusive. Many novels not mentioned in this chapter have touched peripherally upon epilepsy, and I have focused solely on English-language literature and English translations of world classics. It would be a Herculean task to include all the literature in all languages where epilepsy has made an appearance, and I am not alone among those who have tried to review the subject and ended up merely scratching at the surface. However, on the basis of my chosen selection I hope that a few meaningful conclusions can be drawn.

Peter Wolf, a Danish neurologist who is a specialist in the field of epilepsy, has made a career-long study of the way that seizures have been portrayed in both English-language and world literature.[100] He has catalogued how epilepsy is used by writers to develop plots and to portray vulnerability, weakness and sexuality. He has scoured the literature for what he refers to as 'epilepsy metaphors' that reflect deep emotions, crisis, breakdown, religious experience, and ecstasy. Fiction appears to have gone full circle in its representation of epilepsy. Whereas early writers demonized those with the condition, others provided sympathetic and accurate accounts. As a generalization, contemporary literature seems often to have reverted back to the earlier myths and prejudices, perhaps because the primary aim is to sensationalize and sell books rather than to responsibly inform the reader.

Those authors with a knowledge of epilepsy that has been acquired through personal experience present a more positive picture than those without such knowledge. Among authors who themselves have had epilepsy, some have written openly about it, while others have concealed their condition due to feelings of shame. Many authors who have suffered from epilepsy themselves have tended to live isolated lives, and have managed to use their circumstances to enhance their art. A small band of authors have embraced their condition, have freely included characters with seizures in their writing, portraying them in a positive manner, and in doing so have gone a long way towards 'normalizing' the condition and reducing its stigma

---

100 Wolf P (2016) Epilepsy and metaphors in literature. *Epilepsy & Behavior* 57, 243–246.

CHAPTER 5
Epilepsy in works of art and in artists

It is probably in Christian Renaissance works that the negative perceptions of epilepsy are most clearly expressed. Such preoccupations centred upon demonic possession and the need to 'cast out' the demon and make the possessed person 'clean'. This was illustrated by using symbolism, and required skill in depicting a twisted torso or face. The challenge to pictorial art was in representing an evolving process, namely the seizure, in a static form, namely the painting. Ladino and her colleagues conducted a comprehensive search of articles and reviews focusing on artistic depictions of epilepsy.[101] They classified these within the following periods: Greek, Early Christian, Renaissance, early Latin American, modern, and contemporary. The methodology used by Ladino and her colleagues to search Western medical databases inevitably resulted in a cultural bias, with an overemphasis on Western Christian religious art and an under-representation of the depiction of epilepsy in Eastern pictorial art. Here we shall explore the presentation of epilepsy in pictorial art using Ladino's epochs, but we shall aim to spread our net a little more widely. Inevitably, however, far from being a systematic review, the following account must be viewed as a personal and highly selective appreciation of the depiction of epilepsy in art.

---

[101] Ladino D, Rizvi S and Téllez-Zenteno JF (2016) Epilepsy through the ages: an artistic point of view. *Epilepsy & Behavior* 57, 255–264.

Greek art

Asclepius, one of Apollo's sons, was the god of medicine in ancient Greek mythology. He shared with Apollo the epithet *Paean* (meaning 'the Healer'), and his followers were known as Therapeutae. The rod of Asclepius – a staff with a serpent entwined around it – remains a global symbol of medicine and healing to this day. It was believed by the ancient Greeks in particular that medical conditions could be cured by sleeping in the god's temple overnight. Asclepius would then appear to the patient in a dream and offer advice on how to achieve a cure. The ancient Greeks also believed that a person could develop seizures as a result of upsetting Selene, the moon goddess. They considered epilepsy to be a condition that resembled death, especially in the post-seizure state, when the individual appears motionless and breathing is barely perceptible. The hyacinth was one of the spring-flowering plants regarded by the Greeks as representing renewal and recovery from such a state, and it came to symbolize the escape of the goddess Persephone from the underworld. The word hyacinth is derived from the Greek name 'Hyakinthos'.[102] According to Greek mythology, Hyakinthos was a beautiful young man and lover of the god Apollo. While he and Apollo were taking turns at throwing and catching the discus, Hyakinthos was struck on the head by the discus and fell to the ground, dying. Apollo would not allow Hades to claim the youth, and instead made the hyacinth flower from his spilled blood, thus saving him from hell. Since that time the hyacinth has appeared as a symbol both of rebirth and of resolution of seizures. An example of the use of this Greek symbolism can be found in the *Book of Characteristics*, a fifteenth-century manuscript believed to have been written by the English Franciscan monk Bartholomew, also known as Bartholomew the English. Although there is little definite Greek art (other than the hyacinth) relating to epilepsy, there is much that suggests the condition, including the depiction of a frenetic dance in which one of the dancers is held by two others who have placed their hands upon her head. The placing of hands in such a manner was recommended in order to control seizures. Although one can never be certain whether the artist's intention and our interpretation are one and the same, and indeed this is the fundamental appeal of pictorial art, this could well be a depiction of a seizure.

Early Christian and Renaissance art

The European Renaissance spanned the period from the fourteenth century (i.e. the late Middle Ages) to the seventeenth century. However, the earliest example of epilepsy in

---

102 Mann MW (2012) The epileptic seizure and the myth of Hyakinthos. *Seizure* 21, 595–596.

Middle Ages art dates back to the twelfth century, and curiously is about treatment rather than exorcism.

The *Epilepticus Sic Curatubitur* (which can be translated as 'The way to cure epilepsy') can be found in the British Library, and was donated by **Sir Hans Sloane** (1660–1753), an Irish physician and collector (his huge collection, bequeathed to the British nation, led to the foundation of the British Museum). The anonymous author included a painting of trepanation and cauterization (see Figure 9), which is the first known artistic impression of epilepsy surgery. Trepanation involves making a hole in the skull, and cauterization is the practice or technique of burning a part of the body, and is described in the *Hippocratic Corpus*. The treatment illustrated is based upon mystical and superstitious beliefs that opening the skull would cause the demons, gases, or disease-causing humors to escape. Cauterization was based on the same beliefs

The treatment of epilepsy was also documented by the Turkish surgeon and artist **Serefeddin Sabuncuoglu** (1385–1468). Sabuncuoglu was the author of the first illustrated surgery atlas, *Cerrahiyyetü'l Haniyye* (*Imperial Surgery*), which describes the treatment of conditions such as epilepsy. The book, which contains many detailed illustrations by Sabuncuoglu, was banned under Islamic law because of its depiction of the human body. Colour illustrations were used to describe surgical techniques for epilepsy, such as cautery to cleanse the body of evil spirits. Sabuncuoglu suggested that, before resorting to surgery, the use of herbal mixtures that produced unpleasant odours should be tried first, followed (if this was unsuccessful) by burning or cauterization of the forehead that involved 'shaving the hairs in the frontal region; afterwards one should cauterize the cranium and repeat two times this procedure with iron cauter near the hairline at the middle between the eyebrows'.

As mentioned earlier, the Franciscan monk known as Bartholomew the English is credited with the authorship of the fifteenth-century *Book of Characteristics* in which the Greeks' hyacinth appears in the chapter entitled *Serious Scourge the Physicians Call Epilencie*. The manuscript contains a miniature that depicts a young man who has fallen to the ground as a result of his seizure (see Figure 10). He is shown lying on the grass, frothing at the mouth. The title of the chapter and the illustration leave the reader in little doubt that this is epilepsy. The young man's hat lies on the ground next to him, indicating that the fall happened without warning. In the foreground there are two hyacinth flowers, which symbolize recovery from the seizure. Indeed, seizures have been interpreted as a symbol of death and resurrection by some authors.[103] According to the text *Nature and Its Symbols*,[104]

---

103 Mann MW (2013) The epileptic seizure and the mythology of death in Christian painting. *Epilepsy & Behavior* 28, 303–304.
104 Impelluso L (2004) *Nature and its Symbols*. The Paul Getty Museum, Los Angeles, CA.

the hyacinth symbolizes prudence, wisdom, mourning, and renown, but its presence and context in the *Book of Characteristics* clearly point to its symbolic role in epilepsy.

Les Très Riches Heures du Duc de Berry (*The Very Rich Hours of the Duke of Berry*) is a lavishly decorated Book of Hours containing prayers to be said at certain hours of the day. It was commissioned by John, Duke of Berry, in around 1410, and is probably the most important illuminated manuscript of the fifteenth century. The book took nearly 100 years to complete, and was illustrated by the Limbourg brothers, three Dutch miniature painters from the city of Nijmegen. They used extremely fine paintbrushes, and their work along with the text is on display at the Musée Condé in Chantilly, France. The brothers left the book unfinished and unbound when they died, and the illustrations were completed by a number of other artists from their workshop.[105] The miniature illustrated in Figure 11 is perhaps one of the earliest depictions of Christ driving out an unclean spirit. The woman is held with her arms outstretched and her legs buckled, and the spirit is shown symbolically as leaving through the head of a dragon.

The painter and draughtsman **Hieronymus Bosch** (1450–1516) was born Jheronimus van Aken in the Dutch town of Hertogenbosch, from where he took his name. He became so popular in Spain that he was referred to as 'El Bosco'. The psychiatrist Carl Jung described Bosch as the 'master of the monstrous'.[106] His painting *The Cure of Folly* (also known as *The Extraction of the Stone of Madness*) (see Figure 12) hangs in the Prado Museum in Madrid. It is regarded as one of the earliest paintings of surgery, and is claimed by many to depict epilepsy treatment. The surgeon in the painting is performing a trepanation or craniotomy against the will of the restrained patient, while a disinterested woman, wearing a nun's habit and balancing a book on her head, looks on. Sprouting from the surgical incision is a tulip flower. The calligraphic inscription around the painting reads '*Meester snijt die keye ras/Myne nam is Lubbert das*' ('Master, cut the stone out quickly, my name is Lubbert Das'), and offers a clue to the meaning. Lubbert was a Dutch nickname for a simple, foolish person and, with what seems to be some reluctance, the patient appears to be asking the surgeon to remove the stone from his head. The stone in question was, according to popular belief at that time, known as the 'stone of folly' or 'stone of madness', and was thought to be a cause of mental disorders or 'folly'. The imagery of a surgeon, barber-surgeon, or 'quack' making a hole in a patient's head and plucking out a foreign body in order to cure that person of such conditions occurs frequently throughout the medical art of the late Middle Ages.

William Schupbach, from the Wellcome Institute for the History of Medicine, has reviewed the whole question of 'the cure of folly' in a detailed article that draws upon this

---

105 Pognon E (1987) *Les Très Riches Heures du Duc de Berry*. Liber, Geneva.
106 Jung CC (1964) *Man and his Symbols*. Aldus Books, London.

painting by Bosch, as well as many other artists' interpretations of the same theme.[107] He quotes the Persian physician **Rhazes** (*c.* 854–825), who denounced quacks who pretended to cure epilepsy by making an incision in the scalp and then producing a stone that they were already holding in the palm of their hand. Dutch medical literature suggested that mental illness and brain disorders such as epilepsy were caused by these stones, and that this played literally into the hands of the Dutch and Flemish practitioners, who fabricated surgical procedures. Such quackery associated with the illusion of stone removal was known as 'palming'. This practice of removing or attempting to remove the stone of folly from a patient's head was continued from the Middle Ages right up until the seventeenth century in Flanders, France, and other northern European countries. Was there any rationale for offering this treatment to those with epilepsy as well as to the insane? Medical texts had by this time provided post-mortem evidence that epilepsy could be associated with the presence of foreign bodies inside the skull. It was also believed that an odour or spirit within the head could cause epilepsy. During the Middle Ages, when there were so many theories and superstitions about what caused epilepsy, patients with the condition would have formed a significant target group for those practising surgery or quackery. The 'Cure of Folly' or '*La Pierre de Tête*' became the subject matter of a host of Dutch and Flemish painters from the fifteenth century to the seventeenth century. Among the best known of these are *The Surgeon* by **Jan Sanders van Hemessen** (*c.* 1550) (Prado Museum, Madrid), an untitled '*pierre de tête*' painting by **Pieter Huys** (1561) (Museum of Art and Archaeology of Périgord in Périgueux), and *Cutting Out the Stone of Madness* by **Pieter Bruegel the Elder** (*c.* 1550) (Hotel Sandelin Museum, France). Van Hemessen, Huys, and Bruegel the Elder all depict the same procedure, namely the removal of a stone from the head of a restrained patient, in the presence of nurses, assistants, and assorted onlookers. Van Hemessen's *The Surgeon* (see Figure 13) is one of his most famous works. It shows the surgeon homing in on his target with his knife, while surrounded by surgical specimens that he has successfully removed from other patients. The impression that the painter gives of this surgeon is of someone who has scientific knowledge and a professional approach, rather than a charlatan. The person standing beside the surgeon is perhaps the next patient on the operating list, and his hand-wringing may be a sign of anxiety about what is to follow. The final example is *The Quack* by **Benjamin Cuyp** (1645) (Kelvingrove Museum and Art Gallery, Glasgow), a less well-known Dutch landscape painter. The term 'quack', which means a medical imposter, has a Dutch origin, being a shortening of the Dutch word *quacksalver*, which was used to describe a person who attempted to treat others using false cures or knowledge.

---

107 Schupbach W (1978) A new look at The Cure of Folly. *Medical History* 22, 267–281.

It is interesting to speculate why so many painters chose such apparently obscure subject matter. Schupbach suggests that the stone extractions were theatrical performances, farces, or tableaux, and that these paintings were never intended to document the actual surgical procedures, but rather to depict the drama and sham that surrounded the enactments. Medical and art historians have disputed whether the sham operations depicted in the 'stone of madness' paintings reflect real events, or whether they are allegorical. Whatever the case, some of them must depict people being treated for epilepsy as well as for a host of other mental and physical disorders.

Perhaps the strangest portrayal of epilepsy treatment is a drawing by **Pieter Bruegel the Elder** (1525–1569). He was one of the most significant Dutch and Flemish Renaissance painters, specializing in landscapes and peasant scenes, which earned him the title 'Peasant Bruegel'. After his marriage to Mayken Coecke, the daughter of the painter Pieter Coecke van Aelst, he went to live in Moolenbeek outside Brussels. Here there was a tradition that involved dancing epileptic people over a bridge to the church of St John on St John's day. The belief was that if they were danced over the bridge to the sound of bagpipes, they would be free of seizures until they repeated this ritual the following year. Based on Bruegel the Elder's drawing (possibly lost) or copies by the artist Hendrik Hondius, his son **Pieter Bruegel** (also known as Bruegel the Younger) produced the wood panel painting, *Pilgrimage of the Epileptics to the Church at Molenbeek* (see Figure 14). This painting is also known as *The Dance of St John or St Vitus*. It depicts figures dancing wildly, with the original drawings apparently showing people calling on demons and collapsing to the ground. It is through the Elder's original drawing, and copies by his son, that we gain this disturbing image of those with epilepsy possibly mixed with hysteria. Here we see two women in distress supported by men. They appear tormented and seem to be being dragged along against their will. The women's suffering is evident, and they appear to be writhing, in as much as a static picture can convey this. Their clothing suggests that they are peasants. Other authors such as Robert Bartholomew[108] argue that the Bruegels were depicting dancing mania rather than genuine epilepsy. Dancing mania was a social phenomenon that was documented in Europe between the fourteenth century and the seventeenth century. It involved large groups of people, sometimes thousands at a time, dancing erratically until they collapsed from exhaustion. The mania affected men, women, and children. It predominantly affected poor rural peasant communities, with people dancing for hours, often naked, provocatively and orgiastically. Bartholomew noted that observers of dancing mania who refused to participate were sometimes treated violently. It is unclear whether the Bruegels' painting and drawing were

---

108 Bartholomew RE (2001) *Little Green Men, Meowing Nuns and Head-Hunting Panics: A Study of Mass Psychogenic Illnesses and Social Delusion.* McFarland, Jefferson, NC.

depicting dance mania or epilepsy. The painting is entitled *The Pilgrimage of the Epileptics*, but it is not known who gave the painting that title. However, despite all this uncertainty, on the basis of its title alone this painting merits a place in our portfolio of epilepsy in pictorial art.

The Italian painter **Raffaello Sanzio da Urbino** (1483–1520), better known as **Raphael**, can be credited with the most famous of all Renaissance paintings believed to illustrate epilepsy. The *Transfiguration of Christ* became known to a generation of epilepsy physicians as the first illustration, or frontispiece, in William Lennox's classic textbook, *Epilepsy and Related Disorders*.[109] The name 'Raphael' means '[he whom] God has healed', and some authors have rather fancifully suggested that this, his final painting, is linked to his own health. It depicts the figure of a child, who many writers refer to simply as the 'epileptic boy'.

To summarize the background to the painting, the Transfiguration is an event described in the New Testament, in which Jesus takes three of his apostles – Peter, James, and John – to a mountain to pray. On the mountain Jesus becomes radiant in glory, the prophets Moses and Elijah appear before him, and the apostles hear the voice of God proclaiming Jesus' name.

Giulio di Medici, the future Pope Clement VII, commissioned the painting from Raphael, who died (aged 37 years) before its completion, and it was subsequently placed at the head of his funeral bier. It is now in the Vatican Museums, Rome, with a copy in St Peter's Dome, and a painting with the same theme by another artist is in the Prado Museum in Madrid. The painting is divided into two parts. The upper part depicts the Transfiguration and the lower part, which was unfinished by Raphael, shows the scene immediately before the healing of the boy. This lower section is based on the following passage in the Bible: 'Teacher, I brought my son to you, because he has an evil spirit in him and cannot talk. Whenever the spirit attacks him, it throws him to the ground, and he foams at the mouth, grits his teeth and becomes stiff all over' (Mark 9, 17–18). The boy's father is supporting him, and is wearing a green robe (this colour symbolizes hope). The boy appears to be having a seizure, as his limbs are stiff and twisted, his mouth is open, his lips have a bluish colour, and his eyes are directed to one side. As far as it is possible for an artist to do so, Raphael seems to have painted a static image of a dynamic seizure. The distorted shape of the boy's body is considered by some to represent the cross on which Christ was crucified. Dieter Janz[110] argues that the painter wanted to provide a link between the transient form of death during the epileptic boy's seizure, and Christ's suffering, death, and resurrection. Some authors have

---

109 Lennox WG (1960) *Epilepsy and Related Disorders*. Little, Brown & Company, Boston, MA.
110 Janz D (1986) Epilepsy, viewed metaphysically: an interpretation of the biblical story of the epileptic boy and of Raphael's Transfiguration. *Epilepsia* 27, 316–322.

argued as to whether the boy is coming out of or still having a seizure.[111] Realistically we can never do more than speculate about such details and the painter's intentions.

St Valentine has long been associated with and regarded as the patron saint of epilepsy. Evidence to support this comes from European pictorial art and in particular a fifteenth-century woodcut (see Figure 1). The situation is confused somewhat by the fact that there were three Valentines, in the third, fifth, and eighth centuries respectively. To complicate matters further, the German pronunciation of St Valentine is 'St Fallentin', which itself may create a false link to the 'falling illness'. It is not known for certain which Valentine is the patron saint, although Valentine of Terni seems to be the most likely candidate, and probably over time two of the Valentines became referred to as one individual. The woodcut shown in Figure 1 was kept at Ruffec Priory in France. It is hand-coloured and shows two pilgrims with offerings standing over two people who could simply be asleep, although the bottom figure appears to be twisted. A painting by Hans Georg Geigerfeld (1675) shows St Valentine standing over two people, one of whom is unconscious and foaming at the mouth, while the other has a protruding tongue. Similar paintings include the altarpiece of Bartholomäus Zeitbloom (1455–1515) entitled *Saint Valentin of Terni blesses a man with the falling sickness*. A ceiling painting dated 1740 from Germany shows demons being expelled from the mouth of a child with possible epilepsy, and there are many other examples. Kluger and Kudernatsch, working at an epilepsy centre in Vogtareuth in Germany, have undertaken an exhaustive review of all European art in which St Valentine is associated with possible epilepsy.[112] They reviewed 341 paintings and sculptures from 14 different European countries in which St Valentine appeared, and of these they identified 127 artworks, spanning the fourteenth to nineteenth centuries, that appeared to depict epilepsy. Epileptic patients of all ages, genders, and social classes were represented, along with many different types of seizure. Their attempt to classify seizures on the basis of static images seems somewhat unrealistic, but for all its flaws their study clearly demonstrates that St Valentine is the saint most strongly associated with the condition. More than 40 other saints are linked to epilepsy through art – for example, St Severein and St Vitus. The twelfth-century altarpiece *Saint Severin of Noricum drives out the "falling sickness demon" from a young woman* shows a prostrate young woman being restrained while a priest stands over her with a book (possibly a Bible) in his hand. A fleeing devil can be seen above the red hat of one of her restrainers. Symbols of evil (e.g. monkeys, pigs, crabs, dragons, blackbirds, clouds) are found throughout medieval paintings of possible seizures. Thus a clear message is being conveyed to the worshipping public, namely that epilepsy is a tainting condition

---

111 deToledo J, Ramsay RE and Marsan CA (1996) The lunatic and his seizure. *Neurology* 47, 292–293.

112 Kluger G and Kudernatsch V (2009) St Valentine – patron saint of epilepsy: illustrating the semiology of seizures over the course of six centuries. *Epilepsy & Behavior* 14, 219–225.

associated with the devil, and it can only be cured by the church. This is most evident in the biblical paintings of the 'casting out of the possessed'.

Let us now look at art depicting Jesus and his driving out of unclean spirits. Of course we cannot assume that all unclean spirits are related to epilepsy, just as we can only speculate about the intended message of the artist. The possible association with epilepsy depends upon the posture and countenance of the person who is having evil spirits exorcised. In many depictions the individual appears to be having a seizure, although it could just as easily be argued that their body posture is caused by psychiatric illness or hysteria.

The New Testament contains 25 references to Jesus casting out demons, and so has provided plenty of material for artists to illustrate. In the Gospel of Mark (1:23–28), Jesus is in Capernaum and enters a synagogue where there is a man with an unclean spirit. The man cries out '"What business do we have with each other, Jesus of Nazareth? Have You come to destroy us? I know who You are – the Holy One of God!" And Jesus rebuked him, saying, "Be quiet, and come out of him!" Throwing him into convulsions, the unclean spirit cried out with a loud voice and came out of him.' An unattributed painting that accompanies the verses is titled *Jesus Drives Out an Evil Spirit From a Man in Capernaum*, and shows a kneeling man being touched on the forehead by Jesus. Although the biblical passage mentions convulsions, the artist has not depicted these. The illustration from a German Bible of 1720, again unattributed, is entitled *Jesus Driving Out an Unclean Spirit* and is reproduced in Owsei Temkin's *The Falling Sickness*.[113] Here there can be no doubt that a seizure has been captured for all to see. The subject is being held down by two attendants who appear to be forcibly restraining him. His head and upper body are arched backwards, while his arms and one leg are extended and his mouth is gaping open. There is even a hint that his eyes are rolling backwards. The image is clearly that of a generalized tonic seizure. Other paintings of 'casting out' are less graphic in their depiction, and much depends upon the symbolism within the story that is being told. There are striking similarities between Christian and Hindu illustrations of the casting out of unclean spirits or demons. Krishna, a major deity in Hinduism, was the god of love and compassion, and was often called upon to exorcise demons. In paintings of Krishna exorcisms, the same black devil can be seen emerging from the mouth of the cleansed or cured person.

Votive tablets had a significant place in Christian worship from the seventeenth century onwards. They often consisted of simple paintings that explained why a sick person might seek help from a specific saint. The process would initially involve undertaking a vow and lighting a votive candle on behalf of the sick person. The paintings would then take the

---

113 Temkin O (1971) *The Falling Sickness: A History of Epilepsy from the Greeks to the Beginnings of Modern Neurology*, second edition. Johns Hopkins University Press, Baltimore, MD. p. 88. See also Rosenthal O (1925) *Wunderheilungen und arztliche Schutzpatrone in der bildenden Kunst*. F. C. W. Vogel, Leipzig. Table 21.

form of a religious image giving thanks for a miracle or favour that the vow and prayers had delivered. This was a particularly common practice in Mexico, where it was introduced by Spanish colonists. The ritual, already common in Europe, was one in which paintings could be produced to give thanks for a whole range of answered prayers, from surviving an avalanche to surviving a cart accident. The votive tablets *Girl with the Falling Sickness* (*c.* 1510) and *Child with Epilepsy and its Parents at Altötting, a Place of Pilgrimage in Bavaria* are simple artworks offering up thanks for the miracle that has been performed.

The social disadvantages of people with epilepsy were chronicled by **Thomas Harman** (*fl.* 1547–1567), an English writer who described the lives of beggars in his *Caveat or Warning for Common Cursitors* (1566). As a magistrate he was obliged to enforce Henry VIII's laws against beggars. In his book, his descriptions were accompanied by drawings illustrating the lives of the less fortunate as well as those who mimicked illness in order to beg. He referred to such people as 'Counterfeit Cranks', and noted that some pretended to suffer from the falling illness of epilepsy, wearing dirty clothes and carrying soap with them to enable them to give the illusion of foaming at the mouth, as well as carrying false testimonials from their alleged parish priest.[114] One particular culprit, Nicholas Blunt, is illustrated half-naked in dirty rags with his face smeared with fresh blood. Such images provide an important window into sixteenth-century perceptions of epilepsy, although they cannot be considered pictorial masterpieces. Rather they were the precursors of the art of social commentary that was to become perfected by both the text and the illustrations of Charles Dickens' novels.[115]

Sir Peter Paul Rubens (1577–1640) was a Flemish artist who painted classical and biblical scenes in the Baroque style. Knighted by Charles I of England, he was also a painter, a revered scholar, and a diplomat. In 1600 he travelled to Italy, where he studied the works of the Italian masters, including Michelangelo and Leonardo da Vinci. In 1602 he was employed by the Spanish Duke of Mantua, who had a renowned art collection, and from there he travelled to Spain as a diplomat to the court of King Philip. Both in Spain and in Rome he would have encountered the works of Raphael, especially his *Transfiguration*. Rubens' own painting, *The Transfiguration of Christ* (*c.* 1605), is in the Museum of Fine Arts in Nancy, France. It is one of three paintings completed while Rubens was employed by the Duke. Here the 'epileptic boy' is shown again in the arms of his father. The contact with Jesus is less evident, as their respective gazes do not meet. The boy's right arm and leg are extended and appear to have stiffened, but his head is turned away towards his father, and his eyes seem to be directed away from him (see Figure 15). It appears likely that Rubens is

---

114 Salgado S (1972) *Cony-Catchers and Bawdy Baskets; an Anthology of Elizabethan Low Life.* Penguin, Harmondsworth.
115 Text is available online to subscribers to Early English Books Online (EEBO), and page images of an 1814 reprint of the 1573 edition can be accessed using Google Book Search.

illustrating a seizure, but whether deliberately and knowingly, or merely as a consequence of copying Raphael's stage scene or tableau, is uncertain.

Epilepsy also features in two versions of Rubens' *The Miracles of St Ignatius of Loyola*, although it is unclear whether this reflects a personal knowledge of the condition or simply a general observation of epilepsy. St Ignatius of Loyola (1491–1556) was a Spanish Basque theologian who co-founded the Society of Jesus (the Jesuit religious movement). William Lennox goes so far as to suggest that St Ignatius himself may have had epilepsy, citing as evidence an autobiographical account of hallucinations and episodes of unconsciousness.[116]

Both versions of the painting (1617 and 1618) take the form of oil on canvas *modellos* for altarpieces, and depict a woman in a convulsive state undergoing exorcism. The first version was painted for the high altar of the Jesuit Church of Antwerp in Belgium, and is in the Kunsthistorisches Museum in Vienna, and the second version is in Genoa, Italy. In both paintings Rubens captures the spectacle of the exorcism, with St Ignatius standing aloft with one hand raised as he banishes the demons. The demons take the form of a horned beast and a fiery dragon. At the saint's feet are a man who has already been cleansed and a woman undergoing the process of exorcism. Her mouth is wide open with her tongue protruding, and she is tearing at her hair and clothing. Her eyes are wide and turned upwards. The previous 'patient' is lying on the ground half-naked with his face twisted, his eyes turned upwards, and with foam coming from his gaping mouth. Some authors have interpreted these postures as being indicative of a hysterical state, whereas others view them as a convincing portrayal of epileptic seizures. Ultimately it is for the individual observer to interpret the artist's intentions. It appears to this observer that both the man and the woman are having seizures. To others, such as James Harris,[117] psychiatric disorders such as schizophrenia seem to be a more plausible explanation for those afflicted by demons. Harris points out that exorcism was formally accepted by the Catholic Church under Pope Paul V in 1614, before Rubens' paintings were completed.

Early Latin-American art

The Incas called epilepsy the 'wind (air) of the dead' or 'disease of the dead'. The Mayas referred to it as 'pseudo death', and the Aztecs described their various treatments for epilepsy as medicine 'for the dying'. The Aztecs arrived in Mexico in the twelfth century, and remained the dominant culture there throughout the fourteenth, fifteenth, and sixteenth centuries. Their capital, Tenochtitlan, became Mexico City after they were defeated by the Spanish

---

116 Lennox WG and Lennox MA (1960) Epileptics of worth and fame. In: *Epilepsy and Related Disorders*. Little, Brown & Company, Boston, MA. pp. 700–711.
117 Harris JCO (2014) Exorcism: The Miracles of St Ignatius of Loyola. *JAMA Psychiatry* 71, 866–867.

conquistadors under the command of Herman Cortes in 1521. Their religion was based upon the worship of their gods, and incorporated human sacrifice. They included deities from other religions in their religious worship, and their calendar was filled with festivals. They regarded the universe as divided into upper and nether worlds, with gods and religious symbols for each world. Their gods were neither good nor bad, but rather a mixture of the two. Their medical treatment was based upon the use of medicinal plants, and knowledge of it was passed down from father to son. As in Europe, epilepsy was regarded as a sacred illness that required treatment with herbs and magic. These treatments were recorded in the *Codice de la Cruz Badiano*, a compendium of Aztec medicine written in the early sixteenth century at the request of the Spanish conquerors.

Art was an important element of Aztec civilization, whether it took the form of clothing and jewellery to display their wealth, or painting, sculpture, music and poetry to celebrate their many gods and festival days. The Aztecs had no written language, and instead conveyed knowledge and stories by means of drawings made in codices (manuscript books). These drawings used rich colours and very precise linear contours, usually without any depth. Coral, clay, chalk and stone were commonly used materials, often in combination with bird feathers, gold, silver and copper. Although the names of the artists have long been forgotten, in their time they were feted and commissioned by the wealthy and by nobility.

The Aztec goddess **Tlazolteotl**, a lunar deity, has become associated with epilepsy in almost the same way as St Valentine in Christian religion. Tlazolteotl is one of the most complex Aztec goddesses, and can be easily identified in sculptures and illustrations by her bitumen-blackened mouth, clown's hat, and broomstick, and the fact that she is often in the squatting position for giving birth. Her name is derived from a word meaning 'garbage' or 'filth', and she was the pardoner of all that was unsavoury, including illnesses. She could only give absolution once in the lifetime of each person who needed her services. Tlazolteotl was not just a pardoner but also a provoker in that she could pass on diseases as well as cure them. By eating dirt or excrement she would draw out the sins of those who had confessed, and by regurgitation she could pass these back to others and cause them to convulse. Her blackened mouth is thought to symbolize the ingestion of devils. Just like the ancient Greeks thousands of miles away and centuries earlier, the Aztecs believed that epilepsy could be caught from saliva and repelled by spitting. Ancient Greek and Aztec cultures also shared the belief that epilepsy was a transient form of dying, with recovery from the very brink of death as the event abated. As a moon goddess, Tlazolteotl was regarded as having power over life and death and thus the ability to decide who would recover from such an event. Certainly her role as the Aztec goddess of epilepsy seems to be well established.[118] The most

---

118 Ladino D and Téllez-Zentino JF (2016) Tlazolteotl: the Aztec goddess of epilepsy. *Epilepsy & Behavior* 57, 60–68.

famous painting of the goddess in action is held in the Vatican Library in Rome, and has been used as the logo of the Mexican branch of the International League Against Epilepsy (ILEA). The brightly coloured painting appears in the *Borgia Codex* or manuscript, and shows the goddess regurgitating into the mouth of an individual. Although many consider this to be an illustration of the transmission of epilepsy, it can more rationally be interpreted as the passing on of an unspecified illness by the goddess of epilepsy. Further evidence of Tlazolteotl's place in epilepsy art is provided by the more recent paintings of her in this role by the Mexican artists Eduardo Urbano Merino and Frida Kahlo.

Vincent van Gogh and epilepsy

Before we move on to consider Van Gogh and epilepsy, some important myths need to be laid to rest. The name of **Leonardo da Vinci** (1452–1519) appears on many lists of 'famous people with epilepsy',[119] as does that of **Michelangelo** (1475–1564), who merely suffered from fainting when it was hot. Indeed the long lists of famous people with epilepsy that can be found on many websites as a result of internet searches are often extremely inaccurate. The suggestion that Leonardo da Vinci had epilepsy is based mainly on the fact that he would often shake when angered! His illegitimacy, personality, sexuality, mirror writing, and failure to complete works have also all been cited by those keen to make a diagnosis. Walter Isaacson, in his book *Leonardo Da Vinci: The Biography*,[120] makes no reference to seizures, fits, or blackouts, and the Chicago neurologist John Hughes in his meticulously researched review[121] attributes Da Vinci's occasional shaking episodes to 'angst and spasm of furious sensibility'.

The question of whether or not Van Gogh had epilepsy certainly merits a discussion of the evidence available. However, here again caution is needed, as over 150 physicians have suggested a total of 30 different diagnoses for the artist's various health problems. His name also appears on most of the above-mentioned lists of famous people with epilepsy.

Vincent van Gogh (1853–1890), the Dutch Post-Impressionist painter, was born into an upper-middle-class family at Groot-Zundert in southern Holland. His father was the pastor of a Dutch Reformed church in a particularly Catholic part of the country. Vincent was one of five surviving children, and his youngest sister, Wilhelmina, was incarcerated for much of her life with a diagnosis of schizophrenia. His brother Theo, who supported him throughout his life, suffered from depression, and another brother, Cornelius, committed

---

119 See, for example, www.epilepsytoronto.org/about-epilepsy/learn-about-epilepsy/famous-people-with-epilepsy/
120 Isaacson W (2017) *Leonardo Da Vinci: The Biography*. Simon and Schuster, New York.
121 Hughes JR (2005) Did all these famous people really have epilepsy? *Epilepsy & Behavior* 6, 115–139.

suicide. During the last decade of his life, Van Gogh produced over 800 oil paintings (landscape, still life, portraits, and self-portraits), many of them characterized by the use of bold colours and frenetic brushwork. His suicide at the age of 37 was the culmination of years of mental turmoil, illness, and poverty.

Vincent did not complete a formal education, but instead left school at the age of 15 to work for a firm of art dealers in the Hague. He was transferred by his firm to London, where he remained for about two years before leaving his position, probably due to a combination of factors, including a failed romantic infatuation, an inability to manage his personal finances or the commercial side of his occupation, and a tendency to argue with clients about the merit of their purchases. I think we can safely assume that he was fired. There followed a period of profound religiosity in the artist's early twenties, which has been outlined by Dietrich Blumer.[122] During this period Van Gogh became a social recluse and was increasingly concerned with religion. After failing his theological studies he became an unqualified evangelist in a poverty-stricken mining town in Belgium, but was eventually dismissed because of his dishevelled appearance, his demeanour, and his inappropriate and excessive charitable acts. At the age of 27, only 10 years before his death, he decided to become a painter and applied to art school, only to be rejected. By this stage he was an agnostic and entirely supported by his faithful brother Theo. The only hint that something might be amiss was his somewhat unusual personality. Indeed his mother, with whom he was now living, said that she was 'so afraid that wherever he goes and whatever he does, he will spoil everything by his peculiar behavior and queer ideas'.[123] Van Gogh then went to Paris to stay with his brother Theo, who was now working as a successful art dealer, and it is around this time that the first indications of epilepsy symptoms begin to emerge. Van Gogh was in his early thirties and was experiencing episodes of sudden fear and loss of consciousness. He was also drinking absinthe (a distilled highly alcoholic drink made from medicinal herbs, and regularly consumed by Bohemian writers and artists) and smoking to excess, and becoming increasingly unkempt and argumentative. Absinthe was known to induce hallucinations, and it was also thought to provoke seizures.

In 1888, just two years before his death, Van Gogh moved to the warmer climate of the ancient Roman town of Arles in the south of France. Here he was to produce over 300 oil paintings at a frantic pace. He rented the now famous 'Yellow House', and invited other artists such as Paul Gauguin to stay with him as guests and help to set up his somewhat grandiose vision of a 'Studio of the South'. Gauguin's stay was to find a permanent place in Van Gogh's history. An absinthe-fuelled argument led to Gauguin leaving, pursued by Van Gogh holding

---

122 Blumer D (2002) The illness of Vincent Van Gogh. *American Journal of Psychiatry* 159, 519–526.
123 Hughes JR (2005) A reappraisal of the possible seizures of Vincent Van Gogh. *Epilepsy & Behavior* 6, 504–510.

an open razor. Giving up the chase, Van Gogh returned to the Yellow House, where he cut off the lower part of his ear. Eventually the local inhabitants of Arles became so disturbed by his behaviour that a petition was successfully raised to have him committed to the Saint Paul de Mausole asylum for epilepsy and mental disorders, on the outskirts of Saint Rémy-de-Provence. It was here that the somewhat uncertain diagnosis of epilepsy was made by the asylum director, an elderly semi-retired clinician called Dr Peyton. On the basis of this diagnosis, Van Gogh was prescribed potassium bromide. He returned to the asylum voluntarily the following year in a psychotic state, experiencing religious and paranoid delusions and auditory hallucinations. By now he was swinging between manic and depressive modes indicative of a bipolar disorder. At this point he may also have started to receive treatment with digitalis.

Van Gogh was a prodigious letter writer, and it is in his personal correspondence, especially his letters to his brother, Theo, that the strongest evidence for a diagnosis of epilepsy can be found. A six-volume edition of his correspondence was published recently,[124] and the Swiss neurologist Fabienne Picard has identified within this work evidence that he feels 'makes the diagnosis of epilepsy indisputable', from 1888 (when Vincent was 35 years old) onward.[125] Picard cites letters written not only by Van Gogh but also by the clinicians. There are references within the correspondence to the episodic nature of attacks, concern about tongue biting, fatigue and sore throat on recovery, and Van Gogh's fear of having an attack, falling into the hands of the police, and being 'forcibly carried off into an asylum'. Nowhere, however, is there a clear description of what an epileptologist would unequivocally recognize as a seizure. In May 1890, Theo wrote to his brother, advising him not to travel alone, and commenting that 'in any event on the day you have decided to come here you absolutely must be accompanied during the entire journey by someone you trust'. Picard also quotes from the admission notes of the asylum director, Dr Peyton, which state that Van Gogh 'is suffering from acute mania with hallucinations of sight and hearing, which may have caused him to mutilate himself by cutting off his ear ... based on all the above I consider Mr Van Gogh is subject to attacks of epilepsy, separated by long intervals'. The published correspondence also reveals for the first time a family history of epilepsy.

Although Picard is convinced by the evidence, others are less so, and over the years many alternative physical and mental diagnoses have been suggested to explain Van Gogh's tragic life experiences. Possible psychiatric explanations have included borderline personality disorder and bipolar disorder, and suggested physical causes have ranged from fainting during episodes of near starvation to lead poisoning and the 'royal illness' of porphyria. To this author, epilepsy seems to be the most likely diagnosis, and many of Van Gogh's personality traits

---

124 Jansen L, Luijten H and Bakker N (2009) *Vincent Van Gogh: The Letters*. Thames and Hudson (in association with the Van Gogh Museum and the Huygens Institute), London.
125 Picard F (2011) Vincent van Gogh's epilepsy. *Epilepsy & Behavior* 22, 414–415.

could be explained by Geschwind's controversial epileptic personality syndrome, including his emotional volatility, depression, hyposexuality, religiosity, and hypergraphia (as evidenced by six volumes of correspondence). It was the great French neurologist and epileptologist Henri Gastaut who first raised the question of whether Van Gogh had epilepsy,[126] so perhaps he should have the last word here. He was convinced that epilepsy was indeed the correct diagnosis, and he suggested that the seizures had initially been triggered by alcohol.

Van Gogh's death had just as much pathos as his life. He had been discharged from the asylum in May 1890, and was abstaining from alcohol, free from the presumed seizures, and working furiously. On 27 July 1890 he went out into the fields with his paints and a revolver and shot himself in the lower chest. He then staggered back to an inn, where he told friends that he could not bear life any longer. The decision was made not to remove the bullet, and he died two days later. If it is accepted that Van Gogh indeed had epilepsy, he is yet another tragic statistic demonstrating the high risk of suicide in those who have the condition.

In an article entitled 'The science of art', V. S. Ramachandran proposes the following theory: 'Van Gogh's epileptic seizures in his temporal lobes may have actually strengthened neural connections between his visual object and face area and the amygdala, nucleus accumbens and other brain regions involved in gauging the emotional significance of what's being viewed. Such a heightened attention and emotional response to visual images may have made him a more accomplished artist – his seizures enabling him to "attend" to certain critical dimensions more than you or I.'[127] This in-depth analysis, which claims that the disorder gave the painter some sort of advantage compared with other people, assumes that the diagnosis of epilepsy is correct, as does the observation made by other writers that Van Gogh's unusual perception and use of colour can be explained scientifically by the possibility that he was taking the drug digitalis, which was often given to patients with epilepsy. Studies have shown red–green visual impairment in approximately a quarter to a third of people taking digitalis, with a quarter also showing tritan colour blindness, which results in their confusing blue with green, and yellow with violet. This might possibly therefore have given Van Gogh yet another artistic advantage resulting from his epilepsy. However, the evidence that he was ever treated with digitalis is based on the fact that it was used to treat mental conditions, and that he painted one of his doctors (the above-mentioned Dr Peyton) holding a foxglove, from which the drug is derived. Finally, even if Van Gogh was taking digitalis, this would only have been for the last year or so of his life, and so would have had little effect on his artistic output as a whole.

---

126 Gastaut H (1956) Vincent van Gogh's disease seen in the light of new concepts of psychomotor epilepsy [article in French]. *Annales Medico-Psychologiques* 114, 196–238.

127 Ramachandran VS and Hirstein W (1999) The science of art: a neurological theory of aesthetic experience. *Journal of Consciousness Studies* 6, 15–51.

Modern and contemporary art

Modern art refers to works produced from the 1860s until the 1970s, and reflects the gargantuan cultural, social, and industrial changes which occurred during that period. Traditional art from the Renaissance was replaced by the creed of experimentation. There was also a move away from the narrative paintings that told their story through the use of symbolism, and towards the depiction of scenes for their own sake as a chronicler of the times. Art no longer needed to depict a biblical or mythological story, but could instead focus on nature, the urban environment, and social activities, and with this came abstract art. **Contemporary or postmodern art** refers to works produced in the late twentieth century or in the twenty-first century. Contemporary art is the art of the present day, and its cultural and global diversity reflects the shrinking and technologically advancing world. Art has become more explicit in what it purports to convey. Therefore if a contemporary painting is about epilepsy we are told as much and left in no doubt about the matter. The Renaissance painters provided an ambiguous image that viewers interpreted on the basis of their own notions and experiences, whereas now we can be more certain about whether or not it was the artist's intention to paint an epilepsy-related work. This change in attitude to the pictorial depiction of epilepsy has been made possible by modern and contemporary art providing a more liberal perception of the condition, far removed from the biblical concepts of cleansing and sin. This has coincided with an era in which artists with epilepsy have begun to be open about their condition, and to depict it pictorially.

One of the most notable and widely recognized modern paintings of epilepsy is *The Red Curtain* (*c.* 1965), also known as *Homage to Vincent Van Gogh*, by an anonymous German painter. There are at least three other paintings entitled *The Red Curtain*, but none of them deal with the subject of seizures. This iconic painting symbolizes how epilepsy can disrupt life for anyone who has the condition, and it has become the symbol of the Bonn-based Michael Foundation,[128] the oldest private foundation for people with epilepsy in Germany. The vivid backdrop of the red curtain and what lies beyond tantalizes the observer and suggests danger (see Figure 16). The birds that are just visible against the background of blue sky may be significant as symbolizing evil, or alternatively they could be a homage to Van Gogh's *Wheat Field with Crows*, which, despite common belief, is almost certainly not his last work. In pictorial art the crow is widely regarded as an image of negativity, being symbolic of death, the devil, or misfortune.[129] In the foreground, Van Gogh lies in a convulsive posture with his arms drawn up and his legs apparently kicking. His eyes stand out black and open, and

---

128 www.stiftung-michael.de
129 Impelluso L (2004) *Nature and its Symbols*. The Paul Getty Museum, Los Angeles, CA.

beside him lies a chair from which we can assume he has just fallen. Curiously, his palette lies beside him undisturbed, as if to suggest that despite what has happened, his most important tool remains unaffected and is awaiting his recovery so that he can resume his work when the seizure has been overcome. In fact, the artist responsible for this painting was someone with epilepsy who assisted at art therapy classes.

Van Gogh was not the only artist who probably had epilepsy, and indeed in the case of other modern and contemporary artists there is perhaps less diagnostic uncertainty. **Edward Lear** (1812–1888), the English illustrator, musician, and poet, has already been mentioned in Chapter 4 in relation to his writings and the shame he felt about his condition. However, he was also an accomplished artist with epilepsy. He lived abroad and alone for much of his life, and travelled throughout Europe, the Middle East, and India. He produced large numbers of watercolours and oil paintings that, through their sales, gave him a financial independence that his writings could never have achieved. He finally settled in San Remo, Italy, in his 'Villa Tennyson', with only his faithful cat Foss for company. In addition to his epilepsy, his eventual near blindness combined with hearing impairment exacerbated his sense of isolation and sadness. Jenny Uglow's recent biography of Lear[130] outlines the conflicting feelings of a celibate gay person who was ashamed of being an 'epileptic' and who, although he had a brilliant mind and was constantly fascinated by life, was doomed to live – like many people with epilepsy – in the shadows. Neither his writings nor his paintings and illustrations give any hint of his epilepsy. One of his best-known oil paintings, *The Plains of Lombardy from Monte Generoso* (1880), is in the Ashmolean Museum in Oxford.

The prominent landscape painter **George Inness** (1825–1894) has been hailed as one of America's greatest and most influential artists. During a prolific career he produced over 1000 paintings, and became known as the 'Father of the American Landscape'. He was born in Newburgh, New York, the fifth of 13 children. His epilepsy started in his early youth, and significantly affected his training and subsequent career. At the age of 16, by which time the family had moved to Newark, he returned to New York to study engraving, but soon had to abandon this as his epilepsy worsened. Four years later he managed to return to New York for a month to study in the studio of **Régis Gignoux** (1816–1882), a French landscape painter who was active in America, but again he had to return home sooner than planned for health reasons. Inness received no further formal training. He did eventually manage two visits to Europe, and even lived briefly in Rome, but there is no doubt that his epilepsy prevented him from undertaking the travel and the tutoring that he felt he needed in order to develop his early career. In 1868 he became a National Academician, and he spent the final four years of his life in Italy.

---

130 Uglow J (2016) *Mr Lear: A Life of Art and Nonsense.* Faber & Faber, London.

Inness developed a deep interest in the spiritual world and especially in the theories of **Emanuel Swedenborg** (1688–1772), a theologian who believed that even material objects within a landscape possessed spiritual qualities. Inness reflected on this in his *Writings and Reflections on Art and Philosophy*.[131] Such an excessive interest in the spiritual world could be interpreted, along with his prolific output, as part of the 'epileptic personality' (see Chapter 11 for a detailed discussion of this concept). However, this would be to read too much into an interest that was pursued by all of Swedenborg's disciples, whether or not they had epilepsy. There is no detailed biography of Inness – all we know is that epilepsy played a significant role in his life. It is worth remembering that this was a time when a considerably greater social stigma was attached to epilepsy than is the case today, and consequently people with the condition tended to go to some lengths to conceal it.

Giorgio de Chirico (1888–1978) was a Greek-born Italian artist and writer who in his early years founded the *Scuola Metafisica* (Metaphysical School) art movement, but reverted to a more traditional style in the later part of his career. The Metaphysical art movement began just before the First World War and was influenced by several surrealist artists, including **Max Ernst** (1891–1976). De Chirico's own paintings were dreamlike, threatening, and mysterious. He was known to have suffered from a lifelong episodic condition in which he experienced the same symptoms repeatedly. Some authors have suggested that this was an unusually severe form of migraine,[132] and others have proposed that he had temporal lobe or complex partial epilepsy. Both camps agree that his condition influenced his paintings and through them the Surrealist movement. Olaf Blanke and Theodor Landis argue the case for temporal lobe epilepsy,[133] although with customary caution. They base this on a detailed study of de Chirico's copious autobiographical writings. The sheer volume of these writings (as also in the case of Van Gogh) might be a clue in itself, given that hypergraphia (excessive writing) is observed in patients with temporal lobe epilepsy. The writings describe an unusual sensation rising from the stomach, associated with a strange taste in the mouth 'like phenic acid' (phenol), and accompanied by an inexplicable feeling of fear and anxiety. De Chirico was advised to take sedatives, have plenty of bedrest, and adopt a more stable lifestyle. He also described having strange visual hallucinations.[134] These would come on suddenly and resolve just as rapidly, and could take the form of scenes and people. He describes graphically how 'at such moments it sometimes happened that a back wall opened up like a theatre curtain and visions appeared, sometimes terrifying, sometimes sublime or enchanting; there would be the ocean in a storm or hideous gnomes'. This description is highly suggestive of temporal

---

131 Bell AB (ed.) (2007) *George Inness: Writings and Reflections on Art and Philosophy*. George Braziller, Inc., New York.
132 Fuller GN and Gale MV (1988) Migraine aura as artistic inspiration. *British Medical Journal* 297, 1670–1672.
133 Blanke O and Landis T (2003) The metaphysical art of Giorgio de Chirico. *European Neurology* 50, 191–194.
134 De Chirico (1994) *The Memoirs of Giorgio de Chirico*. Da Capo Press, Boston, MA.

lobe epilepsy, and although similar complex visual hallucinations can occur in migraine, they are much rarer in that condition. Blanke and Landis provide an exhaustive review of De Chirico's writings, which hint at the possibility that he had the so-called 'epileptic personality' (a concept that will be discussed later), as evidenced by his hypergraphia. They note philosophical and personal preoccupations manifested as a conviction of self-ability, self-destiny, and the possession of special powers, along with an overwhelming interest in moral and ethical issues. Added to these traits is the hypergraphia. Finally, a diagnosis of epilepsy is supported by the occasional although infrequent episodes of loss of consciousness, and evidence that argues against migraine is provided by the complete absence of any episodes of headache. On the basis of the descriptions in the memoirs and the controversial concept of the 'epileptic personality', it seems highly probable that De Chirico did indeed have epilepsy. In this case, how did the condition influence his art? He made it clear that his visual hallucinatory experiences were transposed to and inspired his paintings. These images were mysterious, often threatening, and commonly took the form of complex superimpositions or inappropriate objects that seem incongruous in the scene in which they occur. An example of this is his oil painting *The Songs of Love* (1914) (Museum of Modern Art, New York), in which a glove appears pinned to a wall alongside a representation of a Greek sculpture. His inflexibility and rigid adherence to repetition and order are also manifested in his work; for example, he produced 18 almost identical versions of the same painting, *The Disquieting Muse*. Much of his copying work was undertaken in the latter part of his life, when perhaps he could no longer access the inspirational imagery. He acknowledged that his own 'mental phenomenon' was often reflected in his paintings, and the evidence that exists suggests that this condition was undiagnosed and lifelong temporal lobe epilepsy.

Sir John 'Kyffin' Williams (1918–2006) was born in Llangefni, on Anglesey in North Wales, and became a painter best known for his works featuring the Welsh countryside and the activities of its farming communities. He studied at the Slade School of Fine Art in London, and became a senior art teacher at Highgate School in the same city. He was subsequently appointed President of the Royal College of Art, and was knighted in 1999. Such a career could hardly have been envisaged in 1941 when he was invalided out of the army because of epilepsy. Williams showed no particular artistic or general academic ability at school, and left to join the army as a member of the Royal Welsh Fusiliers. In his autobiography, of which there are two volumes, *Across the Straits*[135] and *A Wider Sky*,[136] covering different periods of his life, he recalls his first seizure. This occurred when he was 19 years old, after a regimental dinner: 'I don't know when I woke, but I remember lying

---

135 Williams K (1973) *Across the Straits*. Gerald Duckworth & Co. Ltd, London.
136 Williams K (1991) *A Wider Sky*. Gomer Press, Llandysul, Wales.

beside the open window. ... There was a taste of blood in my mouth and my tongue was terribly painful. ... My tongue was in agony, but I got up, dressed and unsteadily made my way downstairs to breakfast.'[137] He was subsequently seen by a neurologist, diagnosed with epilepsy, and started on phenytoin and a mixture of belladonna (deadly nightshade) and a seaweed called Irish moss. This unpleasant-tasting mixture had been prescribed to prevent recurrence, but within six months a further seizure ensued, followed by another, resulting in hospital investigations involving an electroencephalogram and lumbar puncture. It was at this stage that a doctor said to him: 'What are you going to do when you leave the army? ... as you are in fact abnormal. I think it would be a good idea if you took up art.' If such a statement was made today it would rightly result in a complaint, but for Williams it led to the start of a new and rewarding venture.

In 1941 he went to the prestigious Slade School of Fine Art with the intention of becoming an art teacher and being able to live a fairly sheltered life. The Second World War had by now started, and as a result Williams was virtually the only man in his class, the others having being conscripted into the armed services, and by his own admission he was the worst student. His seizures were no longer generalized or grand mal, but had taken on a new form: 'The illness found a new way through minor epileptiform attacks which sometimes numbered as many as nine in a single day.' He describes hearing music: 'symphonies that had never been heard before'. Such musical hallucinations can occur in epilepsy arising in the temporal lobe. There is even a rare inherited form of epilepsy called autosomal dominant partial epilepsy with auditory features (ADPEAF). When this occurs, sounds such as buzzing, humming, or ringing are associated with the attack. The ability of music to trigger seizures (musicogenic epilepsy) or even soothe them (the Mozart effect) will be discussed later.

Despite Williams' openness about his diagnosis, his autobiography provides little information about the true impact of epilepsy on his personal life. He lived alone, and in later life returned to his native North Wales, where Lord Anglesey provided him with a house, and, according to his autobiography, 'ever since he and Lady Anglesey have been concerned for both my artistic and everyday welfare'. John Griffin has studied both volumes of Williams' autobiography, and he comments that the artist had a tendency towards obsessiveness in that he frequently either destroyed his paintings or lamented the fact that he could not choose their purchasers or their final destinations: 'It is unfortunate that I am unable to give my pictures away to people of my own choice.'[138]

Williams described himself as 'an obsessive, depressive, diabetic epileptic, who's apprehensive, selfish, intolerant and ruthless'. This was a harsh self-assessment by a man

---

137 Williams K (1973) op. cit.
138 Griffin JP (2010) Epilepsy—the making of a painter: Sir (John) Kyffin Williams. *Clinical Medicine* 10, 91–92.

whose pupils and friends found him warm, funny, and generous. His various biographies and obituaries in the national press and on the Internet mention his diagnosis of epilepsy, but only briefly refer to its impact on his life. A short biography of Williams on the Big Sky Fine Art website commented on his 'tendency to melancholy', and believed it to be 'exacerbated by circumstance, instinctively feeling that a certain despair and gloom was the logical sequel to his grand mal seizures'.[139] It was also pointed out that Williams felt a close affinity to Van Gogh, 'not least that they were both epileptic'. An obituary in *The Guardian* commented on 'his perception of the difficulties of epilepsy, and perhaps too its stigma, that caused Kyffin not to marry, despite many loves and also engagements, and being denied a wife and family always pained him'.[140] For Williams, epilepsy opened a door to artistic achievement and acclaim, but in my opinion it is likely that at the same time it closed many other doors in his personal life and his relationships with others. We can only speculate as to whether he considered his condition a price worth paying for his creativity.

The Mexican artist **Frida Kahlo** (1907–1954) is one of the most well-known twentieth-century painters. Her own long-term health was poor after she developed poliomyelitis at the age of six, and was involved in a trolley car accident in her teens. She had intended to become a doctor, but after the accident had to abandon this dream. As a consequence of the accident she suffered from chronic pain throughout her life, and she underwent spinal surgery that was unsuccessful, had 28 different corsets made for her, and ultimately had to undergo amputation of one leg. She became addicted to morphine and alcohol, and was chronically depressed. Her father had epilepsy throughout his life, and due to fear of passing on the genetic trait herself, and also because of her pelvic injuries, she was fearful of having children. The following inscription on her painting *Portrait of my Father* (1951) highlights the family history: 'I painted my father Wilhelm Kahlo, of Hungarian-German origin, artist-photographer by profession, in character generous, intelligent and fine, valiant because he suffered for sixty years with epilepsy, but never gave up working and fought against Hitler. With adoration, his daughter Frida Kahlo.' She commented that as a child she would often be present and help to provide first aid when her father was having one of his fits. Perhaps it was this that provided the incentive for her to study medicine before the trolley car accident intervened, and also to collect sculptures of the Aztec goddess of epilepsy, Tlazolteotl.

Contemporary depictions of epilepsy have become increasingly realistic or graphic, and the works of artists with the condition are becoming more widely known to the art world. Rather than epilepsy necessarily being the subject of paintings, there is a now a recognized group of painters with epilepsy who are using their creative skills either to depict their own

---

139 www.bigskyfineart.com/a-welsh-pony-refusing-to-be-led-166
140 Evans R (2006) Sir Kyffin Williams. *The Guardian*, 4 September 2006.

personal experiences of seizures, or to express their artistic ability despite their condition. **Eduardo Urbano Merino**, the painter and sculptor, was born in Mexico City in 1975. His work is best described as figurative and anatomically precise. One of his most well-known paintings entitled *Epilepsy, Leaving Behind the Nightmare*, is on permanent display in the main lobby of the Royal University Hospital in Saskatoon, Canada. It was exhibited during the 30th International Epilepsy Congress in Montreal in 2013, and has been widely used as an illustration in books and journal articles about epilepsy. On the left-hand side of the painting are dark storm clouds and the darker images of neurons or brain cells within them. In the centre is the person with epilepsy, who appears through four superimposed images to be emerging from a seizure into the hands of two doctors, one of whom touches his shoulder as though welcoming him back, while the other appears to be perusing a page of data. The image is one of recovery and hope. Merino's other epilepsy painting, entitled *Tlazolteotl Healing a Child of Epilepsy*, is also on display in Saskatchewan. Here a child in modern casual clothing is having a seizure and being held by his mother while being ministered to by the goddess Tlazolteotl, the Aztec goddess of epilepsy from the artist's native Mexico. The goddess is holding a maize cob, as a symbol of life, in one hand, and a rattle, as if to waken the child from the seizure, in the other. Both paintings tell a positive story and serve to convey the transient nature of epilepsy to a wider public.

'From the Storm', a collection of artworks by 27 artists with temporal lobe epilepsy, opened in Boston in 1992 and toured throughout America and Canada, where it was exhibited at neurology and epilepsy conferences. This sparked a growing interest in the artistic abilities of people with epilepsy. Steven Schachter, a Harvard neurologist, has edited a book entitled *Visions: Artists Living with Epilepsy*[141] as testament to the creative skills of those with epilepsy. It contains an astonishing collection of illustrations depicting what individual artists visualize before, during, and after their seizures, as well as examples of their non-epilepsy-related work. A total of 34 artists have contributed illustrations to the publication, each with their own personal statement. Most of the contributors have epilepsy; others work with patients who have the condition, or have family experiences of it.

In his introduction to the book, Schachter touches upon stigma and misunderstanding, and states that 'what is needed is an emphasis on the abilities and individuality of people with epilepsy'. Among the many outstanding examples of visual art is **Jennifer Hall's** computer graphic entitled *Transcending* (see Figure 17). This series of striking images documents performances from the 'Out of Body Theatre' (1986–1990), a multi-media collage of light projection, robotic marionettes, and live actors. Schachter[142] quotes Hall as saying that 'during

---

141 Schachter SC (ed.) (2003) *Visions: Artists Living with Epilepsy*. Academic Press, Cambridge, MA.
142 Schachter SC (2016) Epilepsy and art: windows into complexity and comorbidities. *Epilepsy & Behavior* 57, 265–269.

these electrical firings, my visions flourish, and I hallucinate indescribable visions. I have felt virtual slivers slicing my throat when I draw the air to describe them. I'm sucked down into the explosion, fumble through the chaos and land disembodied from the intensity'.

Hall describes her work as being drawn from a combination of her temporal lobe and petit mal seizures.[143] She adds that she is interested in how a single event such as a seizure becomes something larger, 'creating a world of other events that emerge when life does not go as expected'. She articulates the difference between the two types of seizure that she experiences, with the temporal lobe attacks manifesting many perceptual feelings whereas the petit mal is solely a loss of awareness, or absence. Hall has experienced epilepsy throughout most of her life, and does not regard it as an illness but as day-to-day experiences that are a part of her functioning life. In her own words: 'rather than thinking of seizures as "altered states", I see them as part of a multiple understanding of myself. This distinction is important for me because it allows for trauma to exist within an operational life, rather than separating and isolating certain events from what we imagine to be ourselves. Seizures are part of the whole of me, that embraces the beauty of a life lived acknowledging that not all the parts are optimized for idealized functionality. This I believe is a critical understanding of the humanist project – imperfection, and even pain, are essential to our lives. I have come to realize that I occupy life imperfectly.' Hall's philosophy allows her to derive something creative from her epilepsy by producing insightful imagery and language that convey what it is like to experience seizures.

One of the contributors to *Visions: Artists Living with Epilepsy*, **Jim Chambliss**, has gone on to develop the 'Creative Sparks' website,[144] which is designed to serve as a positive reminder of the artistic talent of those with epilepsy, to bring about a greater understanding of living with the condition, and to provide insights into what it is like to experience a seizure. 'Creative Sparks' also invites adult artists with epilepsy to submit their artworks for future exhibitions, both online and in galleries.

Conclusion

Pictorial art is a powerful medium for influencing change as well as for chronicling the views and events of the time. Until comparatively recent times it was often the commonest method of communicating a narrative. For example, the role of paintings in promoting religious perceptions and stories is evident to anyone who visits a cathedral, mosque, or synagogue. What can we learn from paintings about the shifting sands of public opinion and knowledge

---

143 Hall J. Personal communication, 2018.
144 www.artandepilepsy.com

of epilepsy? Before the modern and contemporary eras, the person with epilepsy was viewed as unclean, and the saint or god was regarded as the purifier. This is consistent with our knowledge of how people with epilepsy were perceived in the Ancient and Renaissance periods. Christ, St Valentine, and the Aztec goddess Tlazolteotl are all examples of those who had the power to cleanse, and the votive tablets reveal how grateful the recipients of their miracles were. There is no empathy with or understanding of the epileptic – the only message that is conveyed is that they are in the wrong. But do Raphael's *Transfiguration* or Rubens' *The Miracles of St Ignatius of Loyola* truly represent epilepsy? And are paintings of 'the stone of insanity' in fact paintings of early attempts to perform epilepsy surgery? Unless the title of the painting actually includes the words 'epilepsy' or 'epileptic', any conclusions about what is being depicted are bound to be speculative and based on personal interpretation. But is that not one of the greatest appeals of pictorial art? The artist is no longer around to be asked what they intended, and even if their intentions were known, they would not necessarily be the same as what the observer sees in their work. Interpretation also depends upon the experiences and professional background of the observer, as evidenced by specialist journal articles in which the same painting is described by a psychiatrist as showing the classic textbook features of hysteria, and by a neurologist as being indisputably a seizure.

In modern and contemporary art there is no ambiguity. The title of the painting tells us what it depicts, and often the artist is around to tell us what it is conveying. The use of symbolism to describe the narrative has become redundant. Paintings are now more empathetic, consistent with the shedding of much of the mystique and stigma of epilepsy. Now artists with epilepsy are expressing their creativity and using it to convey what it is like to go through the various stages of a fit. Pictorial art has moved from marginalizing epilepsy to informing and educating about the condition in a positive manner. However, such art is not yet reaching a wider audience, and its impact on improving the public's understanding of people with epilepsy is still marginal.

With regard to artists of the past who had epilepsy themselves, we see in the lives of Van Gogh and John 'Kiffin' Williams the same recurring themes of social withdrawal, depression, and loneliness that were also experienced by writers such as Lear and Flaubert. Also apparent are the feelings of shame and stigma, and fear of embarking on marriage and parenthood, as articulated by Kahlo. In addition, we get a glimpse of the 'epileptic personality' in their behaviours. With regard to contemporary artists who have epilepsy, we know of their work through the efforts of Steven Schachter and others, but we know little about their struggles and inner conflicts, as most of those with epilepsy still feel compelled to be reticent about declaring their condition, let alone discussing it in public. This is a recurring theme, and one to which we shall return later in this book.

CHAPTER 6
Epilepsy on the moving screen

Whereas pictorial art does not nowadays reach a particularly wide public – art galleries being mainly visited by art historians, potential purchasers, parties of schoolchildren, and the elderly – the moving picture has considerable influence as a medium for social and public health education. However, it has also depicted people with epilepsy more graphically and in some respects judgementally. In this chapter we shall consider the portrayal of epilepsy in cinema films and on television. My first introduction to epilepsy was as a 10-year-old in a cinema – not in relation to the film I was watching, but to a man in the audience who without warning suddenly started to have convulsions. I can still vividly picture his fellow moviegoers moving to sit further away from him, and the sense of isolation that then surrounded him.

Cinema films

Motion pictures were made possible by the invention of the moving-picture camera by the French brothers Auguste and Louis Lumière. They called this new device the cinématographe (derived from the Greek words *kinema*, meaning 'movement', and *grapheca*, meaning 'drawing'). In 1895 the Lumière brothers became the first to demonstrate to a paying audience photographic moving pictures that were projected on to a screen. Their first film was entitled *Workers Leaving The Lumière Factory In Lyon*, and lasted for 50 seconds. The French theatre director and former stage magician Georges Méliès (1861–1938) became one of the early film directors, and his film *A Trip to the Moon* was the first internationally successful motion picture. In 1888 the American inventor and businessman Thomas Edison (1847–1931), together with his young laboratory assistant, William Dickson, made further modifications to the motion-picture camera, and the following year Edison's fellow countryman George Eastman began to manufacture celluloid film rolls. The stage was set for the explosion of creativity that accompanied the development of the motion-picture industry.

In films, an accurate and compassionate presentation of epilepsy to the public is critically important, as for the majority of viewers this will be the only time they see a seizure or possibly ever encounter a person with epilepsy. This is a heavy responsibility for the movie industry, and we shall now consider the extent to which it has succeeded in achieving this objective. Rather than discussing the different film genres, the types of seizure depicted, or the relationship between epilepsy and the plot, we shall examine in chronological order some selected movies to ascertain how attitudes may have changed with the passage of time.

Surprisingly, seizures were first portrayed on celluloid as long ago as 1901, in the French silent film *Le Déshabillage Impossible,* directed by Georges Méliès. This two-minute film was released in the USA as *Going to Bed under Difficulties* and in the UK as *An Increasing Wardrobe*. It uses the editing technique known as 'substitution splicing' to allow items of clothing to suddenly appear or disappear, giving the impression that they have been put on or removed by the wearer. The simple plot, which is merely a vehicle for clever cinematography, involves an individual's chaotic preparations to go to bed. A bearded man, Méliès himself, walks on to a hotel bedroom set, fully clothed and also wearing a hat and coat. He begins to undress so that he can go to bed, and he puts his hat and coat on a peg. However, they refuse to remain on the peg, and instead keep reappearing on him as if by magic. It seems impossible for him to remove his clothes without immediately finding that he is wearing new ones. The piles of discarded garments grow as the man tries ever more frantically to undress. Eventually, exhausted and agitated, he jumps on to the bed while still wearing a random assortment of garments. The end of the film has not survived, but contemporary promotional material describes its conclusion with the bearded man rolling on the floor and convulsing in an epileptic fit. This seems a surprising element for a comedy film, especially one produced primarily for a young audience. I would speculatively suggest that the entire episode could be viewed as a seizure. The confused imagery depicting an unsuccessful attempt to undress could be a pre-seizure automatism, which culminates in the fit itself. Alternatively, the frantic stress of undressing might have induced the seizure, or perhaps the seizure is used solely for dramatic effect and to provide a neat ending to the short story. We shall never know the director's intention, but even though the most important part of the film – its ending – is missing, this is undoubtedly the first attempt to depict an epileptic fit in a motion picture.

The depiction of epilepsy in films has been the subject of two major reviews – the first by Jennie, Toba, and Lawrence Kerson,[145] a family team of American social work and neurology researchers, and the second by the British psychologist Sallie Baxendale.[146] These reviews provide a useful analysis of the period from the very first motion pictures until the late 1990s and the early twenty-first century, respectively. The Kersons confined their review to English-language films, whereas Baxendale has also included non-English-language films from Europe, and has identified over a 70-year period of cinema more than 60 movies of all genres in which seizures or seizure-like events occur. Neither of the reviews explored Asian, South American, or African films in any depth. Recently, however, Sallie Baxendale has updated her survey of epilepsy at the movies by covering the years 2000 to 2014.[147] We shall use these three excellent studies as our 'rough guide' to the depiction of epilepsy in film, but will also look for omissions and investigate the more recent additions to the cannon by referring to the International Movie Database (www.IMDb.com). This search tool allows us to identify both films and television programmes that include epilepsy or seizures as part of the storyline. Many films are based on successful books, as described in Chapter 4, and I shall not repeat those examples here unless the film provides an additional contribution with regard to epilepsy, or portrays it in a different way to the book. The aim of this personal review is to ascertain whether, over time, the movie industry has portrayed epilepsy in a more enlightened way, or whether it has continued to use outmoded and stigmatizing stereotypes as a tool for dramatic effect.

Let us start with *To What Red Hell* (1929), an early British 'talkie' that was directed by Edwin Greenwood and based on a play by Percy Robinson. Originally a silent film, to which sound was added later, it stars the actress Dame Sybil Thorndike, who plays the mother of Harold Fairfield, an alcoholic. Harold has had an epileptic seizure, during which he has strangled a prostitute. With the help of his aristocratic mother he conceals the crime. Jim Nolan, the victim's boyfriend, is wrongly arrested, convicted, and sentenced to be hanged. A scene depicting Jim in the death cell with a priest is missing from the surviving film. Only at the last minute does Harold, the real killer, come forward to confess to the crime and then seek redemption through suicide, and Jim narrowly escapes the death penalty. The storyline highlights all of the old prejudices with regard to violence, alcoholism, criminality, and epilepsy. Harold is clearly bad news. A review by the *New York Times* in 1929 raised the question of whether a drunken epileptic had a moral right to have a part in the plot of any film.[148]

---

145 Kerson JF, Kerson TS and Kerson LA (1999) The depiction of seizures in film. *Epilepsia* 40, 1163–1167.
146 Baxendale S (2003) Epilepsy at the movies: possession to presidential assassination. *The Lancet: Neurology* 2, 764–770.
147 Baxendale S (2016) Epilepsy on the silver screen in the 21st century. *Epilepsy & Behavior* 57, 270–274.
148 Marshall E (1929) London Film Notes; *To What Red Hell. New York Times*, 6 October, 1929.

Walt Disney's animated film *Snow White and the Seven Dwarfs* (1937), which was released by RKO Radio Pictures, is based on one of the fairy tales by the German brothers Jakob and Wilhelm Grimm (the 'Brothers Grimm'), and was the first full-length animated feature film. Of the seven mining dwarfs – Doc, Grumpy, Happy, Sleepy, Bashful, Sneezy, and Dopey – it is Dopey who has attracted the interest of epilepsy specialists. Bernard Dan and Florence Christiaens[149] make the case for Dopey having a condition called Angelman's syndrome, of which seizures are a component. These authors draw attention to Dopey's lack of speech, although he has a good understanding of speech and is able to communicate through gestures and mime. They also point out his unsteady hopping gait and the tendency for his limbs to jerk. Finally, in the film he appears to have a generalized seizure while asleep. It is striking that these are the features of a syndrome that was not formally described until nearly 30 years later, by Harry Angelman in 1965. However, the inspiration for Dopey must have come from somewhere, and was perhaps modelled on a real-life individual with an as-yet-undescribed medical condition. Certainly it is possible that this is the first depiction of a fit in an animated film. There is no corresponding character in the original story by the Brothers Grimm, so we can only assume that the inspiration for Dopey came from the imagination or personal knowledge of one of the eight original film-script writers. Dopey's name is pejorative, but he has a loveable nature and is the favourite dwarf of child audiences. With regard to the portrayal of a seizure, it is unlikely that this film had any significant positive or negative impact on the perception of epilepsy.

The British film *A Matter of Life and Death* (released in the USA as *Stairway to Heaven*) was directed by Michael Powell and Emeric Pressburger and released in 1946. Although the word 'epilepsy' is never used, in some respects this is a positive presentation of the condition, with a surprisingly accurate depiction of seizures that indicates some inside knowledge. Michael Powell, who also co-wrote the script, had a brother-in-law who was a doctor and who might have provided the medical details. The part of the film's dashing hero, Peter Carter, a Second World War bomber pilot, is played by David Niven. Peter is shot down, parachutes to safety, lands in the sea, and is washed up on a beach and found by June, an American radio operator, with whom he falls in love. It becomes apparent that he is only on Earth because of a mistake made by a messenger who should have guided him to the afterlife. Peter resolutely refuses to allow this mistake to be corrected, as he does not want to enter the afterlife; the term 'heaven' is never used. He now develops seizures, which take the form of an unusual smell resembling fried onions, followed by loss of awareness. These symptoms are typical of temporal lobe epilepsy arising in the smell centre or insular cortex of the brain. He also develops worsening headaches, and is seen by Frank Reeves, a local doctor, who

---

149 Dan B and Christiaens F (1999) Dopey's seizure. *Seizure* 8, 238–240.

diagnoses a brain tumour. Peter has to appeal his call to the hereafter at a tribunal, but can only be represented by someone who has died. By chance Dr Reeves is killed in a motorcycle accident, and so can now represent Peter. He states to the tribunal that the mistake that led to Peter remaining on Earth also led to him meeting June and finding a happiness that they both share. The tribunal adjudicates that Peter can stay with June on Earth, and the couple are left to spend the rest of their lives together. This film is basically a fantasy that leaves many unanswered questions. Was the epilepsy caused by the plane crash? If so, it was very sudden, and appeared to occur in the absence of any obvious head injury. Was it due to a brain tumour? If so, how was Peter able to recover and live happily ever after with June? Finally, how much of what Peter imagined to have happened was a consequence of the epilepsy itself? The film almost certainly does depict epilepsy, and there is support for this view,[150] although the cause of the condition is unclear.

The actor and later US President Ronald Reagan (1911–2004) played main characters with epilepsy in two films. *Night Unto Night* (1949), directed by Don Siegel, tells the story of John Gaylord, a former biochemist who has been newly diagnosed with 'the incurable illness epilepsy'. Concealing the fact that he has this condition, he rents a house on the remote Florida coast from the owner Ann, a war widow. In the night Ann hears noises and voices, possibly resulting from John's epilepsy, that she believes are messages from her late husband. After John has developed a romantic attachment to her, he consults a doctor who tells him that his condition will steadily worsen. The ensuing guilt and lack of hope of any cure lead him to contemplate suicide. This film's portrayal of epilepsy is entirely negative, dominated by the hopelessness of John's situation and the imminent failure of his relationship with Ann. The screenwriter, Kathryn Scola, well known for her controversial scripts, worked on more than 30 films during the 1930s and 1940s, but has no known family links to epilepsy, and the condition only features in this one film.

The Winning Team (1952) is a biographical film directed by Lewis Seller and set in the early twentieth century. Ronald Reagan plays the part of a baseball player, Grover Alexander, who has retired from the game due to ill health and alcoholism, but then has the opportunity to make a glorious comeback. At the end of the 1909 season, 'Alex the Great' is struck by a baseball and wakes up in hospital three days later. He seems to have made a good recovery, until he starts drinking. He then goes off to France to fight in the Great War. After being exposed to shellfire he develops seizures. It is uncertain whether these have arisen from the earlier head injury, alcohol misuse, shellfire, or a combination of all three factors, although the latter seems most likely. He has a further seizure during a game and is told by a doctor that he needs to adopt a quieter lifestyle and that he should return to farm work. He

---

150 Friedman DB (1992) A matter of fried onions. *Seizure* 1, 307–310.

resumes drinking, and a downhill spiral ensues. He joins a circus as an idiot savant answering questions on baseball. His year of redemption comes in 1926, when he joins the St Louis Cardinals, plays in the World Series, and wins the game.

The real Grover Cleveland Alexander (1887–1950) was in his time an icon of the baseball game, and married and divorced the same woman twice. His ill health due to epilepsy and alcoholism was well known, as was the fact that he was a phenomenal pitcher whose many records still stand today.[151] Ronald Reagan had some issues with the film script, and at the insistence of Warner Bros the word 'epilepsy' never appears in it. It would seem that Warner Bros. Entertainment Inc. did not want a baseball legend to be associated with seizures, despite the fact that it was common knowledge that he had epilepsy. During the film, which also featured Doris Day as Grover's wife, there are no depictions of an actual fit.

There are two versions of the film *Cleopatra*. There is no mention of epilepsy in the earlier version, made in 1934, whereas in the later version, made in 1963 and directed by Joseph Mankiewicz, Caesar's epilepsy has become central to the plot. This version, which is just over three hours long, tells the story of Queen Cleopatra of Egypt and her dealings with the all-powerful imperial Rome. Mankiewicz's script is based on Shakespeare's play, and the epilepsy theme is probably derived from that work. The film, equally famous for its romantically linked stars Elizabeth Taylor and Richard Burton, is in two parts. The first part tells the story of Cleopatra and Caesar, up to Caesar's death, and the second part tells the story of Cleopatra and Anthony. It is at the very beginning of the film that Caesar's epilepsy is depicted. Cleopatra is initially spirited to Caesar by Ptolemy, her brother (and co-regent of Egypt), wrapped like a gift in a rug that unfurls before him. Soon after this, while she is secretly spying on him, Cleopatra witnesses Caesar having a fit, and she helps him to recover from it. Caesar then tells her that 'one day it will happen where I cannot hide, where the world shall see me fall. I shall tumble down before the mob. I shall foam at the mouth and they will tear me to pieces.' In another scene he shakes violently while holding her in his arms. Caesar's epilepsy is mentioned by those plotting against him, when he requests to be made an emperor, as an exploitable vulnerability. A 1963 *Hollywood Reporter* review of the film[152] highlighted the depiction of epilepsy, stating that 'Rex Harrison's Caesar is crisp, humorous, authoritative. Caesar's epilepsy is shown, and this is an illness difficult to portray and maintain the image of the sardonic conqueror.' The film depicts Caesar as a genius who, despite being flawed by his epilepsy, is successful and feared. Clearly the condition has not held him back, although we can assume that he has tried to conceal it.

---

151 Kavanagh J (2001) *Ol' Pete: The Grover Cleveland Alexander Story*. Diamond Communications, South Bend, IN.
152 www.hollywoodreporter.com/news/cleopatra-1963-movie-review-754694

Mel Brooks' comedy *The Twelve Chairs* (1970) was the first film to illustrate the use of a feigned seizure for the purposes of criminal gain. The use of such a 'scam' has been repeated in several subsequent movies, most notably *Drugstore Cowboy* (1989), an American film directed by Gus Van Sant. Based in Russia during the Revolution in the 1920s, the plot of *The Twelve Chairs* centres around a collection of extremely valuable family jewels that has been concealed in the seat cushion of one of twelve dining chairs in order to prevent it being found by the Bolsheviks. An impoverished aristocratic relative who returns to the family home after the death of the owner finds that the chairs have been expropriated by the communist government and then sold individually, so he sets about the laborious task of locating them one by one. When he and his partner in the search, who is a manipulative con artist, find that none of the twelve chairs contain the jewels, the aristocrat collapses to the ground, feigning an epileptic seizure. This well-rehearsed ploy enables the con artist to implore passers-by to give generously to the apparently stricken man, with the words 'epilepsy my friends, epilepsy, the same disease that struck down our beloved Dostoevsky'.

Seizures that have been deliberately feigned in order to manipulate others or deliberately avoid awkward situations have certainly been portrayed in films, but seizures caused by non-epileptic attack disorder (NEAD) (see page 8) can have a different shade of meaning altogether. Attacks that appear to be epileptic but are more likely to have a psychological basis are depicted in several films, the best-known examples being *The Witches of Salem* (1972), directed by Dennis Azzarella, and *The Crucible* (1996), directed by Nicholas Hytner. The screenplay of *The Crucible* was adapted by the American writer Arthur Miller from his play of the same name. Both films are based on historical events relating to the witch-hunting trials in 1692. Several young girls experience seizures, hallucinations, loss of speech, and pain that are regarded by the local community as evidence that they have become bewitched by the devil. There is clearly a morbid public appetite for the story, given that so many different versions of the tale have been created over the years.

The American science fiction film *The Andromeda Strain* (1971), directed by Robert Wise, includes a central character, Dr Ruth Leavitt, who is attempting to conceal her epilepsy. After a space satellite has returned to Earth, nearly all the residents of a nearby town in New Mexico are found dead as a result of becoming infected by what is assumed to be an alien biological life form. A team of scientists, including Dr Leavitt, who is the only woman member, investigate the deaths. A seal in their top-secret laboratory breaks, setting off an alarm and releasing the strain. Leavitt freezes at the site of the flashing red alarm light and falls to the ground, having a seizure and foaming at the mouth. Help is sought and it is believed that she has become infected by the Andromeda strain, until she explains to those who are assisting her that it is only her epilepsy. The team physician, Dr Hall, states that 'Leavitt had a seizure. Epilepsy. A red light flashing at 3 per second brought on a fit.' When he is asked by a colleague why Leavitt had never mentioned her health problem, the physician replies that 'Probably no top lab would have had her if they knew. Insurance, prejudice and all that crap from the Middle Ages.' This is a most insightful portrayal of epilepsy. We can assume that Leavitt has photosensitive epilepsy, as Dr Hall alludes to the critical light trigger of 3 flashes per second. As Leavitt is the only woman in the team, it can be assumed that she was compelled not only to overcome gender prejudice, but also to avoid mentioning the other issue, namely her epilepsy, which would have further impeded her career. Given her laboratory workplace, the observations about insurance are very accurate. This film highlights the dilemma that is frequently faced by people with epilepsy. If Leavitt had declared her condition she would never have been employed in the first place, and therefore she has to run the risk both of being found out, and of being uninsured if she becomes involved in an accident. She would also be culpable if, as a result of a seizure, she injured or endangered a colleague. Finally, the physician's strong words about prejudice and reference to the Middle Ages indicate his empathy with Leavitt's circumstances. We do not learn Leavitt's fate. The question of whether she keeps her job or loses it remains unanswered. Amazingly, this understanding portrayal of epilepsy in *The Andromeda Strain* is adapted from the book of the same name by Michael Crichton, who in his novel *The Terminal Man* did so much to perpetuate the stereotype that people with epilepsy are violent (see Chapter 4). It should be noted that it was not Crichton but Nelson Gidding who wrote the film's screenplay.

In 1973, Martin Scorsese directed and co-wrote the film *Mean Streets*, which starred Robert De Niro and Harvey Keitel, who at that time were unknown but would go on to become household names. Based in the 'Little Italy' neighbourhood of Manhattan, the story follows Charlie (Harvey Keitel), a young Italian-American man, as he tries to juggle his conscience and Catholicism with his life and activities among the gangs of New York. He works as a money collector for his uncle, a gangster called Giovanni, and spends much time saying Hail Marys to seek absolution from his sins. He has empathy for those in debt, including his best friend Johnny Boy (Robert De Niro), and tries not to be too hard on them when collecting their dues. Johnny Boy is unaware of the hazards of owing money to Michael, a gangster loan shark, and instead lives for the moment, spending money that he does not have, regardless of the consequences. Charlie tries to keep Michael off Johnny Boy's back, and to make Johnny Boy more responsible as well as protect him. Charlie has an affair with Teresa, Johnny Boy's cousin. Because Teresa has epilepsy, no one – including Johnny Boy – approves of this relationship, which is seen as an obstacle to Charlie's advancement in the criminal world. Teresa loves Charlie but knows that because of her seizures and the disapproval of Giovanni, his uncle, she is viewed as a burden and will eventually lose him. She is intelligent and beautiful, but because of her condition she is also friendless and socially excluded. On one occasion when she is trying to separate the arguing Charlie and Johnny Boy she starts to have a seizure, and her mother rushes to her aid. Giovanni believes Teresa to be 'sick in the head', regards her as tarnished goods, and insists that his nephew Charlie must end the relationship. His attitude to epilepsy is harsh and uncaring, as demonstrated by the following extract from the filmscript:

Giovanni: This Johnny Boy is like your mister Groppi … a little crazy. It's nice you should help him out because of his family and our family but watch yourself. … Don't spoil anything. His whole family has problems … his cousin, the girl who lives next door to you …
Charlie: Teresa.
Giovanni: The one who's sick, right? In the head.
Charlie: No, she's got epilepsy.
Giovanni: Yeah. That's what I said, sick in the head.

Teresa makes it to the door and opens it quickly. Johnny Boy grabs her to keep her from leaving. Charlie rushes towards them and pulls Johnny Boy away. By now, they are halfway down the hall.

Johnny Boy: (*shouting*) Charlie … I always wondered about her … What happens when she comes? Does she get one of those fits? Eh? That would be something to see.

Johnny Boy is interrupted by Charlie's fist as it lands a solid punch on the right side of his head. Teresa screams and rushes to separate them.[153]

As pressures mount, Charlie has to make a decision, and does not like any of the options. He tries desperately but unsuccessfully to reconcile the disparate parts of his life, and there is no hope of a good outcome. This film shows no sympathy for Teresa and her epilepsy. It is an unflinching portrayal of the harsh, unforgiving, male-dominated environment that the characters inhabit. It depicts Teresa's epilepsy as a personality flaw, and promotes the message that it is unwise to take on such an unnecessary burden by becoming involved with a person who has the condition. The fact that Teresa and Charlie love one another is

---

153 From the script by Martin Scorsese, Mardik Martin, and Ethan Edwards.

regarded as irrelevant. This is a world where only the fittest survive, and choices have to be made in that context. Scorsese and his colleagues need make no apology for the script, as it reflects accurately the place and time in which it is set. In fact, the shocking nature of the attitudes that are depicted might well have a positive effect in causing viewers to question the acceptability of such views.

The Canadian film *The Apprenticeship of Duddy Kravitz* (1974) is based on the book of the same name (see Chapter 4) by Mordecai Richler, who also wrote the screenplay. Two television adaptations have also been created, one in the 1960s and one in 2005. With the author as screenwriter, the film follows the book very closely. Duddy Kravitz, the footloose son of a Jewish Montreal taxi driver and part-time pimp, is always struggling under the expectations raised by the success of his older brother, a medical student. He works in a hotel and falls in love with Yvette, a French-Canadian, Catholic fellow employee. Duddy embarks on various unsuccessful financial ventures and through these meets the kindly Virgil, a pinball-machine salesman and poet who has epilepsy. Unwisely and illegally, Duddy employs him as a driver, and Virgil subsequently has a seizure while driving, resulting in an accident that leaves him paraplegic. Duddy is racked with guilt and Yvette, who blames him for what has happened, leaves Duddy in order to care for Virgil. Virgil has an idealistic dream of uniting all the people in the world who have epilepsy through an organization that would be akin to the National Association for the Advancement of Coloured People.

This film conveys three messages about epilepsy. First, a person with epilepsy – in this case Virgil – can be good, kind, and gentle. Second, driving with active epilepsy is hazardous and illegal, but is a risk that is sometimes taken in order to gain employment. Virgil understands his limited employment prospects when he says to Duddy 'I can't help it; that's the way I was born. Life is no bowl of cherries for a guy like me. Would you take a chance on me as a waiter or driver?' Finally, there is Virgil's positive vision that people with epilepsy could form an international organization to campaign for their rights along the lines of existing organizations that strive for racial equality.

The American film *One Flew over the Cuckoo's Nest* (1975), directed by Miloš Forman, was adapted from Ken Kesey's book of the same title (discussed in Chapter 4). Kesey was not one of the screenwriters, and the film is not completely true to the original. Set in the early 1960s, it tells the story of an Oregon criminal, Randle McMurphy (played by Jack Nicholson), who, while serving a prison sentence for statutory rape of a teenager, decides to fake insanity in order to be transferred to what he perceives to be the relative long-term comfort of a psychiatric hospital. It all ends badly, with McMurphy being subjected to lobotomy, and shortly afterwards being suffocated by a friend as an act of mercy. The inmates with epilepsy, Jim Sefelt and Bruce Fredrickson, are accurately transferred from book to film.

Let us now consider a film in which a seizure appears only briefly but has considerable impact. *1900* (1976), directed by Bernardo Bertolucci, is an epic account of class struggle and the rise of the Fascist Party in Italy in the first half of the twentieth century, as seen through the eyes of two friends. Alfredo (played by Robert De Niro), who is the son of a landowner, and Olmo (played by Gerard Depardieu), a peasant, are both born on the same day in 1900. Like many of Bertolucci's other movies (e.g. *Last Tango in Paris*) this film was controversial, and the censors made drastic cuts to many of the scenes from the original version. One such scene, which has been retained in some versions, is the *ménage a trois* with Alfredo, Olmo, and Neve, who is described in the film's cast list as 'an epileptic woman', and plays no part in the storyline other than being included in a scene with the two men that is designed to shock the viewer and denote a strengthening of the bond between the two friends through their shared experience.

Alfredo and Olmo pick up Neve, a prostitute, and take her back to her house so that the three of them can share a bed. The scene results in Neve experiencing a full-blown convulsion, and she is immediately abandoned by the two men.

Alfredo: *[all three are lying naked in bed: Alfredo takes a glass of wine]* Drink some wine, eh?
Neve: *[pushes the glass away]* No, please, no.
Olmo: *[looks annoyed at Alfredo's persistence]* She doesn't want it.
Alfredo: *[forces the wine into her mouth]* Drink, you little whore.

[Neve swallows, but soon goes into a seizure]

Alfredo: What the—?
Olmo: *[realization appears on his face]* Oh no, she's an epileptic!

Neve's mother suddenly appears on the scene as the two men dress rapidly and flee. The cruel treatment of Neve in this scene culminates in her being discarded, her only function having been to enable the two men's rite of passage and promote their bonding, homoerotic or otherwise. Here epilepsy, prostitution, the forced consumption of alcohol, and a sense of worthlessness are combined in one brief, shocking moment. Bertolucci appears to view epilepsy merely as a condition that can be sensationalized in order to achieve dramatic effect.

Seizure: The Story of Kathy Morris (1980) is a CBS television movie that portrays a true story about epilepsy. Kathy Morris (played by Penelope Milford) was a promising 22-year-old New York singer who had trained at the Manhattan School of Music, during which time her seizures first started. She underwent surgery to treat them, but unexpected swelling of her brain led to the operation being abandoned, and she spent the next six weeks in a coma. She then underwent several further operations and prolonged rehabilitation. The film describes how she learned to read and write again, as well as her relationship with her brusque doctor (played by Leonard Nimoy). It is a dispassionate account of how she regained language skills, becoming multilingual once more, and even sang in public again and played a cameo role in this very film about her. Sadly, she died around seven years later at the age of 29. The plot focuses more on facing up to and overcoming the physical disability caused by the surgery than on the seizures and the challenges of living with epilepsy. The film is notable for its accuracy and compassionate depiction of the main character, and it demonstrates what can be achieved – when writers research their material thoroughly – in terms of educating the wider public about specific medical conditions.

Fight for Life (1987) is a television film, produced by the ABC network, which, like *Seizure*, aimed to present epilepsy in a positive light. The storyline resonates with more recent media reports of successful campaigning by parents for their children to have licensed access to cannabis in order to control a specific type of epilepsy. However, in this film, based on actual events, the drug in question is sodium valproate (Epilim), which at that time was licensed for use in the UK but not in the USA. An Ohio-based optician and his wife fly to England to pick up the drug for their 6-year-old daughter. The US Food and Drugs Administration (FDA), which is the body that approves drugs for usage, has yet to approve the licensing of the drug. Therefore, by bringing the drug back into the USA the parents are breaking the law and forcing the issues of licensing and availability. By engaging the media to help their campaign they are successful in getting the drug approved for all who need it. This film highlights the positive impact of 'people power' and of the willingness of the media and the public to campaign on behalf of children. Sadly this is a rarer outcome when campaigning for adults.

Both *Seizure* and *Fight for Life* demonstrate that films made for television can convey important public education messages which the big-screen movies are less likely to engage with, given cinema's overriding concern with box-office takings, ratings, awards, and the preference for subjects that will appeal to the widest possible audience. The television film industry is far less constrained by these factors, and can thus address health and social issues in such a way that conditions such as epilepsy can be depicted freely.

Let Him Have It (1991), a British film directed by Peter Medak, tells the true story of Derek Bentley, a 19-year-old boy with epilepsy and learning difficulties who falls in with a gang led by a younger teenager, 16-year-old Christopher Craig. Craig carries a Colt revolver, whereas Bentley has been given only a knuckleduster and a knife. During the course of a warehouse robbery both boys are cornered by the police. Bentley ambiguously shouts out 'Let him have it, Chris!', and in response Craig fires his gun, wounding one police officer and killing another. Both boys go on trial for murder. Craig, because of his young age, is sentenced to life behind bars, whereas Bentley is sentenced to death because of his involvement in the policeman's death. In January 1953, despite a public outcry and the family's pleas for mercy, he is executed within one month of being sentenced. The interpretation of his words, 'Let him have it, Chris!', which could just as easily have meant 'Hand over the gun' as 'Open fire', resulted in the loss of his life.

The film highlighted the most shocking aspect of the case, namely Bentley's background, and also depicted him receiving a royal pardon around 40 years later. Bentley had worked briefly as a garbage man before losing his job, becoming unemployed, and drifting into a life of petty crime. His seizures started at around the age of 15, and during one event he nearly choked to death. By the age of 16 his mental age was considered to be no more than 10, and at the time of his arrest his IQ was found to be 77. Around the time of the onset of his epilepsy he underwent an electroencephalogram (EEG), which was reported to be abnormal. He never underwent brain imaging, as computed tomography (CT) had not yet been developed. At his trial he appeared in front of the notorious Lord Chief Goddard. Goddard forwarded to the Home Secretary the jury's recommendation for clemency, but he damningly added that he himself 'could find no mitigating circumstances' for converting the death penalty to life imprisonment. The appeal failed, and on the day of Bentley's execution there were demonstrations outside Wandsworth Prison, where he was initially buried before being subsequently re-interred in the family grave. The speed of his execution suggests the level of public disquiet and the perceived need to administer the punishment and resolve the case as soon as possible.

The film shows the 'establishment' at work following the death of a policeman in the line of duty. The part of Bentley is played by Christopher Ecclestone, who brilliantly captures the inner torment and uncertainty of a young man who has endured a long history of epilepsy and academic failure. Bentley wants to make friends in order to avoid the isolation that his condition brings, but his fatal mistake is in choosing the wrong ones. Although the film does not depict seizures, it is sympathetic to epilepsy, portraying Bentley as a victim of the circumstances that the condition and his learning difficulties have thrust upon him.

The Australian film *Romper Stomper* (1992), written and directed by Geoffrey Wright, is based in Melbourne and tells the story of a gang of violent neo-Nazi skinheads who attack anyone who is not white, or indeed who differs in any way from what they view as 'normal'. After they have assaulted a group of Vietnamese teenagers, the tables are turned when a group of armed Vietnamese men force them to retreat. The neo-Nazi gang is joined by

Gabrielle, a white girl with epilepsy, after her affluent but abusive father has had her drug-addicted former boyfriend beaten up. Gabrielle soon embarks on a relationship with the leader of the skinhead gang. One reviewer, on noting how Gabrielle helps the gang to evade justice, has speculated that her epilepsy is a sign of her impurity. Early in the film, her father, Martin, questions her about her epilepsy treatment:

Martin:	Have you been taking the phenytoin?
Gabrielle:	Yeah.
Martin:	Where is it?
Gabrielle:	I don't know. I'm busy.
Martin:	You haven't, have you? Seizures been bad? No. You've got a bloody chemist's shop here. The one drug you really need you don't bother with.

In the final scene she is referred to as a 'mental bitch' as she has a seizure while lying beside a dead skinhead. The TV remake of *Romper Stomper* (2018) picks up the story 25 years later, by which time the lives of many of the gang have been transformed. Gabe (Gabrielle) in particular has turned her life around and is now a successful businesswoman whose epilepsy seems to have mysteriously disappeared. Whether this is because it has spontaneously remitted or because getting rid of it was viewed as the necessary removal of a perceived impurity is open to conjecture. Perhaps the scriptwriters decided that success and epilepsy do not play well together, or maybe they simply had not researched Gabrielle's past medical history thoroughly enough, so were unaware of her epilepsy.

The independent film *Simple Men* (1992), directed by Hal Hartley, was nominated for the Palme d'Or prize at the Cannes Film Festival. It tells the story of two brothers who are united in their hunt to find their father, an anarchist who once tried unsuccessfully to blow up the Pentagon, and who has been on the run for 25 years. The older brother has a criminal past and the younger one is a philosophy student. One of the supporting characters in the film is Elina, a Romanian girl with epilepsy, who is possibly the girlfriend of the missing father. In the concluding scenes of the film she has a major seizure, which is very accurately depicted. Elina, who has been displaced from her country of birth, is portrayed as exotic but mysterious, and as cold, unemotional, and remote. The portrayal of her epilepsy contributes to the sense that she is alienated and stands somewhat apart from the others. The fact that she is beautiful may have been used in the film to convey a more acceptable kind of vulnerability.

The Canadian film *Mesmer* (1994) tells the story of the eighteenth-century German physician **Franz Anton Mesmer** (1734–1815), who used unorthodox healing practices based on his theory of 'animal magnetism' and his encounter with a young blind concert pianist. Interestingly, those who responded to Mesmer's treatments were generally troubled, impressionable young women. In 1843 the Scottish physician James Braid used the term 'hypnosis' to describe Mesmer's techniques, which gives us a clearer contemporary understanding of what his treatments involved. However, the film strays away from the facts. The pianist Maria Theresa Paradies had been blind since the age of three, but had nevertheless gone on to memorize so many concertos and cantatas, as well as composing three cantatas herself, that by the age of 18 she had gained widespread acclaim. She was the daughter of a wealthy businessman, and it is believed that he raped her repeatedly when she was a child.

The film depicts her having a seizure while playing at a concert in Vienna. Mesmer rushes to her aid, calms her down, and subsequently appears to help her to cope with her epilepsy while at the same time, despite being married himself, becoming romantically involved with her. In reality his aim has been to cure her blindness and, following an accidental blow to the head, her vision does indeed seem to have been temporarily restored. However, it later worsens again, and their relationship leads to a scandal, resulting in Mesmer being banished from Vienna by the medical authorities, and thereafter establishing himself as a favourite at Court in Paris. The film appears to suggest that the seizure – whether it was a single occurrence or one of many – is the least of Maria Theresa's problems, and that her blindness, for which Mesmer pursues a cure – is her main health challenge. The introduction of the seizure in the context of childhood sexual abuse raises the question of whether the director had unwittingly portrayed one of the first examples of non-epileptic attack disorder to be depicted on the cinema screen. There are parallels here with the film *Simple Men*. Again, the addition of seizures to the storyline about a vulnerable, impressionable young woman accentuates her vulnerability and makes her easy prey for Mesmer's machinations.

Deceiver (1997) is an American psychological thriller directed by Jonas Pate in which a murder suspect appears to fake his own death from a seizure. James Wayland is not only the heir to his father's textile company, but as a fiercely intelligent Ivy League graduate of Princeton University he has the world at his feet. He is the prime suspect in a particularly gruesome murder case in which a prostitute's body had been found sawn in half. The two investigating police officers have problems of their own – one is having marital difficulties and the other has gambling debts. They are no match for Wayland's intelligence and ability to manipulate and exploit weakness in others, and also one of them seems to have been acquainted with the victim. Wayland, who is portrayed in the film as having temporal lobe epilepsy and being addicted to absinthe, is eventually given a lie detector test. At this point he requests to be allowed to take his drug treatment, carbamazepine, as stress can bring on his seizures. This is the first the police officers have heard about the epilepsy, and they suspect that the request for medication is a ruse to beat the lie detector. Wayland explains that if he has seizures he can behave in a violent and unpredictable manner. He then manages to turn the interview around, exposing one policeman's infidelity and the other's gambling debts, and even suggesting that the officer who knew the victim might himself be the killer. The police now seek the advice of a psychiatrist, who tells them that 'people with temporal lobe epilepsy make your skin crawl for a reason. If you think he is being seized, even if you suspect it, you treat him like a strange dog in an alley.' The interrogation continues, as do the mind games. Wayland confesses that he had a fight with his father, went to the prostitute's house, drank heavily with her, and then went out to get more beers. He claims that on returning to the house he witnessed someone rushing out. Rather than giving chase he went inside and found that the prostitute had been strangled. In desperation – fearing that he would be an obvious suspect – he sawed her body in half and left it in a nearby park. The film then switches abruptly to Wayland in the custody cell reaching for a bottle of black pills which are not the same as the epilepsy medication that had been shown earlier. After taking the pills he has a convulsion, dies, and his body is taken to a funeral home where his father is waiting. The final scene cuts back to the park, where Wayland is seen talking to another prostitute, and one is left to assume that he has faked his own death.

There are several important points about the portrayal of epilepsy in this film. First, Wayland's manipulative personality, violent tendencies, and abuse of absinthe are all portrayed as being linked to his temporal lobe epilepsy. Indeed, the film might be regarded as using his seizures as a way to enhance the image of him as a bad, spoiled rich kid. Second, epilepsy may be serving as the reason for the otherwise inexplicable dysfunction of a young man with the world at his feet. Third, even if Wayland did commit the murder, it is surprising that his epilepsy and associated memory lapses are not introduced as an explanation for him sawing the victim in half. Fourth, the psychiatrist's opinion of people with epilepsy is that they should be treated like 'a strange dog in an alley'. Could that have been a commonly held view at the time when the film was made, in the late 1990s? Finally, at the end of the film, if the seizure and death are genuine, this is sudden unexplained death in epilepsy (SUDEP). If they are not, the fit has been fabricated for gain, just like that in *The Twelve Chairs*. Overall, then, the portrayal of epilepsy in *Deceivers* does not advance our understanding of epilepsy, but instead reinforces the old negative stereotypes.

The Bone Collector (1999), a psychological thriller directed by Phillip Noyce, offers a much more positive depiction of epilepsy in its main character, Lincoln Rhyme, a former detective. The actor Denzel Washington gives credence to and a sympathetic portrayal of the character's disability. After an accident in a tunnel, Rhyme is left quadriplegic, able to move only his head and one finger. He also has seizures and, fearing that these might leave him in a vegetative state, he is considering assisted suicide when a case comes in that grabs his attention. Someone is abducting people in a taxi and then killing them and leaving them to die in very sadistic ways. The rate at which these crimes are being committed is increasing, and Rhyme is faced with a challenge that gives him new purpose. Unusually for a film portrayal of epilepsy, the seizures are seen from Rhyme's own perspective, graphically conveying his fear that they will lead to a vegetative state. Rhyme eventually solves the case, and his value, despite his disability, is reaffirmed, he finds redemption, and all thoughts of suicide vanish. Although this is by and large a positive portrayal of epilepsy, there are a couple of caveats. Rhyme's fits are depicted as having been caused by a demonstrable event, namely his accident in the tunnel, thus 'sanitizing' the condition. Also the viewer is more likely to feel empathy for Rhyme's quadriplegia than for his epilepsy in this story of overcoming adversity.

The Lost Prince (2003), a British television drama written and directed by Steven Poliakoff, is set in the early years of the twentieth century. It tells the true story of how King George V and Queen Mary hid their youngest child, Prince John, from the general public in order to conceal his epilepsy and their embarrassment about his condition. When, at an early age, he is diagnosed with epilepsy and autistic learning difficulties, the medical experts recommend that he should live at Sandringham, one of the royal country estates, well away from the public eye. Referred to as the 'Lost Prince' or Johnnie, he is looked after by his devoted nurse, 'Lala' Bill, at Wood Farm, a remote farmhouse on the estate. During this imposed isolation the major historic events of the early twentieth century – the First World War and the Russian Revolution – pass him by. The emotional coldness with which the royal family refused to provide a refuge for their fleeing Russian cousins parallels their disowning of Prince John. Only the Queen, through a sense of honour, visits him occasionally, and it is his nurse who is solely responsible for his upbringing and emotional development.

As John's cousins are deposed from one European throne after another, he leads a simple and reclusive life, with intermittent company and emotional support provided by his older brother, Prince George (who would eventually become King George VI). From 1916 onward there are no photographic records of him, although he did very occasionally attend royal functions. On 18 January 1919, after a severe seizure, John died in his sleep at Wood Farm. Towards the end of his life, as his condition worsened, his siblings stopped visiting him, apparently because it upset them to see his attacks becoming more severe, prolonged, and frequent.

There is no official biography of Prince John, and the scriptwriter, Steven Poliakoff, had to depend on very limited access to the Royal Archives. He depicts John's parents, the King and Queen, as being caring beneath their Germanic stiff upper lip, and he implies that John's life was more carefree than that of his brother, Edward, who was being prepared to succeed to the throne. The film reflects the era with regard to attitudes to epilepsy, and indeed some years after John's death the British Epilepsy Association stated that there was nothing unusual in the parents' decision to conceal their child from public scrutiny. They also commented that at that time it was quite usual for people with epilepsy to be separated from the rest of the community and to live in epilepsy colonies or mental institutions.

The Exorcism of Emily Rose (2005), an American supernatural horror film directed by Scott Derrickson, and *Requiem* (2006), a German film directed by Hans-Christian Schmid, are both based on a true story about a 17-year-old German girl, Anneliese Michel, and the treatment that was inflicted upon her in order to rid her of epilepsy and her mental health problems. At the age of 16, Anneliese had been diagnosed with temporal lobe epilepsy, depression, and psychosis. She had received treatment in various psychiatric hospitals, but without effect, and by the age of 20 she had become delusional and suicidal. After she had been given conventional medical treatment for 5 years without success, Anneliese and her parents became convinced that she was possessed by six demons, and appealed to the local Catholic bishop for an exorcism. Initially this was refused, but in 1975 two priests were given permission by the Catholic Church to perform the rite. The priests listed Adolf Hitler and Nero among the devils that had entered her and that urgently needed to be removed. One of the priests, on meeting Annaliese for the first time, commented that 'she didn't look like an epileptic' and doubted the diagnosis, despite the fact that the girl had been observed having seizures in the psychiatric hospital and the anti-epileptic drug phenytoin had been prescribed.

The exorcism took place behind the shutters of the family home in a small Bavarian town. Annaliese died nine months later, having endured over 60 rites of exorcism, and weighing just 68 pounds. Both of her legs were broken and she had pneumonia. Her parents and the two Roman Catholic priests were convicted of manslaughter and given a six-month prison sentence, which was later reduced to three years' probation and a fine. The trial attracted media interest worldwide, and led to widespread condemnation of the church's role in the tragedy. The Catholic Church subsequently issued a statement acknowledging that Annaliese was mentally ill and that demonic possession had never occurred.

The Exorcism of Emily Rose is a courtroom drama that is set in America. It follows the trial of a parish priest, Father Moore, who has been accused of negligent homicide after performing an exorcism on a young female college student. The defence lawyer, Erin Bruner, takes on the case in order to gain promotion within her firm, and the priest only agrees to let her defend him if he can tell Emily's full story. The prosecution claim that Emily suffered from both epilepsy and psychosis, whereas Bruner maintains that the young woman was possessed and could never have been cured by conventional medicine, and that Father Moore and the family regarded exorcism as her only hope. Flashbacks show us the onset of

Emily's illness in the college dormitory when she wakens in the early hours with a strange burning smell in her nostrils, followed by hallucinations and a feeling that her body is being compressed. She experiences several further episodes, is hospitalized with a diagnosis of epilepsy, and anti-epileptic drugs are prescribed for her. When she returns home her parents doubt the diagnosis, instead believing Emily to be possessed, and they contact the Church to ask for an exorcism to be performed.

So far a diagnosis of temporal lobe epilepsy has seemed quite probable, given the description of the attacks. However, there is now a twist in that Bruner, the defence lawyer, develops similar symptoms. A supernatural element enters the plot as Father Moore warns Bruner that she may have become the target of the same demons that had entered Emily. An anthropologist who has been called as a defence witness testifies about spiritual possession, and a medical doctor who was present at one of the exorcism sessions is also asked to give evidence. However, the doctor, who believes in demons, is killed in a hit-and-run accident before he can testify. Eventually, after flashbacks to apparitions, voices speaking in tongues, demonic possession, and Emily developing stigmata, Father Moore is found guilty, but he avoids a jail sentence on the recommendation of the jury. Bruner declines the promotion offered by her firm, and she and the released priest visit Emily's grave. Father Moore concludes by saying that, because of what she had to endure, he believes Emily will be declared a saint.

This film does a great disservice to people with epilepsy, as it reintroduces the myth of seizures and demons. Sympathy is shown for Emily not because she has epilepsy and mental health problems, but because these have been inflicted on her by the devil, and her fortitude may be rewarded by her achieving sainthood. The jury do not recommend that Father Moore should be sent to prison as they view him as honourably wrestling with the devil in order to rid Emily of her seizures and psychosis.

Requiem, the German version of this story, was released a year after *The Exorcism of Emily Rose*, and is presented in documentary style. It avoids the dramatic supernatural angle adopted by its predecessor, and tells the true story of Anneliese – in this version called Michaela – whose problems are caused by epilepsy, not by demons. Michaela resists the wishes of her domineering mother and leaves home to attend university. Ashamed of her epilepsy, she is depicted sharing a sorority house with other students, from whom she attempts to conceal the condition by stopping her drug treatment. Her seizures then worsen, and she starts to believe that she is possessed. Two priests become involved, one of whom suggests that Michaela should restart her medication and seek medical help, while the other, younger priest recommends exorcism. Unfortunately the latter recommendation prevails, with tragic consequences. The film sends a clear message that Michaela's situation is entirely the result of her epilepsy – in other words, she is a victim of her condition.

The Last King of Scotland (2006), directed by Kevin Macdonald, is a historical drama film based on the events that took place during the brutal regime of the Ugandan dictator Idi Amin, as seen through the eyes of his personal physician during the 1970s. The young doctor discovers that the youngest of Amin's three wives has been banished because she has given birth to an epileptic son. The prejudice against people with epilepsy that is depicted in the film is an accurate portrayal of attitudes that would have prevailed in East Africa at that time.

Control (2007), directed by Anton Corbijn, is a British biographical film about Ian Curtis, the enigmatic lead singer of the band Joy Division. Based on the book *Touching from a Distance*, written by Ian's widow, Deborah Curtis,[154] the film portrays the pressures of his epilepsy, his mental health problems, his failed marriage, and his decision to hang himself at the age of 23, on the eve of the band's tour to the USA. Ian's epilepsy is poorly controlled, his medication is ineffective, and he is spiralling out of control. In one scene he has a seizure while performing live on stage in front of his audience. Although this film depicts an individual failing to cope with many aspects of his life, including his epilepsy, with ultimately tragic consequences, its main message is a positive one – that a musically talented person with this condition has made a lasting impression on the music world. We shall discuss Ian Curtis in more detail in relation to music and epilepsy in Chapter 7.

My Sister's Keeper (2009) is an American film based on the bestselling book of the same title by Jodi Picoult,[155] and is directed by Nick Cassavetes. Anna has been conceived by in vitro fertilization (IVF) as a genetic match, so that she can become a bone marrow donor for her older sister Kate, who has leukaemia. Kate goes into renal failure at the age of 15, and the now 11-year-old Anna comes under intense pressure from her parents to donate her bone marrow to her sister. She strongly resists this, and seeks advice from attorney Campbell Alexander. He agrees to work as her guardian in suing for partial termination of parental rights. He says that he will take on the case because he has epilepsy and therefore understands her feelings of loss of the right to control over her own body. It transpires that Kate has decided that she wants to die, and that it was she who had urged Anna to refuse to donate her bone marrow. Kate dies with her mother by her side, just as the attorney wins the case. This film portrays a person with epilepsy functioning as a top-flight, highly sought after lawyer. It also provides insights into the feelings that are generated by the prospect of loss of control over one's own body – a situation that is familiar to every person with epilepsy. Finally, it introduces us, for the first time in cinema, to the important role of seizure alert dogs, as Campbell owns one of these.

---

154 Curtis D (2007) *Touching from a Distance*. Faber and Faber, London.
155 Picoult J (2004) *My Sister's Keeper*. Washington Square Press, New York.

Electricity (2014), a British film directed by Bryn Higgins, stars the former model Agyness Deyn in her first major acting role. The glamour of Deyn, who has appeared on the cover of *American Vogue* and modelled for so many major fashion houses, could not be a more stark contrast to the unglamorous subject matter of the film. This harrowing and uplifting adaptation of Ray Robinson's novel of the same name[156] probably represents the first accurate and graphic depiction of epilepsy in a mainstream movie. Because it is such a landmark film in the cinematic portrayal of seizures and their consequences, it will be described in some detail here. When Robinson's novel was first published it was hailed in a review by the *Guardian* newspaper as 'a breath-taking assault on the senses',[157] and the film more than lives up to this description. It centres around Deyn's character, Lily O'Connor. Lily has had epilepsy since early childhood, attributed to an injury sustained after her mother had thrown her downstairs. At the start of the film she is employed as a cashier in an amusement arcade in a seaside resort in the north of England. She arranges to meet one of her young male customers after work, and returns home excitedly to get changed. While she is walking alone along the seafront to meet her date, she becomes increasingly aware of lightning-like images in front of her eyes, and then suddenly falls to the ground as she loses consciousness. At the onset of this attack, Lily's fear, apprehension, and recognition of what is about to happen to her are strikingly authentic, and her auditory and visual experiences are shared by the viewer (e.g. with the screen intermittently appearing blank), as indeed they are in the many subsequent depictions of her epilepsy that punctuate the film. We then see her convulsing, and later witness her gradual recovery as a paramedic takes her back to her flat, where she lives alone. Here, as she undresses and showers, she is seen to be visibly bruised and battered, and her soiled underwear indicates that she has been incontinent. The walls of her flat are covered with self-written messages to reassure her that she is back in her own safe haven. Finally she realizes that she has missed her date and that this much anticipated event, an experience that others would normally take for granted, has been denied her because of her epilepsy.

Later in the film, on hearing that her estranged mother has died, Lily visits the hospital to identify the body. Overcome with anger about the past, including her mother's physically abusive behaviour that caused her to have epilepsy, she slaps the face of her mother's corpse. The film then cuts to Lily and her brother Barry sorting through the possessions in their mother's house. The property has been poorly maintained and is in disarray, but despite this, Barry, a professional poker player, is convinced that the house will sell for a good price. When he proposes that they share the profits, Lily suggests that their long-lost brother Mikey should

---

156 Robinson R (2006) *Electricity*. Picador, London.
157 www.theguardian.com/books/2006/mar/25/featuresreviews.guardianreview17

also receive a share of the inheritance. A flashback to Lily's childhood follows, showing her having a convulsion in the bath while her mother and father are joking drunkenly outside the bathroom door. Mikey rushes past them and pulls her out from under the water, saving her life, a debt that she now feels honour bound to repay.

Lily sets off to London to try to find Mikey, and she books into a hotel using the little money she has so that she can begin her search of homeless shelters. She befriends an impoverished girl whom she meets at a railway station, and generously takes her back to the hotel where she can have a meal, a bath, and rest. Lily then experiences her usual kaleidoscopic visual warning, has a seizure, and wakes up to find that the girl has robbed her of the small amount of money she possessed. Undaunted, she continues to search for her brother. She then has another seizure, this time on the London Underground. The film depicts this alternately through Lily's eyes and through the eyes of the bystanders who are witnessing her convulsions as she lies on the ground. All but one of her fellow passengers turn their backs on her; a woman who is nearby avoids looking at her by fiddling self-consciously with her mobile phone. The viewer then witnesses Lily's fragmented memories of trying to leave the Underground station, being taken to hospital by ambulance, discharging herself from hospital, and returning alone to her hotel bedroom. There she looks in the mirror and sees that she is covered in cuts and bruises. In her handbag she finds the telephone number of Mel, the one passenger who had waited with her until the paramedics arrived. She phones her, and the two women forge a short-lived friendship, which ends when Lily feels that Mel's interest in her is motivated only by her epilepsy and resultant vulnerability, and the sense of control over her that this gives her new friend. This theme of betrayal, exploitation, and abandonment, as well as a sense of unease about the motives of others, persists throughout the film.

After being admitted to hospital Lily undergoes an electroencephalogram (EEG) and is told that her seizures have an occipital-temporal origin (which would explain the visual aura). The neurologist in this scene appears to lack empathy. He insists that Lily's drug treatment needs to be changed, and in a condescending manner he tells her that he will write this information down for her as she might otherwise forget it. At this point Lily loses her temper and demonstrates that there is nothing wrong with her memory, reeling off not only the names of all the drugs that she has taken over the years, but also the doses. She is vehement that she does not wish to switch from her current drug treatment – it is tried and tested and she trusts it. The neurologist refuses to accept her point of view, telling her dogmatically that he knows what is best for her. He then instructs her general practitioner to follow his recommendations to the letter. In despair, Lily decides to stop taking her anti-epileptic drugs altogether. She later goes out to a disco where she has a further seizure, falls and injures her face on the floor, and is again hospitalized. She is seen by the same neurologist, who accuses her of not taking her treatment, and castigates her for staying out late and drinking alcohol. In his opinion it is entirely her own fault that she is in hospital and wasting his valuable time. Her response to him is less than polite, and she then leaves.

Lily eventually finds her long-lost brother Mickey, but for complex reasons is rejected by him. She gives him her contact details, telling him that if he ever does feel ready to meet with her, he only has to pick up the phone. Mickey does receive his share of their mother's inheritance, so to some extent at least Lily's mission has been accomplished. The film ends with Lily returning to the northern town that she had left at the start of her quest. The final scene shows her standing on the beach alone. A young man who is walking his dog passes her, and they exchange smiles. The viewer is left feeling that a new chapter in Lily's life may be imminent, but wondering what course it will take when the young man learns about and eventually witnesses her epilepsy.

The making of this film involved significant expert input from the Epilepsy Society, a major UK epilepsy charity. The picture offers a 'warts and all' portrayal of life with poorly controlled epilepsy, and highlights the remarkable courage and honesty of the protagonist. The seizures are fairly stereotyped, with a flashing, lightning-like visual onset followed by convulsions, and fluctuating confusion on recovery. Facial injuries and bruising to the limbs occur frequently, there is evidence of tongue biting, and incontinence is implied. Despite the emotional nature of the storyline, none of Lily's seizures appear to have been precipitated by stressful circumstances. In fact they always occur unpredictably, and on two occasions when Lily is preparing for an eagerly anticipated event. One wonders what life might have held for the young, intelligent, articulate protagonist if she had not had epilepsy. She strongly resists the neurologist's attempt to change her medication, and when this is nevertheless enforced against her will she finally rebels, flushing her drugs down the toilet and going out for a night on the town.

Lily's neurologist may have expert clinical knowledge of epilepsy but he has very little understanding of the actual impact of the condition on the lives of people like Lily. He is emotionally cold and completely lacking in empathy as he talks down to her on his ward round, surrounded by his fawning entourage. At one stage he asks Lily why she does not wear an epilepsy bracelet to alert the public to the fact that she has the condition. She responds that she does not wear one 'because I am not a dog'. In his view, because she has failed to submit to his instructions and change her drug treatment, anything that befalls her thereafter is entirely her own fault. Yet ultimately it is Lily's courage, decency, and strong personality (all convincingly portrayed by Agyness Deyn) that shine through in this film. She is an independent spirit who has been robbed, manipulated, discarded, and rejected, and yet, although it is difficult to believe that her life will improve, she remains optimistic. *Electricity* highlights the issues of stigma, fear, and vulnerability, and the effects of unpredictability on lifestyle. It is rare in filmic portrayals of epilepsy for such a wide range of issues relating to the condition to be covered so comprehensively and with such profound insight.

This arthouse film conveys to the non-epileptic viewer that no matter how severely people with the condition may be affected, they can still potentially function normally and have the same aspirations as anyone else. Films of this nature, informed by expert advice, can only have a positive effect in educating the public and reducing stigma. Will this film also help people who do have epilepsy? I suspect that the answer to this question is a mixed one. To those who have recently been diagnosed and are just commencing treatment, Lily's story might seem overly depressing. However, to those with epilepsy whose seizures have over many years failed to respond to drug treatment, the film might be reassuring. For such viewers the positive role model provided by Lily's character shows that despite this situation it is possible to lead an independent life, achieve positive things, and share positive experiences. In this context, the casting of a well-known former top model as Lily was a masterstroke. Certainly the production costs will represent money well spent if public attitudes are changed by this film.

As we draw towards the end of this chapter, it should be pointed out that a detailed discussion of public information films and documentaries about epilepsy has not been included, mainly because they do not reach a wide audience. However, their limited influence should not be underestimated, and *Zach: A Film about Epilepsy* (2009) and *What's the Time, Mr Wolf?* (2011) both deserve mention as examples of the genre. *Zach* is a 20-minute US film directed by Christian de Rezendes. It depicts a day in the life of Zachery Smith, who has a severe form of epilepsy that does not respond to drugs, and of his family and school, and his ongoing struggles with epilepsy. *What's the Time, Mr Wolf?* is a 1-hour UK film that portrays an acting workshop whose members have one thing in common, namely their epilepsy. Sadly, such films only influence a small number of people, as most of their viewers are already only too aware of the realities of epilepsy. We shall discuss the depiction of epilepsy in independent films in more detail in Chapter 8.

Toba Kerson, in her studies of the portrayal of the social aspects of epilepsy in movies, has concluded that the condition continues to be associated with fear, secrecy, victimization, possession and the supernatural, and violence.[158] With few exceptions, seizures are used to titillate or terrify the audience, or to enhance the dramatic impact of the plot. In essence they are used as a vehicle to shock. Kerson was based at the Graduate School of Social Work and Social Research at Bryn Mawr, the women's liberal arts college in Pennsylvania, where

---

158 Kerson JF, Kerson TS and Kerson LA (1999) The depiction of seizures in film. *Epilepsia* 40, 1163–1167.

she has maintained a long-term interest in the study of epilepsy in film. She has created an extensive annotated database of films that depict or contain references to seizures,[159] and provided a website report for the film festival at the International League against Epilepsy (ILAE) Centenary celebrations in Budapest in 2009. Kerson suggests that it is up to epilepsy interest groups to monitor and influence the manner in which the movie industry portrays the condition. Only a few films, such as *Electricity*, have been made with the advice and guidance of epilepsy experts, people with epilepsy, and the charities that support them. The major benefits of such an approach are ensuring accuracy and preventing the spread of misinformation and myths. Sadly there is no compunction, apart from the ethical one, for the industry to take notice of the epilepsy lobby.

Sallie Baxendale, in her review of more than 60 films that feature seizures,[160] found a disturbing tendency across all genres of film to equate epilepsy with lunacy, delinquency, and demons. As in literature, those for whom there was a clear physical cause, such as head injury, were heroes (e.g. in *The Bone Collector*), whereas those for whom there was no apparent cause were depicted as either villains or victims (e.g. in *Let Him Have It*). Female characters with epilepsy tended to be either beautiful and vulnerable (e.g. in *Mean Streets* and *Electricity*), or abused (e.g. in *1900* and *The Exorcism of Emily Rose*). False seizures were used for the purpose of deception (e.g. in *The Twelve Chairs*) or robbery (e.g. *Drugstore Cowboy*). Male characters with epilepsy were generally depicted as being mad and/or bad (e.g. *To What Red Hell* and *The Terminal Man*).

When Baxendale reviewed a further 21 films from 2000 to 2014 she found that, with a very few exceptions, the negative stereotypes had persisted.[161] The shining exception is *Electricity*, which demonstrates just what can be achieved with an informed screenplay and the input of expert advice. There is no escaping the fact that seizures are alarming events for both sufferer and witnesses, and will continue to be used for dramatic effect where writers and directors feel that they can enhance the storyline. The relationship between seizures and possession is entrenched in history, so it would not be surprising if period films continue to depict this.

Finally, it is noteworthy that movies made for television, with their smaller budgets and much reduced financial imperative to reward their backers through the box office, are better placed to produce accurate accounts of the human aspects of social care and health issues such as epilepsy.

---

159 Kerson T (2018) List of films depicting or discussing seizures. Personal communication.
160 Baxendale S (2003) Epilepsy at the movies: possession to presidential assassination. *The Lancet: Neurology* 2, 764–770.
161 Baxendale S (2016) Epilepsy on the silver screen in the 21st century. *Epilepsy & Behavior* 57, 270–274.

Television programmes

When discussing the representation of epilepsy on television, it is difficult not to be parochial, given the vast range of programmes and channels available worldwide. Television has enormous potential not only to portray epilepsy appropriately and accurately, but also to educate the public with regard to first-aid management of the condition. A recent Canadian study found that television programmes were alarmingly inaccurate in the way that they depicted basic first-aid treatment, and it recommended that people with epilepsy should lobby the industry to adhere to first-aid guidelines and not simply ignore them. Even more worrying was the fact that the programmes studied were the highest-rated US medical dramas, namely *Grey's Anatomy*, *House M.D.*, *Private Practice*, and the last five seasons of *ER*.[162] It was found that 59 out of a total of 337 episodes showed seizures occurring. Nearly all first-responder first aid was performed by nurses or doctors. The study also identified inappropriate practices, such as holding the person down in order to restrain convulsive movements (26% of cases), or putting an object in the person's mouth to bite on (15% of cases). In only a third of cases was first-aid management undertaken correctly. In *House M.D.*, two doctors were actually shown holding down a small fitting child. The seizures depicted in the television episodes are of interest because they show events that would be more readily identified by the public as epilepsy, with florid convulsions (which accounted for eight out of ten attacks), whereas less easily recognizable attacks, such as temporal lobe epilepsy, accounted for less than 8% of cases.

It seems that screenwriters and directors have opted to conform to the popular view of what a seizure 'should' look like, and in doing so have merely reaffirmed this, rather than broadening the very narrow public image of the condition. Only one psychogenic or non-epileptiform attack was depicted in all the episodes that were studied, whereas in real life it might account for one in ten attacks. Clearly, too, a valuable opportunity to educate the public about first aid for epilepsy has been lost, and in fact much harm could result if the public learned such procedures from US medical soaps. Indeed the inability to convey basic public health first-aid messages accurately in TV medical dramas shows a near negligent lack of care, consultation, and programme research.

The US television drama *Medics* ran from 1954 over a period of two years. The 56 half-hour episodes followed the professional activities of a group of doctors headed by Dr Konrad Styner. *Medics* can claim to be the first medical TV show that paid strict attention to detail. The episode entitled 'Boy in a Storm' involves Robert, a shy 17-year-old with epilepsy, who

---

162 Moeller AD, Moeller JJ, Rahey SR and Sadler RM (2011) Depiction of seizure first aid management in medical television dramas. *Canadian Journal of Neurological Sciences* 38, 723–727.

over the years has been kept concealed and sheltered by his elderly aunt. When she dies he comes to the attention of Dr Styler and his team, whose task is to stabilize his seizures so that he will eventually be fit enough to live a normal life with a caring foster family. The episode addresses not only Robert's epilepsy but also its social consequences in terms of adjusting to an open, less secretive, and less isolated life in the context of crippling shyness. Dr Styner comments that 'An epileptic is not insane, nor is he evil as men have imagined in the past. He is possessed of a disability as logically explainable as a lame leg. But the stigma of fear lives on, a reminder of man's superstitious past. This the doctor must treat, as well as the epilepsy.' This memorable comment is well ahead of its time, making 'Boy in a Storm' a real landmark in the television portrayal of epilepsy. Even today, Dr Styler's lines would be an excellent mantra for anyone caring for a person with epilepsy.

The early US medical 'soap', *Dr Kildare* (1961–1966), ran to 191 episodes and was the prototype for all subsequent US medical soaps. At its height the programme received 12,000 fan letters a week, many of them asking the fictional doctor for medical advice. The two-part episode entitled 'Tyger Tyger' (1964) is a story about Pat Holmes, a smart, able, and beautiful girl who is a keen surfer, although she also has her eye on the good doctor. She is diagnosed with seizures, initially petit mal, that gradually worsen and become major convulsions. She is warned that these could kill her if she continues to surf, but she refuses to give up this activity. By now Kildare has fallen in love with her, and is worried that her determined efforts to carry on with life on her terms will end badly. While Pat is in hospital recovering from a seizure she befriends her young alcoholic roommate and urges her not to let her condition rule her life – a positive philosophy that Pat clearly follows herself. Predictably, she decides to return to her surfing. Kildare follows her to the edge of the ocean to try to stop her, but is too late, and she drowns.

Dr Kildare was a major heart-throb of his time, and the fact that his only real love interest in the whole series was a young girl with epilepsy must have done much to improve the public perception of the condition. Pat is portrayed as feisty, independent, and caring. She is a very positive role model for people with epilepsy who wish to live life to the full and not be hindered by their condition. Finally, the public health warning about the risks associated with seizures while swimming is an obvious and important one.

The Young and the Restless (1973–) is a prime example of how the television industry, in this case Columbia Broadcast System (CBS), and a charity, the Epilepsy Foundation, can collaborate in the interests of accuracy. In 2006 this collaboration involved 20 of the 6000 or more episodes of the long-running US soap, and focused on a character called Victor Newman. It has been the most popular daytime television drama in the USA for 25 consecutive years, with a potentially invaluable opportunity to influence and lead opinion. The programme follows the lives of various families in the fictional Midwestern city of Genoa. The character of Victor Newman, with his infidelity and abuse of his wife, was originally created with the intention of killing him off early in the storyline. However, Victor becomes suddenly transformed from ruthless businessman into charming husband and doting grandfather. He then develops blackouts and hallucinations, and is diagnosed with temporal lobe epilepsy secondary to a head injury sustained in a carjacking incident several months earlier. Fans of the soap who were concerned that the diagnosis of epilepsy meant that the character would be written out of the show were reassured by the actor's return after a short absence.

Initially Victor appears to enjoy the fact that the seizures make him feel uncharacteristically caring towards those around him, and he therefore stops his medication. The seizures then became associated with short episodes of violence, and rather than restarting his drugs he opts to have his epilepsy treated by 'gamma-knife' surgery. He seems to do well thereafter, and is possibly cured, as epilepsy disappears from the plot, although in subsequent episodes he has unexplained episodes of memory loss and a further head injury. CBS announced that it was 'proud to be able to use this forum to raise awareness about epilepsy, and as the story unfolds, viewers will have the opportunity to not only see how Victor himself deals with his diagnosis, but how his family reacts as well'.

The Epilepsy Foundation added that they were 'extremely pleased with CBS's decision to partner with us to help bring epilepsy out of the shadows by associating the condition with one of the network's most renowned programs and famed actors'. However, it could be argued that Victor's epilepsy is made more respectable by giving it a cause, namely a head injury inflicted by thieves. Stopping drug treatment in order to enjoy the effects of the seizures is not a common or advisable situation, nor would many people with epilepsy consider doing such a thing. Moreover, it is misleading to suggest that an apparent cure can be achieved by surgery that would not normally be considered for post-traumatic epilepsy. Finally, even though Victor's epilepsy features in over 20 of the 6000 episodes, it disappears from the storyline as abruptly as it enters it. One cannot help thinking that the Epilepsy Foundation missed an opportunity and should have adopted a firmer position about the representation of the facts. Seizures in this soap are used as much to shock as to educate. For all of the above reasons, this is not a good example of how broadcasters and charities can work for the common good in promoting a realistic picture of epilepsy.

The US family comedy drama *Different Strokes* (1978–1986) tells the story of a New York Park Avenue millionaire who adopts two Harlem orphans. It includes a short episode entitled 'A Special Friend' (1985), in which the two main characters, Arnold and Sam, befriend a street performer only to discover that she has epilepsy. They are confused by this, are frightened to be around her again, and cannot understand the condition. It is only when another major character reveals that she also has the condition that their anxieties and fears are allayed. The episode highlights not only the secrecy and concealment that surround epilepsy, but also the fact that when those affected finally reveal their condition to others, it becomes evident that they are just like everyone else.

Moving forward in time, there is a stark contrast between *Medics*, *Dr Kildare*, and an episode of the HBO television series *The Sopranos*, entitled 'The Two Tony's', in which the ugly face of prejudice against epilepsy comes to the fore. The epilepsy incident occurs towards the end of the episode. The older character, 'Paulie Walnuts' Gualtieri, is henchman to Tony Soprano, the leader of the ruthless criminal DiMeo family in New York. Chris Moltisanti is Tony's keen young protégé. Both men are violent, impulsive, and keen to impress in their desire for self-advancement. Paulie and Chris are arguing over a dinner bill in an Atlantic City restaurant. Because Chris is footing the bill, Paulie has deliberately encouraged the other guest to choose the most expensive options. On leaving, Chris and Paulie confront each other in the restaurant car park. Their waiter suddenly rushes out towards them, confronting them with the miserly tip they have given him. As he is explaining that he has a wife and family to feed, Chris picks up a brick and throws it at his head. The waiter falls to the ground and has a seizure. Chris looks at him and says 'Don't these people know they're supposed to take their medicine, these assholes?' Paulie then glances around to make sure there are no witnesses, before taking out a gun and shooting the waiter dead. Chris immediately grabs the money that they had earlier paid the waiter for the meal.

This bleak and depressing scene and the act of gratuitous violence highlight the mobsters' callous attitude to life – the killing of the waiter while he is having a convulsion is a matter of no consequence to them because he is dispensable. Moreover, the mobsters exploited his seizure in order to recoup their money. The viewer learns nothing about the waiter or who will grieve for him after his death. He is defined only by his lowly employment, his diffident manner, and his epilepsy. *The Sopranos*, which ran from 1999 to 2007, had a worldwide audience of many millions, and thus a potentially huge opportunity to influence the opinions of its followers. Yet this episode is a clear example of epilepsy being used solely for dramatic effect.

Deadwood (2004–2006) is an American Western television series set in South Dakota in the 1870s, and includes real historical characters such as the Reverend Henry Weston Smith, who is also known as Preacher Smith. Although there is no evidence that the real Reverend Smith had epilepsy, the scriptwriters decided to give him the condition, and his fictional demise is attributed to progressive decline caused by a brain tumour, and eventual euthanasia. In real life he was believed to have been killed by Native Americans or criminals who were angered by his campaign against the bars and brothels of Deadwood. In the television series the Reverend Smith rationalizes that his fits are a result of divine intervention. His seizures, including his status epilepticus just prior to his death, are depicted in three of the 36 episodes of the series.

A detailed biography of Smith[163] makes no reference to epilepsy, although it provides an interesting account of how he fought in the American Civil War and briefly studied medicine. One might question why it was necessary to give this colourful real-life character seizures and a brain tumour. The programme's creator, David Milch, is quoted as saying that he based Smith's seizures on suggestions that St Paul (Paul of Tarsus) had temporal lobe epilepsy, and that he incorporated this into Smith's persona as well as giving him a completely fictional cause of death – in the form of mercy killing by suffocation, administered by the main character Al Swearengen, a hotel and saloon owner.

The depiction of epilepsy in long-running television shows is not confined to the USA. The UK soap *Coronation Street* (1960–) is the world's longest-running television soap opera, broadcast six times a week. In an episode in 2010 the local hairdresser David Platt was diagnosed with epilepsy after blacking out behind the wheel of his car. Jack Shepherd, the actor who plays him, has stated that 'epilepsy is a complicated and often misunderstood condition with very little awareness. Shows such as Coronation Street play a really important role in helping to generate awareness. I am pleased that my character may help other young people who are living with the condition.' The Epilepsy Society worked with the programme's production team to ensure accuracy, stating that 'Coronation Street has a huge audience and can provide a great platform for awareness raising around the condition.' David's long-standing persona was not appealing, with his tendency to engage in devious, malicious, and violent behaviour and get away with it, attracting nicknames such as 'Demon David' and 'Psycho Platt'. Thus in a similar way to *The Young and the Restless*, a hitherto undesirable character has been chosen to be the flag bearer for epilepsy.

While driving the car that he has just stolen from his grandmother, David has a blackout and knocks over a man with whom he has previously been seen arguing about a girlfriend. The victim is severely injured and taken to hospital, and David is arrested and charged with attempted murder, despite his claim that he has no recollection of the event. Just before the court case begins he has another blackout. People begin to realize that he has been telling the truth, and when he is diagnosed with epilepsy the case against him is dropped. We know little about his epilepsy thereafter, other than that he subsequently returns to car driving, and he is advised against boxing because of his condition. His old character soon resurfaces when he becomes a suspect in another attempted murder case. His epilepsy appears to be

---

163 Case LD (1961) *Preacher Smith, Martyr: The Story of Henry Weston Smith, Methodist, the Pioneer Preacher in the Black Hills of South Dakota*. Publisher unknown.

controlled on medication, though in a later episode there is a further event. Although the introduction of epilepsy into the script does serve to heighten awareness of the condition, David's character has so many negative attributes that it runs the risk of reinforcing a negative public perception of and attitude towards people with epilepsy.

Beliefs about the association of epilepsy with criminality will be discussed in Chapter 11.

The UK television soap *EastEnders* (1985–), which is set in the fictional borough of Walford in the East End of London, introduced a major character with epilepsy, Nancy Carter, and won praise for its realism and its sympathetic portrayal of the condition. Again there was collaboration between a charity, in this case Epilepsy Action, and the programme makers. Nancy had already become one of the nation's favourite cast members – loyal, stubborn, and always sticking up for the underdog. In contrast to earlier soaps, a likeable, honest character had been chosen to portray a person living with epilepsy. Nancy's first seizure was shown in January 2014 and viewed by 8 million people. Maddy Hill, the actress who played the role of Nancy, expressed concern that she had no knowledge about epilepsy and that her portrayal of a person with the condition might appear disrespectful. To maximize the accuracy of her portrayal of the seizures, she spoke to people with epilepsy, watched video clips of attacks, and was supported by a neurologist (who also had family experience of attacks) who talked her through the seizures. As a result, the depiction of Nancy's seizures was convincingly realistic, as was the portrayal of the social consequences of the condition. Nancy's epilepsy prevents her from joining the army, and she bemoans the loss of control that she experiences when she has an attack. She resents the limitations that the condition imposes on the activities she would like to engage in, and she believes that in the future she may have to conceal her diagnosis. The programme presents all of these issues, which are so commonly experienced by those with epilepsy, in an intelligent and thoughtful way. However, the casting of able-bodied actors to play the parts of disabled characters is now controversial, with disabled actors advocating that they would be better placed to take on such roles.

Epilepsy Today, the newsletter of Epilepsy Action, stated that 'Nancy's seizures are a brave step for the show and are becoming a dramatic fixture in the EastEnders landscape.' Unfortunately, the reaction of viewers to Nancy's epilepsy has been very mixed. There have been many negative and inappropriate comments on social media sites such as Facebook and Twitter, with some even finding the seizures comical. Sections of the press have fared no better, with one reviewer scornfully commenting that there are now 'so many illnesses on view that characters are competing against each other for the camera and our sympathy, as if to determine who was the most traumatized (apart from us).' Perhaps the actress Maddy Hill should have the last word. She is quoted in *Epilepsy Today* (May 2014) as saying that 'People with epilepsy are pleased it is raising awareness ... but there have been some really horrible ignorant people who have no experience of epilepsy. That's why it's important for shows like *EastEnders* to cover this condition: to help educate people.'[164] Overall, then, *EastEnders* and Epilepsy Action have achieved their collective aims. The popular, positive character of Nancy has brought epilepsy to the public's attention in a realistic, truthful, and sympathetic manner.

Other television soaps, such as *Neighbours* in Australia and *Hollyoaks* and *Emmerdale* in the UK, have incorporated epilepsy into their storylines, but in each case the condition is a consequence of a previous incident or situation, such as an assault, car crash, or flashing lights. Meanwhile the broader, more realistic portrayal of epilepsy with all its social consequences is barely addressed, despite the fact that epilepsy charities have often been consulted with a view to improving the accuracy of depictions of the condition. Seizures also feature in medical soaps such as *House MD*, *Grey's Anatomy*, *Casualty*, and *Holby City*, to name just a few. In most of these, epilepsy is used merely for short-lived dramatic effect, and the affected character leaves the plot as rapidly as they enter it, or else their seizures simply disappear from the storyline. In the majority of cases they are minor parts, whom the main characters either treat or observe.

Conclusion

The depiction of epilepsy in a significant number of films is demonstrated both by the International League against Epilepsy 2009 Budapest film festival and by Toba Kerson's painstakingly compiled database which lists the many examples. Both she and Sallie Baxendale, her fellow chronicler of films that portray epilepsy, have shown how ancient beliefs and myths as well as gender bias have influenced how and why epilepsy has been introduced into the storyline of films. Women with epilepsy are generally portrayed as vulnerable and deserving of sympathy, whereas men with the condition, unless they have developed epilepsy as a result of an accident or serving in a war, are flawed and often criminal. These stereotypes have stood the test of time, as evidenced by their continued use. Just as in literature, in film, the sudden insertion of a seizure, whether genuine or contrived, can be guaranteed to gain the audience's attention or to cement their opinion, for good or ill, about a particular character. It is in the films made for television, with their smaller budgets and lack of pressure for box-office success, that the most accurate portrayals of the health and social issues associated with epilepsy are to be found.

---

164 www.epilepsy.org.uk/news/features/epilepsy-east-end-63966

Among the television soaps, only *EastEnders* has an ongoing storyline involving a main character who is young enough to be likely to remain in the narrative for a long time to come, and thus to continue to present the epilepsy message from new angles. Epilepsy organizations collaborated in the making of episodes of both *The Young and The Restless* and *Coronation Street*, yet the final result was very disappointing. The characters who were scripted to have epilepsy were unattractive, the facts surrounding their seizures were inaccurate, and the storyline was not sustained after the initial dramatic impact of the depiction of epilepsy had faded. We have to go back to the early medical programmes, specifically *Medics* and *Dr Kildare*, to find the most positive portrayals of the understanding and compassion of doctors who are caring for those with epilepsy.

It has been suggested that although they are unable to censor, the medical professions and those with epilepsy need to be vigilant about preventing the perpetuation of negative stereotypes, which then raises the question of how this could be practically achieved. There should be a more robust mechanism in place to ensure that misrepresentation of disability is addressed with the same zero tolerance as the misrepresentation of gender, race, and sexuality. There are bodies such as the UK Equality and Human Rights Commission that could intervene, but complaints from those who are disabled about discrimination are rarely forthcoming. With a few notable exceptions, the portrayal of epilepsy in the movies remains unacceptably negative, and those who misrepresent the condition for dramatic effect and commercial gain should be identified and held to account. The movie industry has its own award-giving bodies, such as the Academy Awards (the Oscars) and Emmy Awards, and these need to be lobbied in cases where films are deemed to be medically inaccurate or prejudicial. The 'Me Too' campaign has demonstrated the effectiveness of this type of action. Any medical condition that is depicted on the moving screen should be scrutinized both by those with the condition and by those who advocate on their behalf, and the same scrutiny applied as for issues of race, gender, and sexuality.

CHAPTER 7

Epilepsy in music and the theatre

Epilepsy in music and in musicians

There is a bidirectional relationship between music and epilepsy. First, music itself may have an effect on seizures and their treatment. In the UK, the neurologist Melissa Maguire has written an extensive review of this subject,[165] and also refers to the scholarly book *Music and the Brain: Studies in the Neurology of Music*, edited by Macdonald Critchley and R.A. Henson.[166] Second, epilepsy can influence musicians and the music that they create. *Musicophilia*, an anecdotal and readable account by the writer and neurologist Oliver Sack, describes how a range of brain conditions, including epilepsy, can affect the appreciation and creation of music, not only by skilled musicians but also among the general population.[167]

Let us start by considering the physiological relationship between music and epilepsy. Music – unlike literature, visual art, and film – has been shown to have a measurable effect on brain activity, and a potentially positive influence on seizure control. The term 'music therapy' refers to its application across a wide range of health conditions. The British Association for Music Therapy (BAMT) points out that, in addition to the social benefits of playing a musical instrument or being a member of a choir, music can have a direct effect upon both mental health and physical illnesses. The many conditions that they list include autism and brain

---

165 Maguire MJ (2012) Music and epilepsy: a critical review. *Epilepsia* 53, 947–961.
166 Critchley M and Henson RA (1977) *Music and the Brain: Studies in the Neurology of Music*. Heinemann, London.
167 Sacks O (2007) *Musicophilia: Tales of Music and the Brain*. Picador, London.

injury, and there is both quantitative and qualitative research to support such claims. There are two types of music therapy: *active* therapy involves participation in making music, and *receptive* therapy involves listening to music. In the USA, the therapeutic benefits of music were first officially recognized in the 1940s. University training programmes were subsequently established, and the National Association for Music Therapy (NAMT) was formed.

In fact, the positive effects of music on health have been known since ancient times.[168] Historically they were ascribed to music's effect on the soul, until the Scottish physician John Brown (1735–1788) outlined in his publication *Elementa Medicinae* (1780) the theory that all conditions were caused by excessively strong or weak stimuli. This became known as the *Brunonian system of medicine* (named after Brown), and it lent credence to the theory that health could be improved by using music to cause stimulation or relaxation of the nerves. Peter Lichtenthal (1780–1853), a physician and musical composer, described the use of what he referred to as the *Brunonian scale* to determine the doses of music that should be administered for specific conditions, setting this out in detail in his book *The Musical Doctor* (1805).

Johann Sebastian Bach's *Goldberg Variations* is a striking example of music that seems to have a specific effect on insomnia caused by pain. Bach is believed to have written this music for his pupil, Johann Goldberg, to play on the harpsichord to his patron, Count Hermann Karl von Keyserlingk, who experienced insomnia resulting from pain caused by kidney stones. Although many musicologists dispute this story, *Goldberg Variations* is now regarded as one of the most therapeutic passages of music ever composed, and is still recommended for pain and sleep disturbances. Bach's general contribution to the field of music therapy is now widely recognized both by professionals and more widely – for example, with the recent release of an album entitled 'Bach Music Therapy' on Spotify.

There is significant evidence that music can help people with epilepsy. The positive impact of both active music therapy (singing, playing an instrument, or composing music) and passive music therapy (listening to live or recorded music) on individuals who have epilepsy and any of a wide range of associated mental health problems is well documented.

The question then arises as to whether music has a direct effect in either improving or worsening seizure control. In nearly 80 per cent of people with epilepsy, seizures arise within the temporal lobe of the brain. This region also contains the auditory cortex (the hearing area of the brain), which is where the sound produced by music is processed – that is, recognized, remembered, and either enjoyed or disliked. Therefore it is reasonable to assume that epilepsy and music might have a relationship that could be either beneficial, by reducing the frequency or severity of seizures, or detrimental, by precipitating attacks.

---

168 Misic P, Arandjelovic D, Stanojkovic S et al. (2010) Music therapy. *European Psychiatry* 25 (Suppl. 1), 839.

The 'Mozart effect' is one of the most intriguing demonstrable examples of the way music can affect brain activity. Mozart's compositions are so highly organized, in such an architecturally symmetrical manner, that many authors have referred to the mathematical science of his works and have speculated whether the brain physically resonates with them, such that the music can influence the functional activity of brainwaves. A review of the evidence reveals that this is not as fanciful an idea as it might sound. In 1993, Frances Rauscher and her colleagues from the Department of Psychology at the University of Wisconsin were the first to investigate the effect of listening to music on spatial reasoning, and to coin the term 'Mozart effect'.[169] They found that college students who had listened to Mozart's Sonata for Two Pianos in D major (K. 448) for ten minutes showed significantly better spatial reasoning skills than two control groups who had listened to either recorded relaxation advice or to silence. The mean spatial IQ scores of the students who listened to the sonata increased by 8 to 9 points, but the effect only lasted for 15 minutes. These results were quickly disputed when it became clear that other researchers could not replicate the findings. In response to this, Rauscher commented that 'because some people cannot get bread to rise does not negate the existence of a "yeast effect"'. Extraordinarily, the findings were supported by a study of young mice, which showed that animals that had been exposed to the sound of Mozart's music were more successful in finding their way through a maze than animals that had been exposed to the music of the minimalist composer Philip Glass, or to white noise.

The brain areas that are used for the processing of music overlap with those involved in spatial awareness, so there is a logical basis for the view that activation of one will enhance the other. These areas have been mapped by functional brain imaging, initially by positron emission tomography (PET) and more recently by functional magnetic resonance imaging (fMRI), which has shown that they lie in the temporal lobe. The auditory cortex is located in the upper part of the temporal lobe, with rhythm and pitch being processed on the right side and melody on the left side.

The most impressive evidence of a Mozart effect is seen in people with epilepsy. In a study of 29 patients with temporal lobe epilepsy, it was found that after listening to the piano sonata mentioned earlier, 23 patients showed a reduction in epilepsy activity as measured by electroencephalography (EEG).[170] Moreover, additional studies by the same authors showed a reduction in the number of visible seizures. In order to ascertain whether this effect was specific to Mozart's music or whether it applied to music in general, John Hughes and his colleagues at the University of Illinois, Chicago used computer analysis to study a wide range of composers and composition styles. They demonstrated that much of Mozart's music, as

---

169 Rauscher FH, Shaw GL and Ky CN (1993) Music and spatial task performance. *Nature* 365, 611.
170 Hughes JR, Daaboul Y, Fino JJ et al. (1998) The "Mozart effect" on epileptiform activity. *Clinical Electroencephalography* 29, 109–119.

well as some of that by Bach, displayed specific characteristics, although they did not put these similarities to the test in order to determine whether there was also a 'Bach effect' in patients.

Various theories have been proposed with regard to the mechanism whereby some music has an anticonvulsant effect, presumably by influencing the brain's ability to generate seizure activity. Some propose that the synchronized pattern of music might decrease excitability directly, by targeting the brain area from which the epilepsy arises, whereas others suggest that it is the activation of more widespread brain regions that has a suppressant effect. Finally, dopamine, a chemical that functions as a neurotransmitter (messenger) in the brain, is thought to have a role in activating seizures, and it has been shown that exposure to music increases the levels of this chemical. Clearly, though, in view of the many different theories about the Mozart effect, further research is needed.

In 2015, at the 123rd Annual Conference of the American Psychological Association, one session was dedicated to the topic 'Music and the Brain: Can Music Help People with Epilepsy?' Christine Charyton and her colleagues from Ohio State University had recorded the brainwaves of people with and without epilepsy who had listened to Mozart's piano sonata, followed by 10 minutes of silence, followed by John Coltrane's 'My Favourite Things'. They found that brainwave activity synchronized more with the music in people with epilepsy than in those without the condition, and clearly this effect was not just confined to the music of Mozart. This research appears to provide further evidence that music influences brain activity, particularly in those with temporal lobe epilepsy. Charyton concluded that although music can never replace current treatments, there may be a role for its use in conjunction with them to help to prevent seizures.

Paradoxically, music can in very rare instances actually cause seizures. This phenomenon, termed 'musicogenic epilepsy', was first documented in 1937 by the English neurologist MacDonald Critchley (1900–1997):[171] 'F.C, female, aged 25, consulted me in the outpatient department of the National Hospital in 1931. Since the age of 17 she had been subject to attacks of faintness on hearing certain types of music – particularly that produced by a piano or organ. She fancied that classical music was more noxious than dance music.' More recently, *The Zahir* (2005), a novel by the Brazilian author Paul Coelho, featured a character with musicogenic epilepsy who described ecstatic feelings on hearing a particular kind of sound or type of musical instrument.[172]

Only around 200 cases of this form of epilepsy have been described. Although the trigger for the phenomenon may vary considerably from one person to another, it is always the same trigger

---

171 Critchley M (1937) Musicogenic epilepsy. *Brain* 60, 13–27.
172 Coelho P (2005) *The Zahir: A Novel of Obsession*. HarperCollins, New York.

for a particular individual. It can take the form of a specific sound, word, voice, song, singer, instrument, or passage of music. Musicogenic epilepsy most commonly occurs in women who have above average levels of musicality. This form of epilepsy is of the temporal lobe type, and the short delay between exposure to music and the onset of a seizure has led to the suggestion that it is the emotional arousal induced by the music, rather than the actual sound, that is causal. Indeed, even thinking about music can occasionally induce an attack. Critchley suggested that there were two potential mechanisms, one being physiological and the other psychological. In 1947, David Shaw and Denis Hill[173] championed a psychological cause in a detailed case report of a 44-year-old German woman living in London who had been forced to conceal her origins due to fear of reprisals, and whose music-related attacks started during the Blitz. Today, as a result of modern investigation techniques, the possibility of a psychological mechanism can now be discounted. This rare form of epilepsy is managed by drug treatment and the avoidance of triggers. However, the author's personal experience of an individual whose attacks were triggered by the chiming of a clock exemplifies how difficult it can be to achieve avoidance.

Music and epilepsy also interact in various other ways. Studies of the anticonvulsant drug carbamazepine have shown that it has a reversible effect on perception of the pitch of music (a measure of how high or low a note is in a musical melody) and thus upon musicality. This would be a particularly important point to consider if prescribing the drug to a musician. None of the other commonly used anti-epilepsy drugs appear to have this effect. Given the importance of the temporal lobe area in the perception of sound, temporal lobe surgery would be expected to affect both musical skills and music appreciation. As a general rule of thumb, surgery to the right side is associated with impaired recognition of tunes, and surgery to the left side is associated with a reduced emotional response to them. Pitch and rhythm can also be affected.

Finally, the seizures themselves, especially if they are of temporal lobe origin, may have a musical component. Auditory hallucinations may rarely occur during a seizure, and musical sounds (over and above grunting) in the form of humming or (very rarely) singing may be produced.

Composers and musicians

Much has been made of the absence of epilepsy among composers and musicians, implying that something inherent in the epilepsy itself prevents the development of musicality. Dale

---

[173] Shaw D and Hill D (1947) A case of musicogenic epilepsy. *Journal of Neurology, Neurosurgery & Psychiatry* 10, 107–117.

Hesdorffer and Michael Trimble studied the links between musical creativity and epilepsy, and reported that they were unable to find any evidence of musical composers with the condition.[174] They rebutted the claims that Handel, Beethoven, Schumann, Berlioz, and Tchaikovsky had epilepsy, and they argued that the seizures experienced by Haydn and Mussorgsky were caused by strokes and alcohol, respectively. In fact the only composer whom they conceded might have had epilepsy was Chopin. However, their conclusions need to be weighed against the historical period in which all of these composers lived, when medical documentation was scarce, and those who had epilepsy went to great lengths to conceal it. In view of this, Hesdorffer and Trimble's statement that the lack of association between musical creativity and epilepsy provided 'a gateway to understanding facets of the relationship between the brain and creativity' seems misjudged. Moreover, their conclusion that 'the failure of people with epilepsy to provide elevated music may link to the sheer intellectual demands of the task', and the dismissive manner in which they excluded popular music from the debate, appears elitist and condescending.

Frédéric Chopin (1810–1849), the Polish composer and virtuoso pianist, is best known for his solo piano works and his piano concertos. Plagued by ill health throughout his short life (he died of tuberculosis at the age of 39), he experienced visual hallucinations that some authors have suggested were caused by temporal lobe epilepsy.

In the summer of 1848, in the middle of a performance at a private concert in Manchester, Chopin suddenly rose from the piano and left the room. His own very revealing account of this episode, in a letter to the daughter of his former lover George Sand, was quoted by Manuel Caruncho and Franciso Fernández in their paper on Chopin's hallucinations:[175] 'A strange adventure happened to me while I was playing my B Flat Sonata for some English friends – I was about to play the [Funeral] March when, suddenly, I saw emerging from the half-open case of my piano those cursed creatures that had appeared to me on a lugubrious night at the Carthusian Monastery [in Majorca]. I had to leave for a while in order to recover myself, and after that I continued playing without saying a word.'

The episode in the Majorcan monastery had occurred around 10 years earlier, and appears to have been a terrifying, although not isolated, event. In her autobiography, *Histoire de Ma Vie* (1848), George Sand described Chopin's repeated sense that the monastery was full of terrors and ghosts, and how, upon returning one night with her children, she found him 'at ten o'clock in the evening pale in front of the piano, with wide eyes and his hair on end. He needed a while to recognize us.' She described further episodes in which he would cry out, with wide eyes, in a strange tone. Chopin had vivid hallucinations in which he was

---

174 Hesdorffer DC and Trimble M (2016) Musical and poetic creativity and epilepsy. *Epilepsy & Behavior* 57, 234–237.
175 Caruncho MV and Fernández FB (2011) The hallucinations of Frédéric Chopin. *Medical Humanities* 37, 5–8.

drowning and fighting off fleshless faces and their icy grip on him. These accounts of his brief but complex visual hallucinations were interspersed with short episodes, often when he was playing the piano, when he would appear to be in a trance. Although no medical records are available, Caruncho and Fernández believe that after exclusion of other causes of short, repetitive, complex visual hallucinations, the written accounts of Chopin's episodes strongly suggest a diagnosis of temporal lobe epilepsy. If he did indeed live with that condition, this would go a long way towards explaining his complex personality. Chopin was regarded as the archetypal Romantic artist, with his introversion, tendency to depression and anxiety, state of perpetual suffering, difficulties sustaining relationships, poor health, and obsessive pursuit of perfection. It is sometimes said that an artist must suffer for his art, but Chopin could well have been suffering for his epilepsy, too.

Although the Russian composer **Modest Mussorgsky** (1839–1881) appears on many lists of famous people with epilepsy, it has also been suggested that his seizures may have been alcohol induced. Whether or not his epilepsy was alcohol related, it was present for much of his artistically productive life. Mussorgsky was born in Tsarist Russia, and initially pursued a military career, despite the early evidence of his musical talent (he was composing by the age of 13). He soon resigned from the army and joined a circle of fellow amateur composers, who included the military doctor Alexander Borodin and the naval cadet Nikolai Rimsky-Korsakov. During the summer of 1859 he was struck down by an unidentified nervous illness, and from then on his life became chaotic. He never married or had a permanent address, instead either staying with family or friends, or living in communes, but all the while he continued to compose. In 1865 he became seriously ill from seizures attributed to alcohol withdrawal (delirium tremens), and such episodes were to recur for the rest of his life. In 1874, his great opera *Boris Godunov* had its first performance at the Mariinsky Theatre in St Petersburg. Thereafter, despite the success of *Pictures at an Exhibition*, many of his works remained unfinished, his drinking became more frequent, and his descent into a chaotic, impoverished lifestyle was accompanied by a decline in his artistic output. Tragically, he died at the age of only 42. Aleksandra Orlova's biography of Mussorgsky describes episodes of sudden collapse (which were assumed to be strokes), followed by sudden recovery, that occurred in February 1881.[176] Viewed retrospectively, these events might well have been seizures. Orlova described how, after he had repeatedly experienced such episodes, Mussorgsky was eventually admitted to the Military Hospital, disguised as one of the attending physician's servants. The doctors concluded that he had not suffered strokes but rather the beginnings of epilepsy, and it was in that hospital, shortly after Ilya Repin had painted the iconic portrait of the composer, that Mussorgsky died in 1881. According to Orlova, the post-mortem report cited liver disease

---

176 Orlova A (1983) *Musorgsky's Days and Works: A Biography in Documents*. UMI Research Press, Ann Arbor, MI.

and inflammation of the spinal cord as the causes of death. Mussorgsky is buried in the Tikhvin Cemetery, St Petersburg, alongside the writer Fyodor Dostoevsky, who also suffered from epilepsy.

The American musician **George Gershwin** (1898–1937) composed music that spanned both classical and popular genres. His most enduring works include *Rhapsody in Blue* (1924), *An American in Paris* (1928), and the opera *Porgy and Bess* (1935). The latter was composed the year after his first epileptic seizure, and two years before he was diagnosed with the brain tumour that eventually caused his death. Although his creative output declined significantly during the final three years of his life, he was still able to turn out classic songs such as 'A Foggy Day (in London Town)' and 'Nice Work if You Can Get It' for the Fred Astaire film *A Damsel in Distress* (1937), and his last song, 'Love is Here to Stay', for the movie *The Goldwyn Follies* (1938).

Gershwin's first seizure occurred in 1934, when he was 36 years old. Gregory Sloop has written an article that not only provides a valuable timeline for the composer's progressive illness, but also reconsiders the specific nature of his brain tumour.[177] Gershwin's seizures would start with him experiencing an unpleasant smell like burning rubber. This is an example of an olfactory hallucination, and has its origin in the olfactory cortex, which is the part of the temporal lobe where smell is perceived and interpreted. Gershwin also developed automatisms in relation to the seizures. These are episodes of automatic involuntary behaviour of which there is no personal awareness. For example, on one occasion he tried to push his driver out of the door of a moving car; on another occasion, having just been given a box of chocolates, he crushed it in his hands and smeared himself with the contents. During the performance of his Concerto in F in Los Angeles in 1937, he experienced the smell of burning rubber and blacked out completely, and during a rehearsal of *Porgy and Bess* he fell off the conductor's rostrum.

There are a number of possible reasons why the diagnosis was not made sooner. Not only was Gershwin considered to be a hypochondriac, but also in an effort to avert baldness he had purchased an electric scalp stimulator, and some had suggested that this machine was responsible for the very strange episodes that he experienced. He complained of headaches, was irritable and depressed, and many of his acquaintances, including his own resident psychoanalyst, believed that these symptom had psychological causes. We do not know how frequently his seizures occurred, how physically and mentally disabling they were, and whether his reduced creative output was due to his epilepsy or other factors. However, it is clear that the hallmark quality of his compositions was maintained right to the end. We now know not only that his seizures originated in the temporal lobe, but also from which

---

177 Sloop GD (2001) What caused George Gershwin's untimely death? *Journal of Medical Biography* 9, 28–30.

particular region of the lobe they arose. However, this diagnosis was not made until the final months of Gershwin's life.

In his biography of Gershwin, Alan Kendall[178] describes the events that led up to Gershwin's diagnosis, and his death at the age of 39. His psychoanalyst, Dr Ernst Simmel, who had for so long attributed the symptoms to psychological causes, finally suspected that there was a physical problem, and in June 1937 Gershwin was seen by Dr Ziskind, a neurologist, who told him that the sensation of burning rubber was due to a childhood nasal infection. On receiving this diagnosis, Gershwin sought a second opinion, and had X-rays taken but declined a spinal tap. By that stage his headaches were more severe, he was frequently dropping objects, and his lack of coordination had started to affect his piano playing. On 9 July, after playing the piano for a short period, he went to sleep. He was never to wake again. He was admitted to hospital for surgery on the temporal lobe, and the neurosurgeon identified and removed a large tumour (which he judged to be highly malignant) from the right temporal lobe, but Gershwin died only hours later, on 11 July 1937.

Gregory Sloop points out that the tumour was not thoroughly examined by the pathologist at the time, and that the three-year history of symptoms was incompatible with a highly malignant growth. Based on an analysis of Gershwin's long-standing medical complaints, he suggests that a history of episodic symptoms extending back over 14 years might have been a manifestation of temporal lobe epilepsy. He also suggests, based on a review of photomicrographs, that an alternative, more slow-growing, type of brain tumour called pilocytic astrocytoma was the cause of Gershwin's protracted terminal illness.

The sadness and irony of Gershwin's life are striking. The man who wrote so much about love and marriage never found a long-term partner of his own. Indeed he had a quite repressed personality, although it is unclear to what extent this reflected the effects of living with epilepsy. If Gregory Sloop is correct in suggesting that Gershwin suffered from epilepsy for longer than is generally believed, it might well have shaped his personality. It is noteworthy that he maintained his musical skills to the end, and many have speculated that had the brain tumour been in the left temporal lobe rather than the right one, this would not have been the case. Gershwin once commented that 'No one believes me when I say I'm sick.'[179] The unusual nature of his seizures must have exacerbated this problem, which is perhaps why he concealed them until it was no longer possible to do so.

Hikari Ōe (1963–) is a contemporary Japanese composer who has both autism and epilepsy. He has little verbal output, impaired vision, and diminished coordination. He has

---

178 Kendall A (1989) *George Gershwin: A Biography*. Harrap, London.
179 Fabricant ND (1958) Gershwin's fatal headache. *Eye, Ear, Nose & Throat Monthly* 37, 332–334.

learned to express his feelings through music, and has mastered the art of music notation. A recording of his chamber music has sold over 1 million CDs and won a prize as the top classical Japanese record of the year. His father, Kenzaburo Ōe, won the 1994 Nobel Prize for Literature for his book, *A Personal Matter*,[180] in which he describes the traumatic effects of having a brain-damaged child on family life, and his eventual acceptance of the situation. Hikari Ōe's seizures started at the age of 15, and have since become progressively worse.[181] He has only produced two albums, and it is not known whether he is still composing. He is probably best described as a composer with autism rather than as one with epilepsy, as it is the former condition that constitutes his main disability. He can also be regarded as a musical savant – a person affected by autism (or other forms of cognitive impairment) who exhibits highly developed skills in a very specific area, such as music or mathematics.

The Canadian singer-songwriter and guitarist **Neil Young** (1945–), one of the most influential songwriters and performers of his generation, lives with epilepsy. He began his musical career as a singer, pianist, and harmonica player in his native Canada, before moving to Los Angeles in the late 1960s, where he co-founded the group Buffalo Springfield and subsequently performed both as a solo artist and as a member of Crosby, Stills, Nash & Young (CSN&Y), and Crazy Horse. He has been successful in a variety of other creative fields, in particular songwriting, including the Oscar-nominated title song for *Philadelphia* (1993), and as an environmental activist, fundraiser, and the co-inventor of control systems for model train layouts. His electronics knowledge led to his involvement in the development of uncompressed musical download technology to improve on the sound quality of the MP3 format.

In his lengthy autobiography, *Waging Heavy Peace*,[182] Young only mentions his epilepsy a few times. The first reference relates to a period in his early twenties when he was travelling through Albuquerque: 'Looking back, maybe I had my first seizure there. I know we went to a hospital emergency room but I don't recall much about what happened to me there.' A short while later he experienced his second attack, which involved a sensation of sickness in his stomach, after which he fell to the pavement and remembered faces looking down at him as he recovered, and a feeling 'like I had just been born and I recognized no one. I didn't really know my own name.' Writing about the effect of the condition on his life, he described how 'for years I lived in constant fear that it was going to happen again. I could feel it in my stomach and then get really scared and withdrawn until it went away.' Despite this, no diagnosis was made, no treatment was prescribed, and he continued to indulge in his lifelong obsession with driving cars, along with excessive alcohol consumption, and experimentation with a variety of drugs.

---

180 Ōe K (1969) *A Personal Matter* (translated from the Japanese by J Nathan). Grove Press, Inc., New York.
181 Cameron L (1998) *The Music of Light: The Extraordinary Story of Hikari and Kenzaburo Ōe*. The Free Press, New York.
182 Young N (2012) *Waging Heavy Peace: A Hippie Dream*. Penguin Group, New York.

Eventually, Young's managers arranged an appointment for him at the UCLA Medical Center, where he recalled how staff 'stuck a bunch of things on my head … and told me to go in this dark room and lie down. Then they wired all the things up, and while I was lying there I could feel these little flashes.' This is a description of an electroencephalogram (EEG) with photic stimulation (the use of a flashing light to test whether his epilepsy was photosensitive). He then commented that 'I still feel those today, kind of like little rushes of something, gusts of cosmic wind in my head. My hearing changes for an instant, and it's hard to describe. Anyway, I live with that, and it's nothing.' With regard to the EEG, he concluded that it 'revealed nothing to my knowledge'. Subsequently, after becoming infected with a sexually transmitted disease he attended a clinic, had a blood sample taken, and immediately experienced a seizure. This finally led to the investigation of his epilepsy in 1966, using an investigation known as a lumbar air encephalogram (LAEG). This was long before the availability of CT brain imaging, and his account of the procedure is graphic: 'It is the most painful thing I have ever been through. Pure torture, where they tie you into a big device, stick a needle in you, and inject radioactive dye into your spinal column.' In fact it is air that is injected, and he does describe the bubbles as causing 'the worse pain ever in the universe'. According to Young, 'None of these tests revealed any new information about my condition. There was no conclusion. The doctor's recommendations were that I not take any LSD.' Thereafter his autobiography makes little reference to his epilepsy, but describes how he continued to drive, to collect cars, and generally to indulge in the rock-star lifestyle. There is no mention of anti-epileptic drug (AED) treatment, and his seizures appear to recede into the background, overshadowed by the development of other neurological problems, such as surgery for a herniated lumbar disc and treatment for a cerebral aneurysm.

Young had suffered from polio as a child, and as a result had experienced the effects of ostracism and stigmatization early in life. One of his sons was quadriplegic and had cerebral palsy, another son had suffered intrauterine cerebral hemorrhage, and his daughter had epilepsy. It is possible that the major health problems of his children made him less conscious of the effects of his own epilepsy on his life. Also the very nature of his occupation meant that epilepsy may have impeded his career very little. It is interesting that he never describes himself as being diagnosed 'epileptic', and indeed the condition is referred to in only one of his compositions, 'Burned', a song that he wrote about having a seizure:

Been burned and with both feet on the ground,
I've learned that it's painful comin' down.
No use runnin' away, and there's no time left to stay.
Now I'm finding out that it's so confusin',

No time left and I know I'm losin'.
Flashed and I think I'm fallin' down
Crashed, and my ears can't hear a sound.
No use runnin' away, and there's no time left to stay.
Now I'm finding out that it's so confusin',
No time left and I know I'm losin'.
Now I'm finding out that it's so confusin',
No time left and I know I'm losin'.
Burned and with both feet on the ground.
I've learned that it's painful comin' down.
No use runnin' away, and there's no time left to stay.
Now I'm finding out that it's so confusin',
No time left and I know I'm losin'.

This 'anthem for epilepsy' suggests a much deeper level of insight into the effects of living with the condition than Neil Young conveys in his autobiography.

Prince Rogers Nelson (1958–2016), better known as **Prince** (or, latterly, 'The Artist Formerly Known As Prince'), was a Grammy-Award-winning American singer-songwriter. It was not until he was in his fifties that he spoke publicly about his childhood battle with epilepsy. In 2009, in an interview with the US talk-show host Tavis Smiley, he said 'I've never spoken about this before, but I was born epileptic. I used to have seizures when I was young and my mother and father didn't know what to do or how to handle it, but they did the best they could with what little they had.' The details of his epilepsy and its treatment are uncertain, and something akin to a state of altered consciousness is highlighted by his comment that 'My mother told me one day I walked in to her and said, "Mom, I'm not going to be sick anymore", and she said, "Why?", and I said, "Because an angel told me so."' Some have noted that his music has an almost hallucinatory character, and have speculated that this was influenced by his seizures. Others have suggested that the title of his most famous album, 'Purple Rain', is an allusion to his epilepsy. 'The Sacrifice of Victor' is one of Prince's few songs that directly mention epilepsy:

I was born on a blood-stained table
Cord wrapped around my neck
Epileptic 'til the age of seven
I was sure Heaven marked the deck.

In June 2016, at the age of 57, Prince died of an overdose of fentanyl, the source and purpose of which remain uncertain. During his lifetime he married twice, and he had one child, who had a severe and ultimately fatal form of Pfeiffer's syndrome (premature fusion of some of the skull bones, which affects the shape of the face and head). We do not know much about Prince's epilepsy or its role in his art, but clearly his artistic and performing skills were undimmed by the fact that he lived with this condition.

Elton John (1947–), the English singer, songwriter, pianist, and composer, is an outstandingly accomplished musician. However, his seizures did not become established until after his musical talent had become apparent. He was playing the piano by the age of three, and was awarded a junior scholarship at the Royal Academy of Music when he was eleven. In his late twenties he developed epilepsy after taking a drug overdose, but there was no decline in his musical creativity. He later commented that he came 'very close [to dying]. I mean, I would have an epileptic seizure and turn blue, and people would find me on the floor and put me to bed, and then 40 minutes later I'd be snorting another line.' Drugs such as cocaine, heroin, and stimulants such as amphetamines and ecstasy (MDMA)

can directly affect the brain, producing seizures that may become a permanent long-term problem even if drug abuse stops.

In Chapter 6 we mentioned the English singer-songwriter **Ian Curtis** (1956–1980) in relation to the film *Control* (2007) that chronicles his life and that of the band Joy Division. He was diagnosed with epilepsy at the age of 22, his seizures were severe from the onset of the condition, and he was unsympathetically told by his doctor that his life would be dictated by the condition, which would require strong treatments to control it. Curtis was initially open about his epilepsy, and joined the British Epilepsy Association, but subsequently became more reticent about it. He remained confident in the ability of the doctors to help, and he embraced changes in his treatment with enthusiasm and optimism. However, the 'rockstar lifestyle', with constant access to drugs and alcohol and irregular hours, and the fact that he began to experience side effects from his treatment led to a deterioration in his condition. Despite the birth of a daughter to him and his wife, he became increasingly depressed. His epilepsy became progressively more severe, until he was having at least two tonic–clonic seizures a week, and he could no longer independently care for his daughter. He admitted to the wife of his record manager that he felt he would soon be unable to continue performing live, due to fear of having a seizure while on stage. Even in the recording studio he was prone to seizures, or he would be discovered on the floor of toilets, and he sometimes sustained head injuries as a result of falling. Much of what we know is based on the book written by his widow, Deborah Curtis,[183] and for as long as possible he kept the cause of his

---

183 Curtis D (2007) *Touching from a Distance: Ian Curtis and Joy Division.* Faber and Faber, London.

symptoms a secret from his bandmates. Peter Hook, the band's bass guitarist, often found Curtis unconscious, but did not know what was wrong or how to help him.

In April 1980, the group performed in front of 3000 people at Finsbury Park in London and, contrary to the clear instructions given before the concert, a strobe light was turned on halfway through Joy Division's set. Curtis immediately fell backwards against a drum kit, had a seizure, and was carried off stage. The following month, at the age of just 23, on the eve of Joy Division's debut North American tour, when Curtis had, to all appearances, reached a high point in his musical career, he took his own life by hanging himself in his kitchen, where he was later found by his wife. It seems likely that a combination of uncertainty about how the group would be received in the USA, marital problems, a fear of flying, and an overwhelming concern about his epilepsy led to this tragic outcome. It also highlights the very real risk of suicide associated with epilepsy (which will be discussed in more detail later).

Without access to his medical records it is not possible to ascertain the type of epilepsy from which Ian Curtis suffered. The seizure episode caused by the strobe lighting at the Finsbury Park concert suggests that he had photosensitive epilepsy, but this normally responds well to drugs, which was not the case here. It is possible that although the seizure was attributed to the flashing light it was not actually caused by it.

The Scottish singer **Susan Boyle** (1961–) came to international attention when she appeared on the TV programme 'Britain's Got Talent' in 2009, and sang 'I Dreamed a Dream' from the musical *Les Misérables*. Her spectacular voice and unassuming appearance grabbed the nation's hearts. However, her success put her under a spotlight that made her visibly uncomfortable. When she was a child she was told that she had brain damage and that it was unlikely she would be successful in life. At school she was referred to as 'simple Susan', and experienced more than her fair share of stigmatization and rejection. She describes how 'At school I used to faint a lot. It's something I've never talked about. I had epilepsy. People in the public eye don't have things like that. All through my childhood they'd say epilepsy is to do with mental function. And now I realize it's not. I was up against all those barriers. It wasn't easy.' More recently she was also diagnosed with Asperger's syndrome, and she subsequently commented 'Now I have a clearer understanding of what's wrong and I feel relieved and a bit more relaxed about myself.'

With regard to the depiction of epilepsy in popular music, the only detailed review currently available is that by Sallie Baxendale.[184] Because it is so readily and widely accessible, popular music provides a major platform for influencing the wider public's perceptions of epilepsy. However, although the lyrics of songs sometimes refer to seizures, the images that they conjure up are frequently neither positive nor helpful. The lyrics of modern songs have

---

184 Baxendale S (2008) The representation of epilepsy in popular music. *Epilepsy & Behavior* 12, 165–169.

linked epilepsy and seizures with madness, ecstasy, learning difficulties, sexual acts, and frenetic dancing. Baxendale also draws attention to the frequent use of epilepsy terminology when bands are choosing a name for their ensemble. She cites as examples 'Seizure', 'Aura', and 'Déjà Vu', while a detailed awareness of the anatomy of the brain would have been required to create other names, such as 'Limbic System' and 'Hippocampal Groove.' A prominent Californian punk band was called the 'Falling Sickness', although none of their songs referred to epilepsy. Clearly the allusions to epilepsy in the names that have been chosen for these groups have much more to do with the impact of the words – conveying sudden danger and unpredictability – than with their actual meaning.

Because of the vast repertoire of popular music and lack of the types of database that are available for the movies, the identification of popular songs that contain lyrics about epilepsy or seizures is problematic. The following review, which draws heavily on the work of Sallie Baxendale at University College London and Toba Kerson in the USA,[185] shows that the imagery in many of the lyrics they have identified is discriminatory but has remained uncensored and unchallenged.

The song 'Let's Get Retarded' by the Los Angeles pop and dance-pop group **The Black Eyed Peas** won the 2004 Grammy Award for the year's best 'rap' performance by a group, and was the first song to sell half a million downloads in the USA. Fourteen years later, the group attempted to distance itself from the song's title by reading out a statement by the band member will.i.am, which declared that 'After over a decade of getting messy, loud, and sick, The Black Eyed Peas no longer wish to get retarded in any way, shape, or form.' The lyrics refer to epilepsy only once, in the following section of the song:

> *Let's get ill, that's the deal.*
> *At the gate, we'll bring the bud top drill. (Just)*
> *Lose your mind this is the time*
> *Ya'll test this drill, Just and bang your spine (Just)*
> *Bob your head like epilepsy, up inside your club or in your Bentley*
> *Get messy, loud and sick.*

With the recurring phrase '*Everybody, everybody, let's get into it, get stupid, get retarded, get retarded, get retarded*' the link in the band's mind between epilepsy and mental retardation is evident. The word 'retarded' comes from the Latin verb *retardare*, meaning to hinder or be slow. The dictionary defines it as being less advanced mentally, physically and socially than

---

185 Baxendale S and Kerson T (2010) Epilepsy and the media. In: Pinikahana J and Walker C (eds) *Social Epileptology: Understanding Social Aspects of Epilepsy*. Nova Science Publishers, New York.

is usual. The term is offensive, pejorative, and has become a school playground taunt for those perceived as different. There can be no excuse for the use of this word in a record that is available to millions. The band eventually issued an apology stating that no mockery was intended, and they changed the title of the song to 'Let's get started'. However, by then the damage had been done, and the band's fortune and reputation had been made.

Nicholas Cave (1957–) the Australian singer-songwriter, composer, author, screenwriter and occasional actor, fronted the rock band Nick Cave and the Bad Seeds. The lyrics of one of his songs tell the extraordinary story of Christina the Astonishing, and attribute her recovery from apparent death to a post-ictal (epileptic) stupor:

Christina the Astonishing
Lived a long time ago
She was stricken with a seizure
At the age of twenty-two
They took her body in a coffin
To a tiny church in Liege
Where she sprang up from the coffin
Just after the Agnus Dei.

Born in Belgium in *c.* 1150, Christina the Astonishing (also known as Christina Mirabilis) was considered to be a saint both during her lifetime and for centuries after her death. At the age of 21 she was thought to have died, and was taken to her local church in an open coffin. At her funeral service she rose from her coffin (from 'the dead') during the Agnus Dei, and lived for a further 53 years. The evidence that she might have had epilepsy is scant, and subsequent episodes of self-mutilation suggest that the episode during her funeral may have been caused by hysteria. However, Cave has for some reason linked this episode from the distant past to epilepsy. The Roman Catholic writer Thomas of Cantimpré (1201–1272) describes Christina throwing herself into burning fires without sustaining burns, and immersing herself in frozen rivers without developing hypothermia, but makes no reference to epilepsy.[186] It is not known what led Cave to revisit the story of Christina. The lyrics do not portray negative or offensive attitudes towards those with epilepsy. However, the lyrics of another of his songs, 'Stoney Lodge', describe a woman in a psychiatric hospital whose seizures result in him leaving her: 'When she starts to fucking seizure I'm a leaving her.' Perhaps he chose Christina's story because of a personal

---

186 de Cantimpré T (1999) *The Life of Christina the Astonishing* (translated by MH King). Peregrina Publishing Company, Toronto.

knowledge of epilepsy combined with his desire to believe that the mysterious Christina had this condition.

The group **Malevolent Creation**, who have described themselves as a death metal band, emerged from Buffalo, New York State in the late 1980s. Over the years the original group members have been replaced, and the band returned with its most recent line-up in 2017. Death metal is a form of heavy metal music with lyrics that are preoccupied with death, destruction, and suffering. Their song 'Epileptic Seizure' perceptively and graphically depicts a generalized convulsion and the resultant suffering:

Convulse, twisted
Falling to the ground
Saliva flowing free
Tasting, choking
Swallowed your tongue
Eyes roll back in your head
Frantic twitching
Multiple spasms
Legs begin to buckle
Face blue, can't breathe
Trying to cry out
Your efforts are useless
Hacking vomit
Want to be free
Just don't want to be seen
Convulse …
Consuming your pride
Cursed by this disease
Those around you panic
Onlookers start to freeze.
Living in fear
Tearing your soul
No cure for this pain
This is your hell
Given at birth
Symptoms take course
Seizure taking over

Consuming ...
Convulse ...

The motivation for, background knowledge, and personal experience that led the group to produce these lyrics are not known, but they are clearly both accurate and uncompromisingly negative.

Baxendale concludes from her review that the links between epilepsy, the supernatural, learning difficulties, and sexual ecstasy in the lyrics of popular music are exaggerated, and that in general they present a depressingly negative and stigmatizing view of the condition. The potential effects that the popular music industry may have on public perceptions (especially among the younger generation) of people with epilepsy should not be underestimated. Equally, the potential benefits of conveying a more positive message should not be ignored. In particular, a few musical artists who themselves have epilepsy have been willing to step into the limelight as role models, and have described living with the condition in more neutral or even positive terms.

Epilepsy in the theatre and in actors

The literature on the depiction of epilepsy and seizures in the theatre is much more limited than that on the condition in music and musicians. Michael Trimble and Dale Hesdorffer have provided a review on epilepsy in the theatre,[187] which focuses mainly on Greek and Shakespearean plays. They trace the representation of 'madness' in the Greek tragedies, highlighting the play *Iphigenia among the Taurians* by Euripides (480–406 bce), which probably represents the first theatrical depiction of a seizure. In this tragicomedy a young shipwrecked sailor is described as 'jerking his head up and down – groaning aloud as his hands shook' and with 'his chin dripping foam – then regaining consciousness'. Seizures also feature in *Heracles*, one of Euripides' later plays. We have already mentioned Shakespeare's portrayal of epilepsy in *Julius Caesar* and *Othello* (see Chapter 5). Shakespeare certainly seemed to be well versed in conditions of the brain, depicting dementia in *As You Like It*, stroke in *Henry IV*, and what would pass as Parkinson's disease in *Henry VI*.

The French physician Jean-Martin Charcot (1825–1893) has already been mentioned in relation to the history of epilepsy (see Chapter 2). His highly theatrical teaching style, which would be completely unacceptable today, included putting patients on display as

---

[187] Trimble M and Hesdorffer DC (2016) Representations of epilepsy on the stage: From the Greeks to the 20th century. *Epilepsy & Behavior* 57, 238–242.

entertainment. Charcot opened the doors of what he described as a 'museum of living pathology' at the Salpêtrière Hospital, Paris to allow the public to observe patients with neurological disorders, including epilepsy and hysteria (he often struggled to distinguish between the latter two conditions). This public exposure increased general knowledge, if not understanding, of the conditions on display, which were subsequently frequently depicted in books, plays, and operas. It also led to the vogue for *gommeuses epileptiques* (epileptic singers) who performed live in the cafés and concert halls of nineteenth-century Paris. Sallie Baxendale and Fiona Marshall have provided an illuminating account of these entertainers who mimicked seizures or hysteria.[188] In addition they describe the originator of the vogue, the café-concert singer **Jean-Paul Habans** (1845–1908) (also known as 'Paulus'), whose performances involved much grimacing and jerking.

The most famous of all the epileptic singer-dancers was **Emilie Marie Bouchard** (1874–1939), an Algerian who arrived in Paris in the early 1890s and adopted the stage name of 'Polaire' (meaning 'Pole Star'). She became known as *la gommeuse epileptique* (the gummy epileptic) and *l'epileptique sauteuse* (the epileptic leaper), and audiences were cautioned against watching her act in case it caused them to have seizures. Her large piercing eyes, flowing black hair, and tiny waist were perceived as giving her a primitive, satanic appearance. Her performances involved screaming, writhing, twisting, jerking, hand twisting, and screaming out loud, and often ended in swooning, loss of consciousness, or ecstasy.

A popular song of that time, entitled 'The Epileptic Parisian', contains the line 'when I hear the music I become epileptic'. Indeed such was the appeal of these performers to the masses that they were captured in paint by the prominent artists of the time. For example, in 1895, Henri de Toulouse-Lautrec produced a poster of 'Polaire' performing her epileptic dance.

To understand the vogue for exploiting epilepsy to enhance the careers and popularity of these performers, and the legacy of this phenomenon, we need to consider one of Charcot's most vociferous critics, the Swedish physician and psychiatrist **Axel Munthe** (1857–1949). In his autobiography, *The Story of San Michele*,[189] Munthe describes in detail Charcot's theatre of curiosities at the Salpêtrière Hospital, where he spent some time as an 'unsupervised medical student' and observed the great French physician, with his 'cruel sensitive lips', at first hand. In particular he witnessed Charcot's riveting weekly stage demonstrations of his patients in front of a public audience. Munthe describes the evenings as 'nothing but an absurd farce, a hopeless muddle of truth and cheating, attended by a public audience full of morbid curiosity'. He also comments that 'the huge amphitheatre was full to the last place with a

---

188 Baxendale S and Marshall F (2012) The epileptic singers of belle époque Paris. *Medical Humanities* 38, 88–90.
189 Munthe A (1928) *The Story of San Michele*. John Murray, London.

hugely diverse audience drawn from all Paris – authors, playwrights, journalists, actors and actresses'. For those who could not attend, the '*Iconographie Photographique de la Salpêtrière*' provided a photographic record of female patients with a wide range of conditions, including epileptic seizures.

Charcot's theatrical presentations undoubtedly had an impact on the culture of the time, and their legacy included the performances of the epileptic singers, representing the fusion of clinic and cabaret. Interestingly, Charcot and his staff were at pains to distinguish between epilepsy and hysteria, and treated them very differently. Those with hysteria became the 'star' patients, possibly because they could be manipulated to 'perform' dramatically at will. They were given much more attention and hospital privileges than the epileptic patients, who were perceived as having a disorder that could not be controlled and was therefore of little theatrical value in Charcot's dramatic presentations.

The epileptic singers and performers were a major attraction of Parisian nightlife for a quarter of a century, but their popularity declined after Charcot's death. There was no longer public access to live 'demonstrations' of physically and mentally ill patients, and neurology and psychiatry were beginning to diverge as two separate specialties, the former dealing with disorders of the brain (such as epilepsy) and the latter with mental illnesses (such as hysteria). However, there was still much confusion among the general public, many of whom continued to perceive epilepsy as a mental illness. There can be no doubt that the *gommeuses epileptiques* had a very negative effect on public perceptions of epilepsy, and the sinister appearance of many of the performers (such as 'Polaire') accentuated its satanic image.

The Innocents (1961), a film adaptation of the novella *The Turn of the Screw* (1898) by the American author **Henry James** (1843–1916), was described by the American film critic Pauline Kael as the best ghost movie she had ever seen. James claimed that he was so scared by his own story that proofreading made him 'so frightened that I was afraid to go upstairs to bed'. In 1950 the British playwright Harold Pinter directed the Broadway stage adaptation, also entitled *The Innocents*, which has since been revived at the National and Almeida Theatres in London.

The story concerns a young governess who has recently been hired to look after a man's young niece and nephew after the assumed death of their parents. The setting is a large country house that soon appears to be haunted by the spirits of two dead servants. The governess, who repeatedly sees the figures of a man and woman (whose history and appearance are known to the elderly housekeeper), is known to suffer from 'turns', which are associated with her hallucinations of seeing people as well as with feelings of dread and familiarity or déjà vu. During one of the attacks she falls to the ground shaking, and loses awareness of what is going on around her. The ghosts are never seen by the children or the housekeeper, but only by the governess. This has led to the suggestion that she was suffering from a neurosis or hysteria. However, epilepsy seems a more plausible explanation for her symptoms. In the relatively recent London revival of the play, directed by the former neurologist Jonathan Miller, the young nephew dies in the arms of the governess as she unintentionally suffocates him during one of her seizures. It has been pointed out that Henry James' brother, William James, was a professor of psychology at Harvard, and that through him not only did Henry James acquire a detailed knowledge of epilepsy, but also he might have met Hughlings Jackson, the pioneering neurologist whose research focused on epilepsy. Such knowledge might explain why the governess's symptoms so closely parallel those of temporal lobe epilepsy. J Purdon Martin, an eminent British neurologist, wrote an article on the subject of the governess and epilepsy, and was adamant that she suffered from temporal lobe seizures.[190] He evaluated her 'turns' in detail, and in particular her description (in the original book, *The Turn of the Screw*) of the final event leading to the child's death: 'I sprang straight up ... it was like fighting with a demon for a human soul ... held out, in the tremor of my hands, at arm's length.'

If it is indeed epilepsy that is depicted, its portrayal is negative. The governess is shrouded in the supernatural, and the final outcome is both disturbing and tragic. Although she is heard narrating the tale many years after the events took place, there is no indication of what has become of her and whether her hallucinatory episodes have ceased.

David Fishelson (1956–), the American playwright and director, is best known as the producer of *Golda's Balcony*, the longest-running one-woman show in the history of Broadway. He has also written and directed plays based on two novels by Fyodor Dostoyevsky, *The Idiot* and *The Brothers Karamazov*, which were discussed in Chapter 4. The stage adaptation of *The Idiot* alludes to Prince Myshkin's epilepsy but, disconcertingly, depicts him lapsing back into idiocy (in other words, epilepsy) as a result of society eventually destroying him through its desire for wealth and power. In *The Brothers Karamazov* the epilepsy theme of the book has been largely ignored.

The Pulitzer Prize-winning play *Night Mother* by the American playwright and novelist **Marsha Norman** (1947–) opened on Broadway in 1983 and remains her best-known work. The play is set in the living room and kitchen of Thelma Gates and her daughter Jessie. In her introduction to the characters, Norman describes Jessie as 'in her late thirties or early forties, pale and vaguely unsteady physically' and comments that 'it is only in the last year that she has gained control of her mind and body, she is determined to hold on to that control'. The two women have lived together for some time, and have developed a shorthand way of communicating, as Jessie talks only a little. The play begins with Jessie asking her mother for her father's old service revolver so that she can end her stultifying and empty life.

---

190 Purdon Martin J (1973) Neurology in fiction: The Turn of the Screw. *British Medical Journal* 4, 717–721.

Jessie sees no future for herself, and because of her epilepsy she only ventures out for her hospital appointments. She is divorced from her husband, and her (absent) son has become a petty thief and drug addict. Her mother responds to the request for the revolver by telling Jessie that 'It must be time for your medication.' She also demeans Jessie by questioning her competence even to successfully shoot herself: 'You will miss. You'll end up a vegetable.'

Thelma then tries to save the situation by telling Jessie the truth about her epilepsy, which was not the result of a riding accident, as Jessie had been led to believe, but had been inherited from her beloved father. As the play progresses we learn the extent of the destructive effect that epilepsy has had on Jessie's life, added to which she is now being told that her father is to blame. She has been unable to find work, her friends and neighbours are avoiding her, her brother has deserted her, and her facial features have been coarsened by the drug (Dilantin) that she has been taking. When Thelma tells Jessie, in relation to the brother's desertion, that 'Your fits made him sick and you know it', Jessie corrects her by saying 'Say seizures, not fits. Seizures.'

Graphic images of Jessie's seizures are provided as her mother describes her 'crumple in a heap like a puppet' like 'someone cut the strings all at once' and 'gagging, sucking air in and out – your mouth bites down and I have to get your tongue out of the way fast' and 'then the jerks slow down and you wet yourself.' In the end Jessie quietly closes and locks her bedroom door, and a shot is heard.

This remarkable play, with its candid portrayal of the tragic aspects of epilepsy, stands alongside the book and film *Electricity* as a realistic account of the feelings of guilt, worthlessness, social isolation, and despair that are experienced by many people with the condition. It is a story that needs to be told over and over again, but there is a positive message, as has been pointed out by Frank Rich, the theatre critic of the *New York Times*, in his review of the play: 'Night Mother – say no to hope? It's easy to feel that way after reeling from this play's crushing blow. But there can be hope if there is understanding, and it is Marsha Norman's profound achievement that she brings both understanding and dignity to a forgotten and tragic American life.'[191]

Performance art was used controversially by the Portuguese dancer and choreographer **Rita Marcalo** to display 'real' seizures to a live theatre audience. In 2008, she received a grant from the Arts Council England to stage a show called *Involuntary Dances* in which she planned to attempt to induce a seizure. Marcalo developed epilepsy in her teens and had around two seizures a year when she was on medication. The process of bringing on a seizure required her to stop her drug treatment, fast, deprive herself of sleep, and be subjected

---

[191] Rich F (1983) Theater: suicide talk in "Night Mother". *New York Times*, 1 April. www.nytimes.com/1983/04/01/theater/theater-suicide-talk-in-night-mother.html

to strobe lighting during the performance. The show was intended to last for 24 hours, and the audience was encouraged to film the resulting seizure on their mobile phones. The planned performance drew criticism on the grounds of its appropriateness and the Arts Council's use of public funds. The Arts Council responded to this by stating that 'The grant supports innovative and regional artists. Her project explores a disability issue.' They offered the reassurance that a risk assessment had been conducted and that medical support would be present throughout.

Writing in the *Independent* newspaper, Jonathan Brown commented on the forthcoming event as follows: 'The audience at the Bradford Playhouse next month will be invited to film her convulsions, which she intends to bring on by a variety of methods including alcohol and staring at strobe lights. She said she will also deploy techniques common in animal testing.'[192] Marcalo defended her show, which had been condemned by epilepsy organizations, stating that 'As someone with epilepsy, the threat of seizure is something I deal with every day of my life. It is an invisible disability but most of us know someone with it. My intention is to raise awareness of the condition by making it visible. People will have their own opinion but I am doing this from an artistic perspective.' She denied that her actions involved any risk, and added 'I am interested in creating work that makes people consider certain things they don't normally think about. It raises questions. I knew it could be controversial but I am doing this because it is personal to me.' Ironically she remained seizure-free throughout the performance, thereby succeeding in demonstrating the unpredictability of epilepsy.

Allan Sutherland, a film maker who had previously tried to induce and film his own seizures, wrote about Marcalo's attempt and the condemnation of it by the epilepsy charities sector: 'Part of the controversy has been about whether the performance is a good way to raise awareness about epilepsy. For disability charities, raising awareness is pretty much synonymous with raising funds. What Marcalo's piece highlights is that adults with epilepsy own their own bodies and have a right to choose what to do with them. It illustrates that we are able to speak for ourselves, and don't need charitable organizations to step in on our behalf.'[193]

A number of film actors with epilepsy have been open about their condition and have generally supported the raising of awareness of the disorder. However, due to the live nature of theatre performances, the relative lack of stage actors with epilepsy is understandable, as the risk of seizures occurring on stage or just prior to a performance would be too great.

---

192 Brown J (2009) Artist to have an epileptic fit live on stage. *Independent*, 20 November 2009. www.independent.co.uk/arts-entertainment/art/news/artist-to-have-an-epileptic-fit-live-on-stage-1824122.html

193 Sutherland A (2009) Epilepsy as live art isn't controversial. *The Guardian*, 20 November 2009. www.theguardian.com/stage/theatreblog/2009/nov/20/epilepsy-live-art-rita-marcalo

Danny Glover (1946–), the American actor, film director, and political activist, had epilepsy as a child but it had remitted by the time he reached adulthood and started his acting career. Therefore, in his case concerns about having a seizure in front of a live audience were probably not a hindrance to his performances. Nevertheless he has become a champion for the North American Epilepsy Foundation, and regularly makes public speeches on the subject of increasing awareness about epilepsy.

Margaux Hemingway (1955–1996), a film actress and fashion model, and the granddaughter of the writer Ernest Hemingway, is believed to have died from an overdose of phenobarbital, which she had been taking to control her epilepsy. There was a family history of suicide; her grandfather and three other family members took their own lives. She had experienced seizures from the age of seven. During her career as a supermodel in the 1970s she had a million-dollar contract with Fabergé. She then went on to pursue a film career, and in 1988 she appeared in her one and only stage production, *The Women*. Throughout her life she struggled with depression, alcohol and drug addiction, and failed relationships, as well as with epilepsy, and she died alone and had to be identified by dental records. The extent of the role of her epilepsy in her eventual social isolation is not known.

The acclaimed Welsh stage and film actor **Richard Burton** (1929–1984), born Richard Jenkins, the son of a coal miner, is now often best remembered for his hell-raising lifestyle and his turbulent relationship with the actress Elizabeth Taylor. There is no record of him having epilepsy in childhood, and the main anecdotal evidence that he suffered from the condition in adulthood comes from Michael Munn's biography of the actor.[194] Munn states that Burton lived in terror most of his life because of what he himself described as 'this thing in my head'. He also comments that epilepsy was never officially diagnosed because of Burton's fear of illness and doctors, and that 'alcohol was a cure of sorts'. Richard Burton's family has been scathing about the accuracy of this biography, which was serialized in the *Sunday Express* newspaper, and indeed Munn's epilepsy 'diagnosis' was based on just one formal interview with Burton, on a film set. An earlier biography by Melvyn Bragg,[195] written with the cooperation of members of Burton's family and with access to his diaries and letters, outlines Burton's many health problems, in particular the destructive effects of his alcohol addiction, but does not mention epilepsy. Bragg does describe Burton 'being found shaking in the wings of the theatre, given a couple of brandies and sent on. Alcohol had been the best medicine at hand.' If the actor did have shaking bouts these seem likely to have been caused by alcohol withdrawal symptoms.

---

194 Munn M (2008) *Richard Burton: Prince of Players*. JR Books, London.
195 Bragg M (1988) *Richard Burton: A Life*. Little, Brown and Company, Boston, MA.

Conclusion

In general, musicians and actors with epilepsy have remained silent or been reticent about their condition unless they have become seizure-free. Contrary to some claims that have been made, partly based on the perceived absence of epilepsy among classical musicians, musical creativity is not incompatible with this condition. Many composers of classical music lived in times when epilepsy was still perceived as a symbol of demonic possession, so were unlikely to admit to having the condition. The lives of present-day musicians and singer-songwriters in the field of popular music in particular are much more likely to be familiar to us, so it is not surprising that larger numbers of these musical artists with epilepsy can be identified. Modern singer-songwriters such as Neil Young, Prince, and Elton John have demonstrated that people with epilepsy can have highly developed skills for both creating and performing music.

There seems to be a relative lack of stage plays featuring epilepsy, although this is probably partly due to the limited research that has been undertaken to identify them. Thus, between Shakespeare's *Julius Caesar* and *Othello* and the Broadway stage adaptation of Henry James' *The Turn of the Screw* there appears to be a gap of around 350 years. *Night Mother*, Marsha Norman's dark and tragic account of the worst aspects of living with epilepsy, highlights the need to help the general public to understand the most devastating outcomes of having epilepsy. Yet it seems likely that, in much the same way as the epilepsy charities condemned Rita Marcalo, they would view the negative aspects of Marsha Norman's play as outweighing its educational value. Finally, it is understandable that a stage acting career may well not appeal to people with epilepsy, due to the high risk of seizures occurring before or just after a live performance.

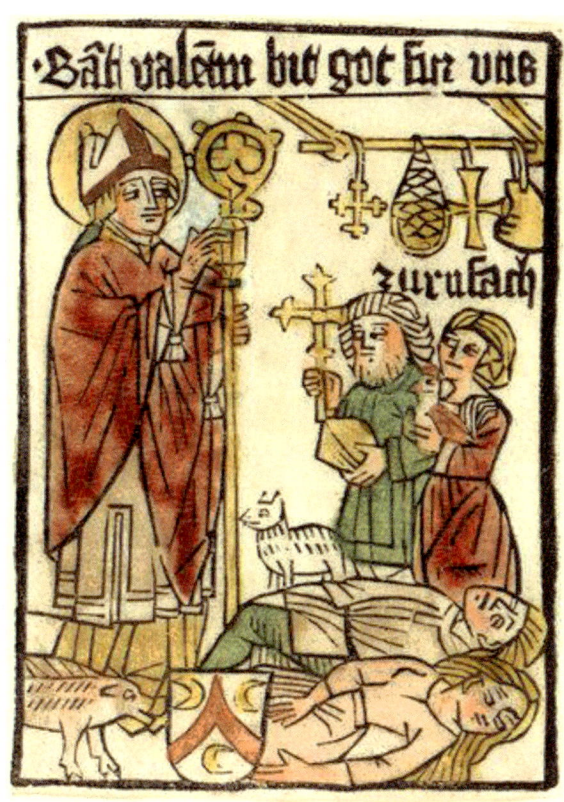

Figure 1. Saint Valentine.
Woodcut by an unknown fifteenth-century German artist. National Gallery of Art. Washington, DC. (1943.3.632)

Figure 2. The homunculus.
A distorted representation of the human body, based on 'mapping' of the proportional areas of the brain dedicated to motor and sensory functions, for different parts of the body. Artist: Ralf Stephan.

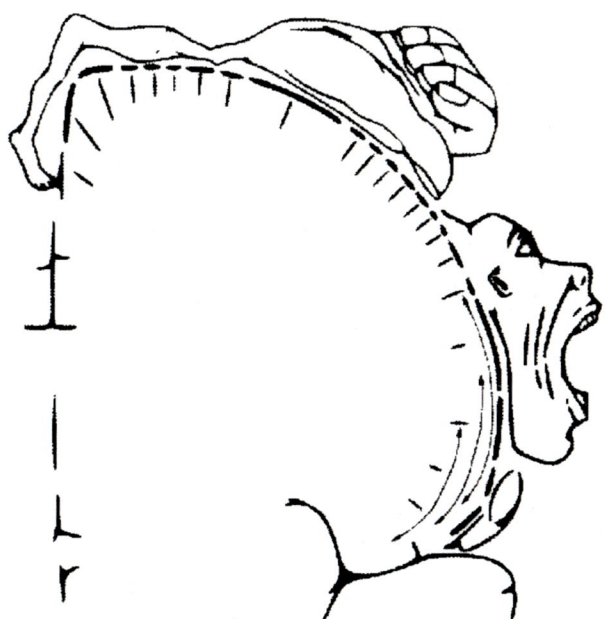

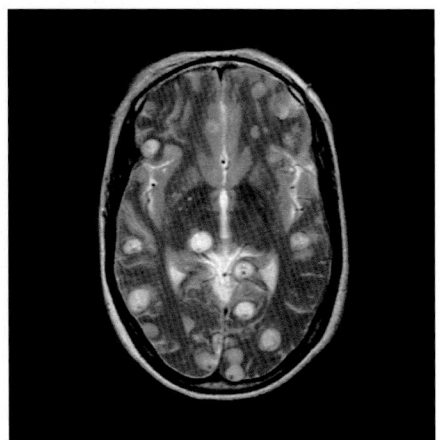

Figure 3. MRI of neurocysticercosis: multiple brain cysts caused by the pork tapeworm (Taenia solium).

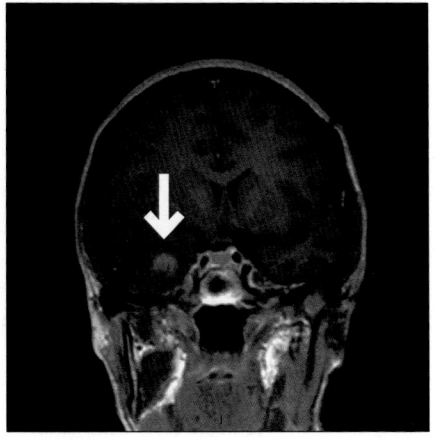

Figure 4. MRI of tumour in the right temporal lobe that is causing frequent temporal lobe (complex partial) seizures.

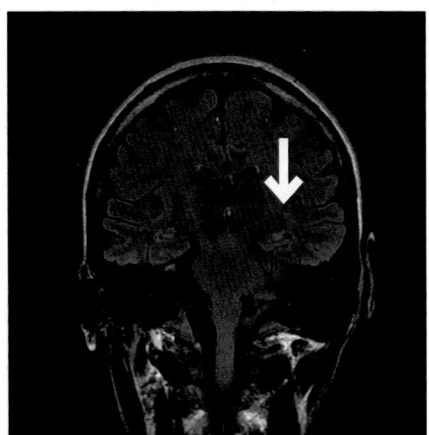

Figure 5. MRI of left-sided mesial temporal sclerosis (MTS) with shrinkage of the deepest part of the temporal lobe.

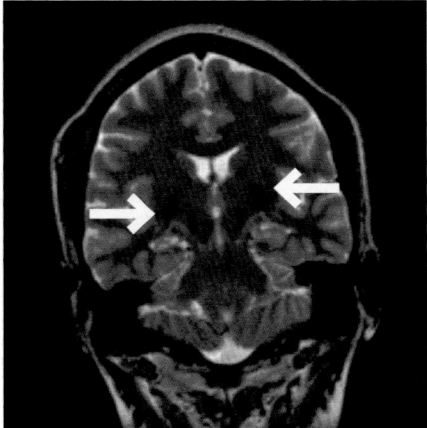

Figure 6. MRI of focal cortical dysplasia (FCD) with islands of the grey matter, normally the brain's outer coat, buried deep within its tissue.

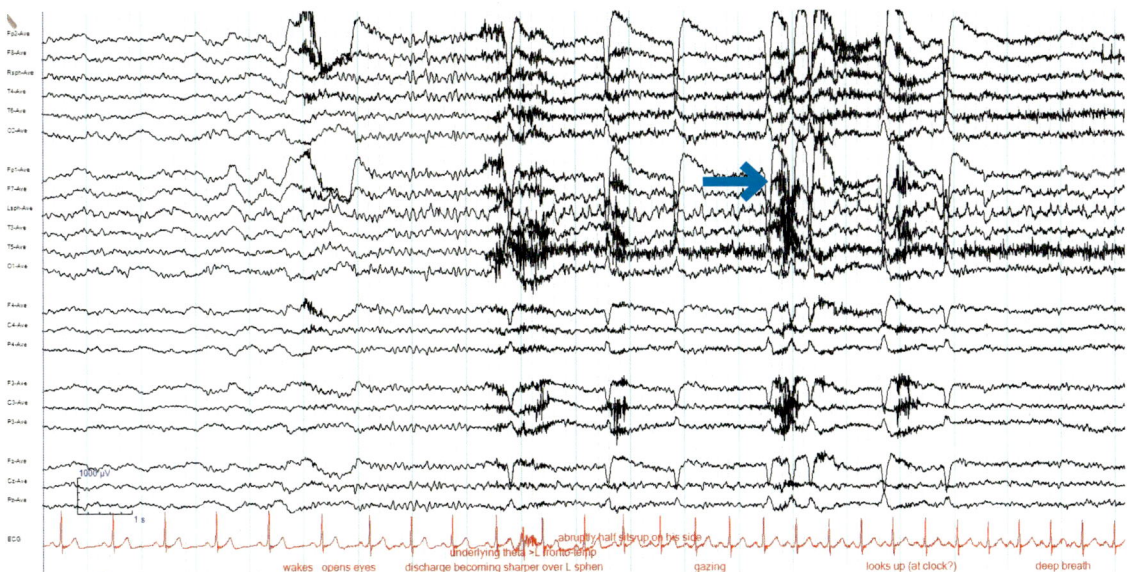

Figure 7. Electroencephalogram (EEG) of focal epilepsy with electrical spikes and waves arising from the left temporal lobe. The red trace at the bottom shows the heart rate.

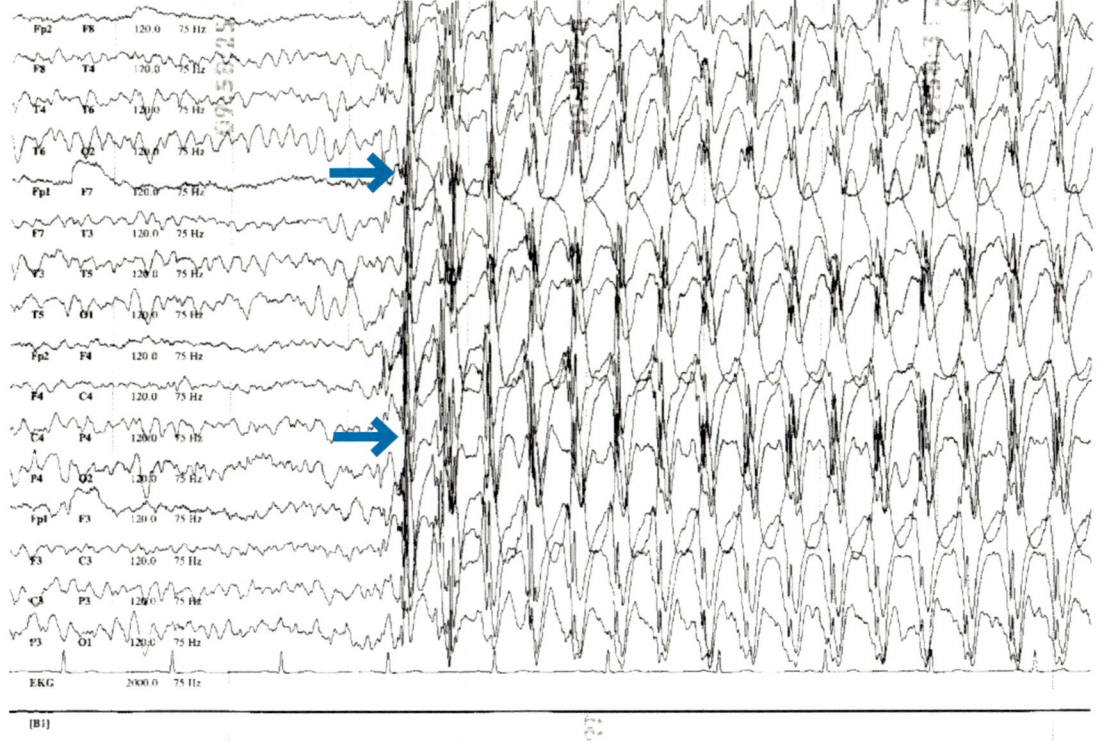

Figure 8. Electroencephalogram (EEG) of generalized epilepsy with electrical spikes and waves arising simultaneously throughout both sides of the brain.

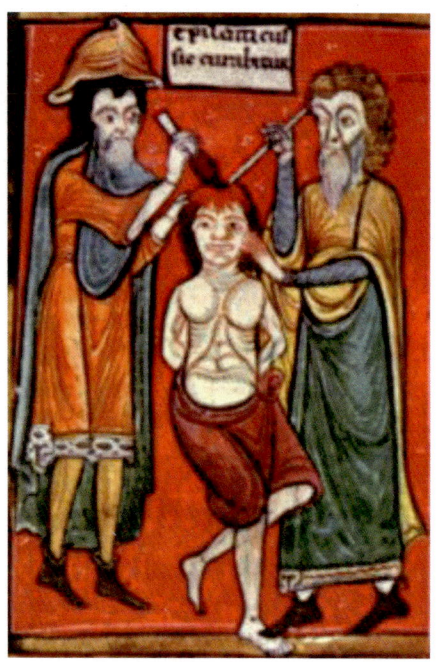

Figure 9. *Epilepticus Sic Curabitur* ('The way to cure epilepsy') (late twelfth century) by an unknown twelfth-century artist. Sloane Manuscript (collection of medical manuscripts), British Library, London.

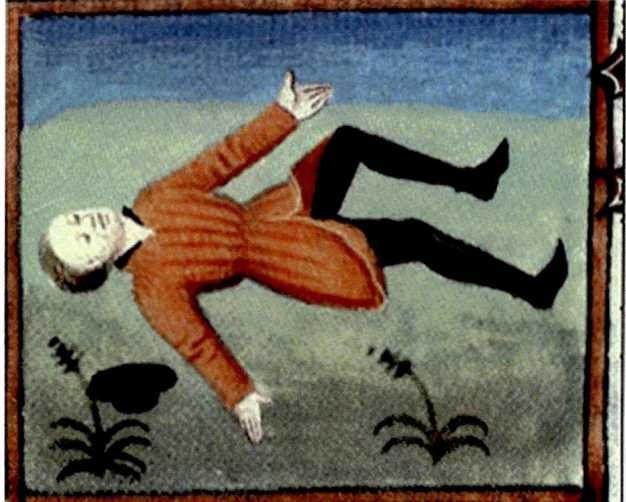

Figure 10. *Serious Scourge the Physicians call Epilencie.* Illustration from the fifteenth-century *Book of Characteristics* by the Franciscan monk known as Bartholomew the English. Bibliothèque Nationale de France.

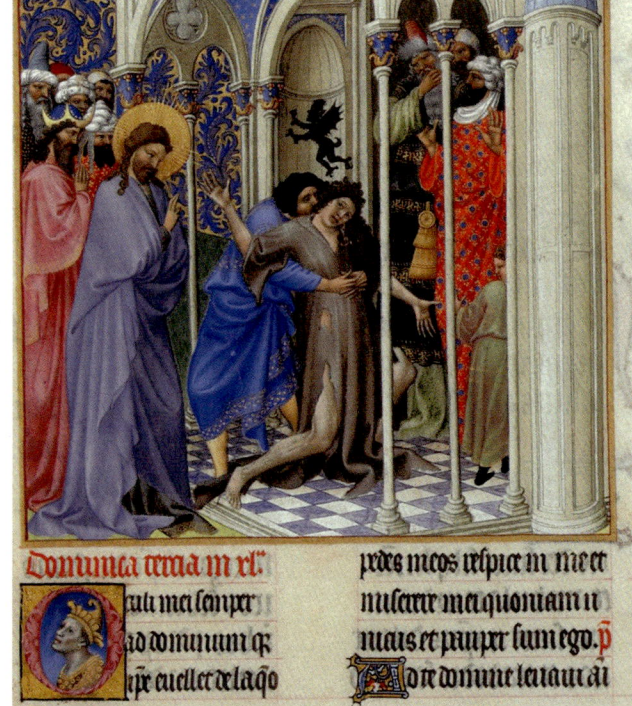

Figure 11. *Les Très Riches Heures du Duc de Berry* (1413–1416). Illustration from the thirteenth-century illuminated manuscript by Herman, Paul, and Jean de Limbourg. Ink on vellum. Musée Condé, Chantilly, France.

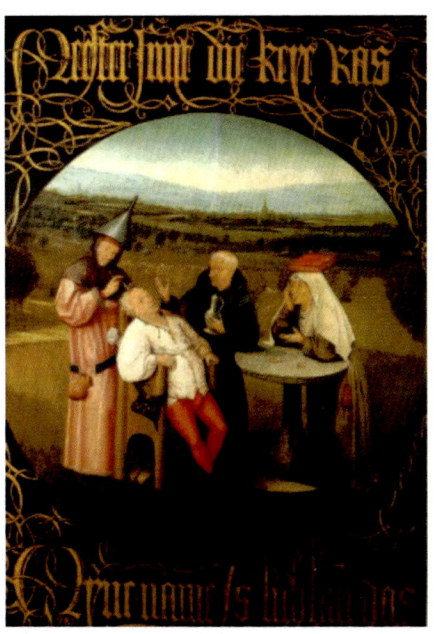

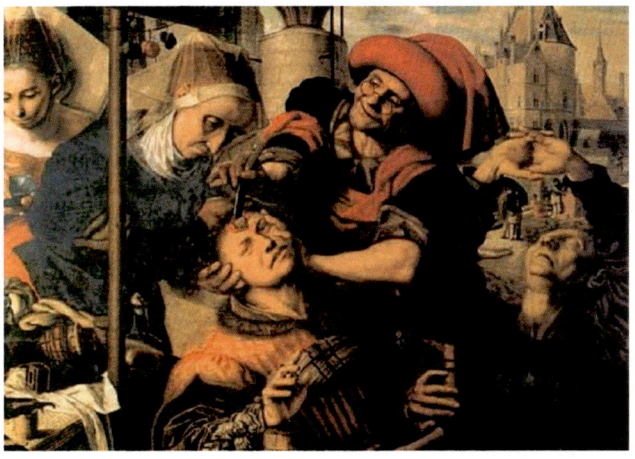

Figure 13. *The Surgeon* (c. 1550) by Jan Sanders van Hemessen. Oil on panel. Museo Nacional del Prado, Madrid.

Figure 12. *The Cure of Folly* (also known as *The Extraction of the Stone of Madness*) (1475–1480) by Hieronymus Bosch ('El Bosco'). Oil painting on board. Museo Nacional del Prado, Madrid.

(Below) Figure 14. *Pilgrimage of the Epileptics to the Church at Molenbeek* by Pieter Bruegel. Wood panel painting. Private collection. In the public domain (location unknown).

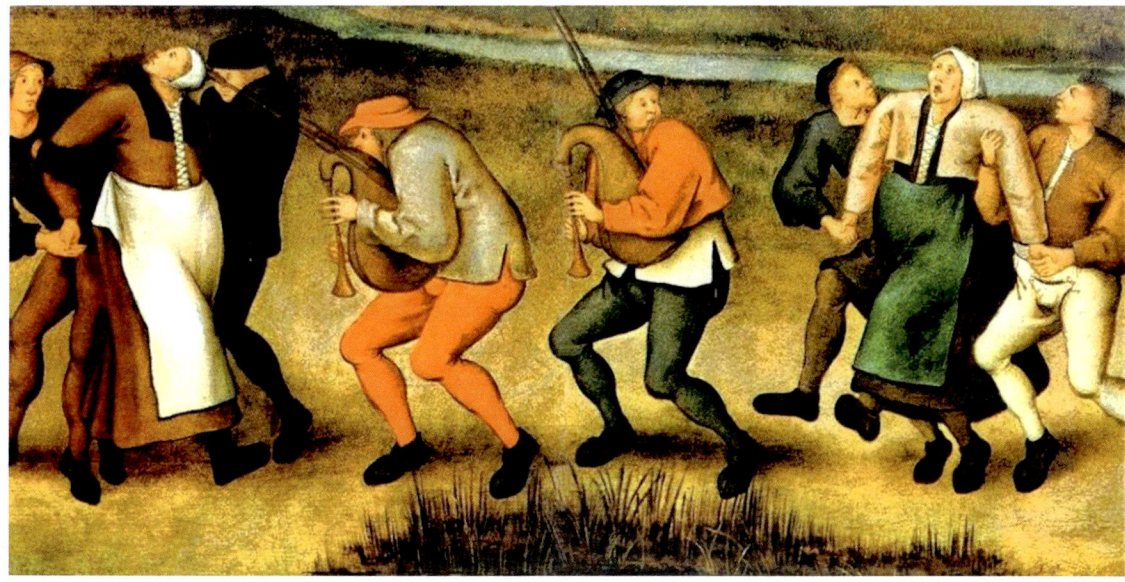

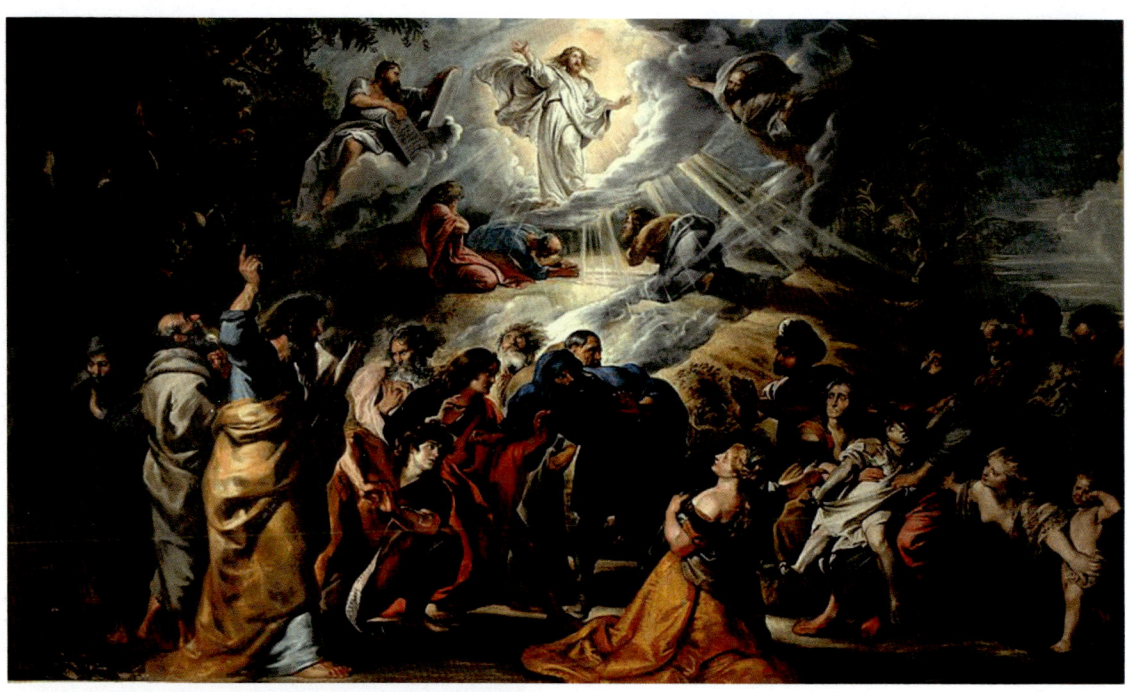

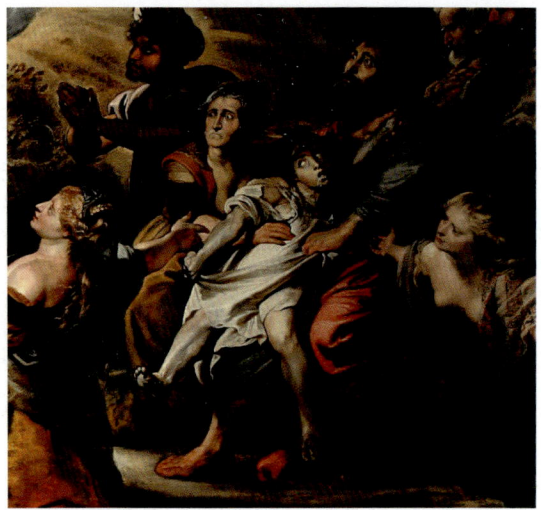

Figure 15. *The Transfiguration* (c. 1604–1606) by Peter Paul Rubens. Oil on canvas. Musée des Beaux-Arts de Nancy.

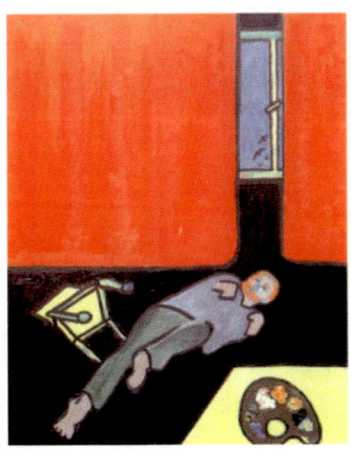

Figure 16. *The Red Curtain* (c. 1965). Anonymous painting. German Epilepsy Museum, Kork.

Figure 17. *Transcending* by Jennifer Hall. Computer graphic.

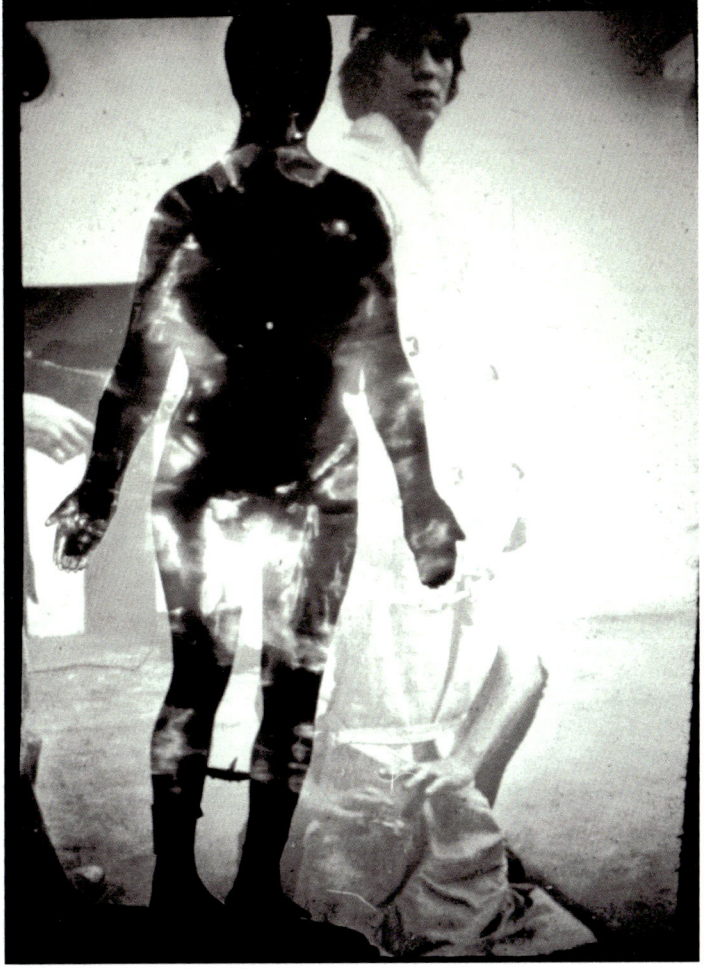

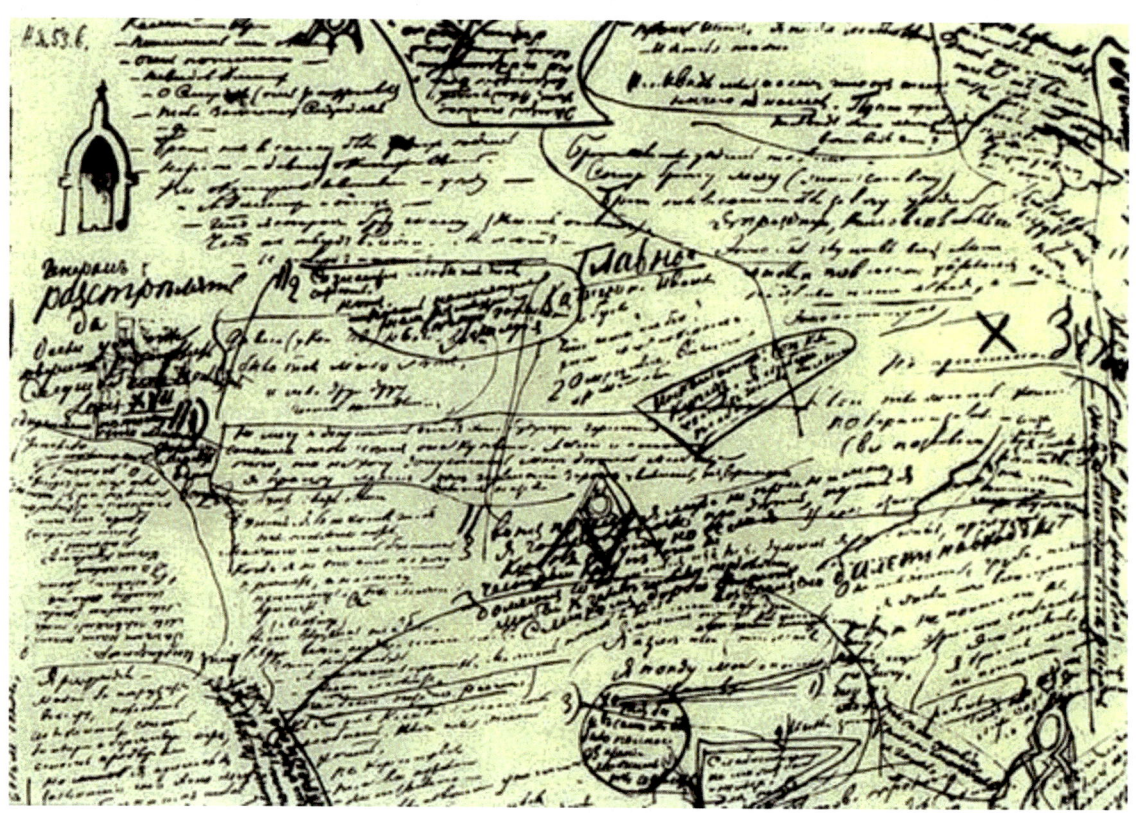

Figure 18. A page from the first draft of *The Brothers Karamazov* by Fyodor Dostoevsky (1880), demonstrating his hypergraphia (excessive writing and doodling).

PART III

Epilepsy in the media

CHAPTER 8
Epilepsy in print, online, and social media

In its landmark document, *Epilepsy Across the Spectrum*,[196] the US Institute of Medicine comments that health information 'of varying accuracy' is widely available and frequently accessed 'in today's crowded media marketplace'. Its long list of potential information sources includes the printed word, broadcasts, online websites, YouTube, and Facebook. In the USA the Kaiser Family Foundation has conducted a survey of the huge changes in the methods used by young people to receive and disseminate information.[197] It identified a dramatic increase in the amount of time spent each day viewing all media, and a decline in the amount of time spent accessing the printed word through books and newspapers.

The increasing role of mobile media, such as smartphones, across all age groups has changed both the manner and speed at which positive and negative perceptions of health issues are received. Such information can now be disseminated to a much larger population.

Moreover, the news media can be manipulated for the purposes of marketing or of influencing political opinion, to the benefit or detriment of perceptions of long-term health conditions such as epilepsy. In the UK a recent study by Ofcom[198] examined which media

---

196 Institute of Medicine (US) Committee on the Public Health Dimensions of the Epilepsies (2012) *Epilepsy Across the Spectrum: Promoting Health and Understanding*. The National Academies Press, Washington, DC.
197 Rideout V, Foehr U and Roberts D (2010) *Generation M²: Media in the Lives of 8- to 18-Year-Olds*. The Henry J. Kaiser Family Foundation, Menlo Park, CA.
198 Ofcom (2019) *News Consumption in the UK*. www.ofcom.org.uk/__data/assets/pdf_file/0027/157914/uk-news-consumption-2019-report.pdf

platforms were most commonly used to access news, and found that television was the most widely used primary source of news information among people over the age of 65 years, whereas the Internet was the main news source for those aged 16–24 years. Overall, nearly one-third of the respondents relied predominantly on their smartphone.

A recent US study conducted by Neilsen Scarborough, an organization that specializes in surveying consumers for marketing purposes, was reported in the American business magazine *Forbes*.[199] It gave a surprisingly rosy picture of the state of hard-copy newspapers, indicating that 51 per cent of readers access the print version alone. This trend was also found among the millennial respondents, boding well for the future of newsprint despite speculation about its imminent demise.

The press and news media

The press and news media are often referred to as 'the Fourth Estate', a term that reflects their independence, freedom, and ability to exert significant social influence. In view of this power, the accuracy of the information that they provide is critically important, especially in relation to complex health issues. This can conflict with the need to inform the public with succinctness, especially when the underlying narrative is complex and a range of different views are held. In this situation, responsible reporters will avoid bias by seeking advice from an expert while they are researching the story. However, if advice is sought from an independently resourced policy group or 'think tank', which then delivers a perspective that reflects the vested interests or political agenda of its funders, bias will creep in. Furthermore, newspapers themselves tend to have an editorial slant on politically contentious issues. An important role of many epilepsy charities is to try to promote responsible reporting by the press of stories about people's experiences of seizures, or advances in treatment.

The UK charity Epilepsy Action provides a 24-hour press office information service that journalists can consult to ensure the accuracy of their reporting. Its Media Press Officer, Claudia Christie (personal communication, November 2018), has reported receiving approximately 100 enquiries per year directly from the press, although she commented that this did not reflect the total amount of press office work done behind the scenes on behalf of people with epilepsy. She also described an example of how the press and charities can work together to ensure accuracy in the reporting of legislation that might potentially disadvantage the disabled. In the UK the Government Department of Work and Pensions

---

199 Fletcher P (2016) Good news for newspapers: 69% of U.S. population still reading. www.forbes.com/sites/paulfletcher/2016/12/26/good-news-for-newspapers-69-of-u-s-population-still-reading/#2bc83f26723c

(DWP) introduced a new scheme termed Personal Independence Payments (PIP) to replace Disability Living Allowance (DLA) as a state benefit for people living with disability. An article in the *Mirror* newspaper reported on the new scheme's assessment process and the delays and traumas faced by the disabled when trying to navigate their way through it.[200] To illustrate this, with Epilepsy Action's assistance, the experiences of a 33-year-old woman with epilepsy were outlined in a disturbing account of someone having to struggle not only with her condition but also with a cumbersome bureaucratic process. This gave the story a focus and impact that increased the public's knowledge and understanding of the situation. There are many other examples of how this collaborative approach can benefit everyone involved, some of which will be discussed later.

Newspaper articles about epilepsy can take a number of different forms. They may tell the story of a person with epilepsy who has suddenly become newsworthy either through a worthy act, such as fundraising, or through a crime or accident that is deemed to be seizure-related. Alternatively, they may outline a new therapeutic breakthrough, or address a lack of healthcare resources alongside the need to ensure the equitable availability of new effective treatments. We can recognize the political persuasions of newspapers through the prism with which they view certain issues. Today, in Western societies, in general the right-wing press is regarded as being supportive of the interests of the powerful, wealthy, and healthy, whereas the left-wing press is viewed as upholding the rights of people of lower socioeconomic status as well as those of the disabled. This suggests that the right-wing press would be more likely to have a negative view of disability and to focus on people whom they feel are not worthy of state benefits (so-called 'benefit cheats') or of support (so-called 'scroungers'), whereas the reporting of healthcare issues in the more liberal press would focus more on medical breakthroughs and positive personal stories. However, the most extreme examples of the press lambasting and demonizing people with disabilities, including epilepsy, came from Nazi Germany between 1933 and 1945, under the dictatorship of Adolf Hitler. The impact of the eugenics movement and compulsory sterilization programmes is discussed in Chapter 10.

Over time there has been a gradual reduction in the use of derogatory language in relation to disabled people. Such language developed as terms that had previously been purely descriptive began to be used as insults. The language of the school playground has made terms such as 'spastic' and 'epileptic' pejorative. It is a matter for concern that such terms. It is a matter for concern that such terms have found their way into press reporting when it is felt that a point is needed to be made. An example of the negative usage of the word 'epileptic'

---

[200] Wynne Jones R (2017) How Chancellor Philip Hammond left the nation's disabled out of the budget. www.mirror.co.uk/news/politics/chancellor-philip-hammond-left-nations-11576182

can be found in the reporting of the arrest, trial, imprisonment, and subsequent acquittal of Barry George for the murder of television presenter Jill Dando in 1999. The shooting of Dando, one of the most popular television presenters at that time, on the doorstep of her home in London shocked the nation. The media reporting of the murder was intense, as was coverage of the arrest of a local man called Barry George around 6 months later. George, a fantasist, had often been in trouble with the police, and complaints had been made against him relating to sexual assault. His neighbours referred to him as 'the local nutcase'. He became a suspect after it was observed that he was inexplicably agitated during meetings with his local housing association officer and his family doctor, and it became known that he frequented a local gun club. He was found guilty of murder at his trial in 2001, and was given a life sentence.

In 2008, George (who was by then 48 years of age) was found not guilty of murder at a second trial, after two appeals and 8 years in jail. The *Telegraph* newspaper (1 August 2008) reported the retrial, and stated that George, 'an epileptic with mental disability, was originally found guilty of murder in 2001'.[201] The *Telegraph* commented that 'his family has always maintained that George, an epileptic with a low IQ and several personality disorders, should never have been charged as he was incapable of carrying out the clinically executed murder of Miss Dando'. The report went on to mention George's 'severely abnormal' brain scans and the evidence of a neuropsychologist who pointed out that George had an IQ of 75 and that there was a family history of epilepsy. The seizures were described in detail, with absence attacks lasting from minutes to hours, associated with shoulder jerks and fluttering of the eyes. The neuropsychologist concluded by stating 'I am sure that Mr George has inherited a gene or genes which predispose him to epilepsy or cognitive impairment.'[202] In the same article he described the results of an electroencephalogram (EEG): 'What it shows are repetitive bursts of abnormal brain discharges that last five to ten seconds, then there is five to ten seconds of normality and then it is abnormal again.' A news item broadcast on the BBC News Channel on 1 August 2008 described George as 'a loner and epileptic who suffers from mental illness'.[203] The forensic evidence relating to a speck of gunpowder that had been found in George's coat pocket, which was central to his initial conviction, was deemed unsound, and furthermore, he had not been placed at the crime scene by any of the witnesses. The press chose to highlight the fact that he was 'an epileptic with mental disability', while barely commenting on the miscarriage of justice that had taken place. During the 8 years for which he was unfairly imprisoned he had become a national figure

---

201 www.telegraph.co.uk/news/uknews/2484841/Barry-George-cleared-of-Jill-Dando-murder.html
202 www.telegraph.co.uk/news/uknews/2440282/Jill-Dandos-alleged-killer-Barry-Georges-mental-ability-in-bottom-one-per-cent-jury-told.html
203 news.bbc.co.uk/1/hi/uk/7536815.stm

of hate, and the world had been informed that thousands of newspaper cuttings of women had been found at his home when it was searched. His brain scan results and IQ were now common knowledge, and yet he was innocent of Jill Dando's murder. There is no doubt that the frequent description of George as 'an epileptic' reinforced public perceptions of a particular personality type being associated with the condition. It seems unlikely that, if George had had, say, asthma or diabetes instead of epilepsy, the press would have stigmatized him on the basis of his health condition in the way that they did. He has also been the subject of subsequent newspaper stories claiming that he stalked several women, and he has been successful in claiming damages from News Group Newspapers, the owners of the *News of the World* and the *Sun*. In April 2010 the Ministry of Justice denied George compensation for the years that he had spent in prison, basing their decision on the definition of what constituted a miscarriage of justice. When this was appealed in the High Court the judges concluded that 'There was indeed a case upon which a reasonable jury properly directed could have convicted the claimant of murder', and compensation was still denied. Despite this, Jill Dando's murder remains officially unsolved.

Nearly four decades earlier, across the Atlantic, Jack Ruby (1911–1967) shot Lee Harvey Oswald (1939–1963), the alleged and untried assassin of President John Kennedy (1917–1963), on 24 November 1963. Two days before the shooting, Oswald, a 24-year-old warehouse worker with communist sympathies, had assassinated the President by shooting him as he drove through the centre of Dallas, Texas, in a motorcade. Oswald was arrested soon afterwards, and was in the process of being transferred from a county jail when Ruby stepped out of a crowd of onlookers and fatally shot him in front of the live television cameras. As a result, graphic footage of the crime was relayed around the world almost immediately. Jack Ruby (born Jacob Rubenstein) was the son of Polish immigrants living in Chicago, and spent much of his youth in care. Poorly educated, he worked as a salesman before learning a trade as an aircraft mechanic in the Army Air Force. He eventually moved to Dallas, where he became a petty criminal and merged into the seamy nightlife of the city. It was at his high-profile trial that the subject of his epilepsy was raised. Ruby seemed to have no motive for killing Oswald apart from the fact that he was deeply upset by the latter's crime. He had no political affiliations, so appeared to have nothing to gain except notoriety. His trial took place in Dallas in spring 1964, after considerable dispute that it should be moved elsewhere to ensure a fairer trial, because of the huge publicity that surrounded the case. Ruby was defended pro bono by the acclaimed San Francisco lawyer Melvin Belli. Belli decided to argue that it was psychomotor (temporal lobe) epilepsy that had caused his client to shoot Oswald while temporarily insane, and it was on these grounds that Belli would ask the jury and judge for leniency. The trial was reported by the national and international media, and the *New York Times* (2 February 1964) stated that 'physical damage to his brain at some point in his life, a defense psychologist has testified, had left Ruby with psychomotor epilepsy which led to periods of automatic reaction, with no control or later memory of his actions'.[204] Epilepsy was now to become central to a court case that would soon be reported around the world.

Ludwig Gutmann, a neurologist based in West Virginia, has provided a unique account of how the defence introduced the medical issues to the court, and in his short article he quotes from the trial transcripts.[205] He describes a visit to his department at this time by Frank Forster, a professor of neurology at the University of Wisconsin. Forster told him 'I've been asked to testify at his trial in Dallas. ... His attorneys maintain that epilepsy is a player, or at least that's what his attorneys intend to establish. ... They say he committed the act during an epileptic seizure and that an abnormality on his EEG taken while he was in prison proves he had one.' Belli's intention in evoking epilepsy was to convince the jury that Ruby could not know the difference between right and wrong if he was having a seizure at the time of the offence. This inability to distinguish between right and wrong is based on the M'Naghten Rules, which will be discussed later. At the trial a host of epilepsy experts were called by both the defence and the prosecution. Professor Martin Towler, for the defence, had no doubt that Ruby had seizures. William Lennox, a key researcher in the development of the EEG, concurred but had difficulty classifying the type of epilepsy Ruby might have. A psychiatrist provided expert opinion on Ruby's personality disorder and his epilepsy, and expressed the view that he did not know the consequences of his behaviour. When Ruby testified, he commented that Oswald 'looked cunning and vicious, like a rat, like a communist'. The collapse of Ruby's defence was ultimately brought about by Frank Forster. "Doctor," the state's prosecuting attorney said, "let me ask you a hypothetical question. Suppose a person were standing on the edge of a crowd, had to make his way through at least one line of the crowd in order to draw a gun and shoot a moving man who is at least ten feet away when he first saw him and was heard to say 'You rat, son of a bitch, you shot the president' and was immediately apprehended and within two minutes said something to the effect 'I intended to kill him' or that 'I hope the son of a bitch dies' and then within three minutes said 'I thought I could get off three shots, but you guys stopped me.' I'll ask you if, in your opinion, that person could have been suffering from psychomotor epilepsy at the time that he did the shooting." Frank Forster said without hesitation, "No."

On 14 March 1964 the jury convicted Ruby of killing Oswald, and sentenced him to death, but the conviction was later overturned. The Appeals Court agreed that Ruby could

---

204 www.nytimes.com/1964/02/02/archives/jack-rubyprofile-of-oswalds-assassin-he-became-a-promoter-while.html
205 Gutmann L (2007) Jack Ruby. *Neurology* 68, 707–708.

not have received a fair trial in Dallas because of the huge publicity surrounding the case, and with Belli's argument that anti-Semitism had been a decisive factor in reaching the verdict (Ruby was Jewish). He died of cancer 3 years later while awaiting a retrial.

The defence that Ruby's epilepsy provided an explanation for the crime reinforced the public perception that people with epilepsy, on experiencing loss of control due to some kind of altered mental state during a seizure, could commit a crime and possibly even kill another human being. Around the world the press, in reporting the trial, gave credence to this idea and had a direct and damaging effect on the public's understanding of epilepsy. It is a matter of great concern that medical professionals could, for a fee, appear as 'expert witnesses' and knowingly argue a case in court to support this argument.

Another area where the press has a strong influence on public perceptions of people with epilepsy is in its coverage of road vehicle accidents and fatalities that are reported to have been caused by people with epilepsy as a direct result of loss of awareness or consciousness. The laws in relation to vehicle driving and epilepsy are discussed in Chapter 10. Here we shall focus on some stories that have been reported by the press, and the manner in which they were presented. In November 2011 a BBC News item reported that, according to the police, 'A driver with a history of epilepsy caused the death of a woman by playing "Russian roulette" with his condition.'[206] The 56-year-old man, who had crashed into four cars while having a seizure, fatally injuring one person and seriously injuring three others (including a 2-year-old child), was sentenced to 6 years in prison. In November 2017 a BBC News item reported that 'A man who continued to drive despite suffering epileptic episodes has been jailed for killing a teenager after blacking out at the wheel.'[207] The news item reported that there had been a note in his medical records about not driving, and that he had been advised to inform the Driver and Vehicle Licensing Agency (DVLA) about his condition, but that the accused denied that his doctor had told him not to drive. The prosecuting lawyer was reported to have stated that 'As an epileptic, the defendant should have told the DVLA of his condition'. It was concluded that it was 'most likely' that he had had a seizure before hitting the teenager. However, the fact that he had not slept for more than 19 hours before the crash, and was then seen driving at high speed on the wrong side of the road, suggests that he had indeed caused death by dangerous driving, but that this was due to factors other than epilepsy. Like members of the population at large, people with epilepsy can commit heinous crimes, but these should not be attributed to their epilepsy.

More recently *The Irish Times* (25 July 2018) reported that a 38-year-old man with epilepsy, who had knocked down a teenage pedestrian and left him with permanent physical

---

206 www.bbc.co.uk/news/uk-england-essex-15790030
207 www.bbc.co.uk/news/uk-england-merseyside-41937209

and cognitive disability, had been jailed for three and a half years. The defendant admitted that he had experienced about half a dozen epileptic seizures over the previous 2 years, and had given incorrect information about his doctors warning him not to drive.[208]

In the USA, the *Daily Beast* (5 April 2018) reported a tragic accident with the headline 'Should epileptics be banned from driving?' (again using the term 'epileptic' pejoratively). The driver allegedly had an epileptic seizure while driving, which resulted in her running over two toddlers, who died instantly. The Mayor of New York, Bill de Blasio, said of the driver 'I wish she was under arrest right now'. The author of the article, Tanya Basu, commented that 'what made the story especially sticky' was the possibility that the driver of the car might have had a seizure, causing her to 'step on the gas instead of brake at the crosswalk'. Alexandra Finucane, senior legal adviser to the Epilepsy Foundation, defended the situation, emphasizing that it was illogical to associate bad driving with epilepsy, and stating that 'Epilepsy, after all, is not reflective of intellectual capability'. In response to the suggestion that all people with epilepsy should be banned from driving, Ms Finucane highlighted the risk of harming a whole group because of one individual, and commented that 'There are enormous consequences here.'[209] However, in the interests of providing a balanced account it should be pointed out that this driver had previously been involved in another seizure-related incident while behind the wheel, and had also run up a dozen driving offences (including ignoring red lights) within a very short space of time.

It is worth considering the manner in which these particularly tragic events, and many others like them, were reported to the public. The message conveyed was that people with epilepsy should not be allowed to drive a car – a potentially lethal vehicle – as they cannot be trusted to declare their condition to the driving authorities, and the resulting risk posed to society by allowing them to drive is unacceptably high. The actual evidence that people with epilepsy are dangerous drivers differs markedly from public perceptions of this risk. A landmark study showed that, among a sample of approximately 44,000 drivers who die in the USA each year, alcohol and relatively young age were much larger contributing factors than epilepsy. In fact, epilepsy was rarely considered to be a factor in fatalities caused by road vehicles.[210] Despite the press media's message, it would be much more sensible to consider whether the young (16–24 years age group) and those with a history of alcohol misuse should be considered unsafe to drive, rather than people with controlled epilepsy. In general, press coverage of issues relating to epilepsy and driving is negative and tends to exaggerate

---

208 www.irishtimes.com/news/crime-and-law/courts/circuit-court/driver-who-hit-teen-during-epileptic-seizure-jailed-for-3-years-1.3576547
209 www.thedailybeast.com/should-epileptics-be-banned-from-driving
210 Sheth SG, Krauss G, Krumholz A et al. (2004) Mortality in epilepsy: driving fatalities vs other causes of death in patients with epilepsy. *Neurology* 63, 1002–1007.

the risks. Legislation is clearly needed, but the majority of people with epilepsy are only too well aware of the risks, understand their responsibility to society, and provide the driving authorities with accurate information about their seizure control.

So far we have focused on the negative aspects of press coverage of people with epilepsy. However, as a result of the input of epilepsy charities into press stories, and their policing of the language used by the media, there have been some significant improvements in reporting, resulting in the press having less negative effects, and sometimes even having positive ones, on the lives of people with this condition. For example, the term 'epileptic' is now used much less frequently than it was in the past to refer to a person with epilepsy, and expressions such as 'brainstorm' are also used much less often. In addition, the assumption that all people with epilepsy are learning impaired has been successfully challenged. In fact, around 30 per cent of people with learning disabilities have epilepsy, whereas six out of seven people with epilepsy have no learning impairments at all.

We shall now consider the role of the press in promoting stories that might actually have a positive effect by improving the situation for people with epilepsy. Such stories may focus on personal achievements, highlight the need for better care, improve public perception, or increase access to new treatments. In June 2018 in the UK the *Metro* newspaper ran an 'opinion' article by Philip Lee, Chief Executive of the charity Epilepsy Action, entitled 'Epilepsy sufferers deserve effective treatment and proper research into medicinal cannabis'.[211] The article was triggered by the stories of two children whose parents had gone to great lengths to obtain cannabis for their sons' epilepsy, and had then taken the matter to the press to gain support for their campaign. This was shared on Facebook, Twitter, and other social media, and resulted in a petition signed by 370,000 people demanding access to cannabis for epilepsy being presented to the then-Prime Minister, Theresa May. The boys' parents had been forced to travel abroad to countries where medicinal cannabis was available in order to obtain the drug and then (illegally) bring it back to the UK. Cannabis plants produce many complex compounds, some of which have addictive properties, and for this reason there was reluctance to sanction widespread access to the drug for medicinal purposes. The parents were not seeking to obtain 'street cannabis', but rather cannabidiol (CBD) oil, one of over 100 cannabinoid compounds that are found in the plant. Clinical trials had already shown CBD oil to be beneficial in treating pain. In September 2018 the *Guardian* newspaper published a video account, under the heading 'Medical cannabis keeps my epileptic son alive', of the journey of the mother of one of the boys to Dubai to pick up her son's treatment.[212] The use of the word 'epileptic' was

---

211 www.metro.co.uk/2018/06/14/epilepsy-sufferers-like-billy-caldwell-deserve-effective-treatment-and-that-means-proper-research-into-medicinal-cannabis-7625992/
212 www.theguardian.com/politics/video/2018/jul/05/billy-caldwells-mother-medical-cannabis-keeps-my-epileptic-son-alive-video

unfortunate, but the story attracted widespread interest, and it accurately informed the public that this was not the normal street cannabis, but a specific medicinal compound that had been effective in these two young children, and which appeared to be life-saving. The newspapers that carried the story highlighted the need for more research into the mechanism by which this specific component of the plant suppressed seizures. Under this intense media pressure, the UK Home Office handed back the cannabis oil that had been confiscated from one of the families, and the Home Secretary issued a licence for treatment to be allowed, as a matter of urgency, in these specific circumstances. The press had not only dealt effectively with this urgent situation, but also called for randomized clinical trials to be conducted so that the true role of cannabis oil could be determined and its active ingredient identified. One could argue that the press had behaved in a more balanced manner than the Government. The Home Secretary had reacted impulsively, whereas the press appeared to have a better understanding of the long-term nature and complexity of the problem, as well as the need for further research. The potential power of the press to bring about change is clearly demonstrated in this case. There is always a need for caution, as press campaigns risk empowering the public as judge and jury on the basis of evidence that may be selectively presented. However, this story demonstrates what can be achieved by responsible, measured reporting of a complex medical issue if informed advice is sought from epilepsy charities and independent experts.

Not surprisingly, given the complexity of the subject, there have been very few in-depth studies of the accuracy of press reporting about healthcare issues, and epilepsy in particular. Around 20 years ago, Gregory Krauss and his colleagues from the Johns Hopkins Epilepsy Centre in Baltimore, USA, in collaboration with the *Washington Post*, looked for stories about epilepsy in English-language newspapers and magazines.[213] They searched a large commercial database (LexisNexis, which contains several thousand English-language newspaper, magazine, and journal databases) for stories published between 1991 and 1996 that contained the keywords 'seizure', 'epilepsy', and the often derogatory term 'epileptic'. The researchers identified 210 stories, of which the majority had been published in newspapers and only a small number in magazines. Two epilepsy specialists reviewed the articles and evaluated them with regard to scientific accuracy, stigmatizing attitudes, exaggerated claims about advances in treatment, and omission of key information. The most frequent storylines were about individuals 'overcoming' epilepsy, advances in drug and non-drug treatments, surgical developments, scientific advances, misdiagnosis, and famous people living with the condition. Only a minority of the stories covered sudden death or sudden unexplained death in epilepsy (SUDEP), employment discrimination, or accidents. Reassuringly, there were

---

213 Krauss GL, Gondek S, Krumholz A et al. (2000) "The Scarlet E": the presentation of epilepsy in the English language print media. *Neurology* 54, 1894–1898.

relatively few stories that associated epilepsy with violent behaviour. Physicians and epilepsy charities were credited with providing key information, and were quoted in around 50 per cent of the articles, while people with epilepsy themselves and their families were quoted in just under 20 per cent. Sadly, almost a third of the stories contained significant inaccuracies. Basic errors were found in 14 per cent of the articles, with exaggerated claims for treatment in 10 per cent. Bias and stigmatizing attitudes towards people with epilepsy were found in only 5 per cent of the newspaper articles. Although this result is encouraging, and perhaps better than expected, prejudiced articles still appear.

The article by Krauss and his colleagues includes examples of both the best and the worst of epilepsy reporting. For instance, in 1994 the new drug lamotrigine was described as being able to 'liberate epileptics' (*Pharmaceutical Business News*, 10 January 1994), while another drug was claimed to 'have made me an epileptic' (*The People*, 24 July 1994). A report of a mother's attempt at euthanasia included the phrase 'epileptic son begged her to kill him' (*Daily Mirror*, 13 December 1995), while the suggestion that epilepsy is related to the supernatural was encapsulated in the words of a report which stated that 'seizures are Zachary's demons' (*Calgary Herald*, 5 October 1996). The word 'demonic' appeared in 6 per cent of the stories about epilepsy, and the term 'epileptic' was used in nearly 50 per cent. Krauss and his colleagues commented that the fear elicited by seizures makes the reporting of epilepsy challenging and contributes to journalistic errors. They concluded that 'physicians and reporters should be aware of both professional and popular biases that influence the print media's presentation of the causes and consequences of epilepsy'. How such a message can be conveyed and sustained is problematic, but a small step forward has been the award of annual prizes by epilepsy charities for the best-informed epilepsy news story. In recent years both the Epilepsy Association of Scotland and the International League Against Epilepsy (ILEA) have adopted this approach.

In 1999 a joint study from Jerusalem, Israel and Ontario, Canada compared the manner in which newspapers in the two countries reported disability issues.[214] A total of 400 newspaper articles that had been published over a 3-month period were accessed. The study confirmed an overall trend towards negative reporting, especially with regard to disabilities such as mental illness and epilepsy, in which there is no visible impairment. The research indicated that the press showed neither empathy nor support for issues relating to these 'unseen disabilities', with little difference found between the two countries apart from a tendency to use more appropriate and less pejorative language in Canada. However, visible physical illness received much more attention and empathy.

---

214 Auslander GK and Gold N Paul Baerwald School of Social Work, The Hebrew University of Jerusalem, Mt. Scopus, Jerusalem 91905, Israel (1999) Media reports on disability: a binational comparison of types and causes of disability as reported in major newspapers. *Disability and Rehabilitation* 21, 420–431.

In 2013, a study by Kimberly Devotta and her colleagues analysed the ways in which the representation of disability in a sample of the Canadian press had changed over a 10-year period (1998–2008).[215] The researchers studied three newspapers, *The Globe and Mail*, the *Toronto Star*, and the *Toronto Sun*, and monitored them over the same 3-month period in the years 1998 and 2008, respectively. After comparing a total of 362 newspaper articles they were able to demonstrate an improvement over the 10-year period, with the 2008 sample showing that the three papers were now more likely to report disability in a positive manner. Disabled people were more sympathetically portrayed, and the complexity of their various conditions and social needs and roles were better understood and expressed.

Regrettably, this progress in reporting was not to be maintained after the arrival of the age of austerity in the UK. Emma Briant and her colleagues from the Strathclyde Centre for Disability Research at the University of Glasgow described the financial downturn of 2007–2008 as the worst economic crisis for 50 years, with 'dire consequences for workers and their families'.[216] They drew attention to the perception among some that high levels of sickness and disability benefits were an obstacle to economic recovery, and that the latter could only be achieved by a reduction in the 'burgeoning welfare burden'. The financial crisis had now begun to serve as an excuse to re-evaluate the benefits system, and to arbitrarily withhold benefits, often from the least able in society, for the greater benefit of the economy and hence 'for the good of all'. The researchers at the Strathclyde Centre decided to investigate how the economic crash had influenced the image of disabled people that was presented by the press. Focusing on newspaper articles published between October 2004 and January 2005, and between October 2010 and January 2011, they studied five national papers that had each traditionally supported the main political parties in the UK, namely the Conservative, Labour, and Liberal Democrat parties. The LexisNexis database was used to identify articles containing the keywords 'disabled', 'disability', 'disabilities', and 'incapacity.' This yielded a total of 713 articles in the 2004–2005 study period and 1015 articles in the 2010–2011 period. They were coded on a scale ranging from a 'bare mention' to a 'dominant theme' in the article. The researchers' analysis of these articles was supplemented by the opinions of focus groups consisting of disabled and non-disabled people. Specific conditions such as epilepsy were included in the articles reviewed, but were not analysed separately.

It was found that by 2010–2011 the number of articles about disability had increased by 43 per cent, and the message being conveyed by the press was shifting from one of

---

215 Devotta K, Wilton R and Yiannakoulias N (2013) Representations of disability in the Canadian news media: a decade of change? *Disability and Rehabilitation* 35, 1859–1868.

216 Briant E, Watson M and Philo G (2013) Reporting in the age of austerity: the changing face of media representation of disability and disabled people in the United Kingdom and the creation of new 'folk devils'. *Disability and Society* 28, 874–889.

sympathy to a highlighting of the financial costs of supporting people with disabilities. The terms 'scroungers' and 'fraudsters' were now being used to promote an image of disabled people as undeserving and untrustworthy, respectively. Fewer stories were being reported about individuals overcoming the hardship and disadvantage associated with their condition. Pejorative words were used more frequently, and the word 'cripple' had re-entered the reporter's vocabulary. The message conveyed by the headline of an article published in the *Daily Express* newspaper in January 2011, namely '75% on Sick are Skiving',[217] risked inciting hatred of people with disabilities. Those articles that showed some compassion for disabled people dealt predominantly with physical (i.e. visible) conditions, and only rarely addressed hidden conditions such as mental health disorders and epilepsy.

The authors of this important study highlighted the influence and responsibility wielded by the media in shaping public knowledge and opinion. They also noted that by tending to demonize people with disabilities the press has played into the hands of the political agenda of austerity, with its emphasis on reducing the state benefits bill rather than risking the introduction of unpopular tax increases. They concluded that 'disabled people have become, for some newspapers, a "folk devil" and this change has been justified by the need to reduce costs in welfare provision as a response to the global financial crises'.

More recently, Joseph Caspermeyer and his colleagues from the Walter Cronkite School of Journalism at Arizona State University have looked at the errors and stigmatizing language found in US newspaper reports about neurological conditions.[218] They used the definition of stigmatization proposed by Erving Goffman, a highly influential Canadian-American sociologist, who described stigma as 'the situation of the individual who is disqualified from full social acceptance'.[219] The authors used the LexisNexis database to search newspapers with a total readership of 6 million in 2003. They identified 1203 articles on 11 major neurological conditions, of which dementia scored most stories, while epilepsy was in sixth place with 114 stories (9.8 per cent of the total). Nearly a third of these articles contained stigmatizing language, with around 50 per cent of this articulated directly by the reporter. In addition, 20 per cent of the articles contained basic errors with regard to prevalence and life expectancy, as well as exaggerated claims for new treatments. Epilepsy was the most stigmatized of the 11 conditions studied, but interestingly was second only to dementia with regard to the number of feature articles (as opposed to news stories) written about it. This would suggest an editorial belief that the public wanted to know more about epilepsy and its impact. Examples of stigmatization included the following quotes: 'A lot of epileptics are not

---

217 www.express.co.uk/news/uk/225311/75-on-sick-are-skiving
218 Caspermeyer JJ, Sylvester EJ, Drazkowski JF et al. (2006) Evaluation of stigmatizing language and medical errors in neurology coverage by US newspapers. *Mayo Clinic Proceedings* 81, 300–306.
219 Goffman E (1963) *Stigma: Notes on the Management of Spoiled Identity*. Penguin Books, London.

going to tell you they have it because they're embarrassed', and the description of a family as 'a bunch of genetically linked paupers, criminals, harlots, epileptics and mental defectives'. The authors concluded that 'neurologic health information continues to be compromised by issues of reporting accuracy', but they did not suggest any possible solutions to this problem.

One newspaper that was not included in Caspermeyer's study was the *Los Angeles Times*. Its online archive can be used to identify published articles containing the keyword 'epilepsy'. Surprisingly, there were only 18 stories over a 10-year period, but in each of them epilepsy was the main focus of the article. Several were about new treatment developments, such as the approval of a new drug, the potential benefit of cannabis, and the role of surgery. There was a cautionary tale about the use of epilepsy drugs in pregnancy and developmental delay, and a story by a board-certificated specialist giving an accurate account of the incidence, nature, and treatment of the condition. These articles were informative and generally accurate. Other stories covered epilepsy as a defence in a murder trial and road traffic accident, the death from a seizure of the Olympic sprint champion Florence Griffith Joiner (Flo Jo), and a campaigning story that outlined the plight of Jerry Kill, head coach of the University of Minnesota Golden Gophers football team. Kill was described as an inspirational person who had worked his way up to a top coaching appointment only to suffer four seizures during games and be told that he should step down from his post because of his epilepsy. In September 2013 the enraged reporter Bill Dwyre wrote that 'it never ceases to amaze how sport can become a morality play and take so many wrong and disgusting turns along the way. Take the case of Jerry Kill. Jerry has epilepsy.'[220] Kill did return to coaching after a break to stabilize his seizures, and indeed was named Coach of the Year in 2014, but after worsening health problems he retired in October 2015. It is unclear how influential Dwyre's article was in Kill's reinstatement, but a very positive message about epilepsy had been conveyed to sports fans by the press.

Toba Kerson, an American social researcher, has made a detailed study of epilepsy and the media. It is hard to disagree with her comment that 'epilepsy continues to be portrayed as associated with victimization, fear, secrecy, possession, supernatural power and violence'. In her book chapter on epilepsy and the media she cites as an example the media coverage of a seizure experienced by John G Roberts, the Chief Justice of the US Supreme Court.[221] The question of his suitability to serve was raised by the fact that he had experienced an epileptic seizure. Yet it seems unlikely that if he had any other acute illness, such as a heart condition, the question of fitness to serve would have arisen. Linda Greenhouse reported in the *New York Times* (30 July 2007) that 'Chief Justice John G. Roberts Jr. was hospitalized Monday

---

220 www.latimes.com/sports/la-xpm-2013-sep-25-la-sp-dwyre-jerry-kill-20130926-story.html
221 Kerson TS (2010) Epilepsy and media. In: Pinikahana J and Walker C (eds) *Social Epileptology: Understanding the Social Aspects of Epilepsy*. Nova Science Publishers, New York. pp. 231–263.

after suffering a seizure at his summer home in Maine, the Supreme Court announced. The episode, described as a "benign idiopathic seizure", was similar to one he suffered 14 years ago, according to the court's press release. Idiopathic means that the cause of the seizure remains unknown.'[222] The earlier seizure had taken place on the golf course, and apart from the fact that he had not been able to drive for a while it had had little impact on Justice Roberts' life. When he was nominated for the Supreme Court in 2005, his earlier seizure had been declared but not considered significant enough to be brought up in public at his confirmation hearings.

This highly publicized press story led to an open debate as to what constituted epilepsy, and whether two seizures 14 years apart justified the use of the term, with even the medical pundits being unable to agree about this. Most damaging of all was the recurring question about the suitability of a person with epilepsy to sit on the Supreme Court, a lifelong appointment, and deliberate on the direction of new legislation. A political analyst on CNN, who showed no understanding of how quickly recovery occurs after a seizure, questioned how long it would take for Justice Roberts 'to get back to normal'. The conversation surrounding this case continued with the right-wing radio show host Michael Savage expressing the view that the Justice's anti-epilepsy medication was to blame for his decision to uphold President Obama's healthcare legislation. Savage was reported as saying that 'neurologists will tell you that medication used for seizure disorders, such as epilepsy, can introduce mental slowing, forgetfulness and other cognitive problems, and if you look at Roberts' writings you can see the cognitive dissociation in what he is saying'.[223] From a confident commentator such as Savage, this would sound plausible to anyone opposed to Obamacare, and would lead them to believe that a person who was taking drugs to control epilepsy could not be professionally competent. High-profile stories such as that of Justice Roberts can do immense damage to the public perception of epilepsy if they are reported inaccurately, especially when even the experts appear to disagree about what constitutes epilepsy.

The Internet

The arrival of the Internet, followed by YouTube, Facebook, and other online resources, has created enormous potential for both benefit and harm. The Internet is now the leading source of health information, and it has been estimated that there are at least 100,000 websites that provide medical information about specific conditions. A study conducted in 2010 showed

---

222 www.nytimes.com/2007/07/31/washington/31roberts.html?mtrref=www.google.com&gwh=7208DAF3875C60C716356E39A8A31977&gwt=pay&assetType=REGIWALL

223 www.businessinsider.com/conservative-radio-host-blames-roberts-epilepsy-for-health-care-ruling-2012-6?r=US&IR=T

that 61 per cent of American adults looked for health information online,[224] and it seems reasonable to suggest that this figure would be much higher today. The Internet may provide accurate data and realistic information for the affected individual and their family, or it may give inaccurate information that raises false hopes, exaggerates the benefits of certain treatments, and stigmatizes the person's condition.

Facebook enables individuals and organizations with a common interest to make contact with each other, and is now, along with Twitter, an essential part of the public face of charities and organizations that address healthcare issues. However, it does not meet the needs of the significant numbers of disabled people who cannot afford a smartphone or computer, or who lack IT or basic literacy skills. Thus the widespread use of digital communications runs the risk of further disenfranchizing and disempowering people with disabilities. For example, the need to complete many of the benefits application forms online can be challenging and intimidating to those who are unfamiliar with the new information highway.

Every epilepsy charity, medical institution, and specialist epilepsy centre is expected to have at least a website, Facebook page, and Twitter feed. The sense of isolation that often results from epilepsy has been partly alleviated by the availability of social media, which enables many people who are living with the condition to tell their stories, share their feelings and experiences, and contribute their knowledge of established and new treatments. However, social media can never be a substitute for the face-to-face contact that many people with epilepsy so desperately need. We shall discuss the issue of social isolation and epilepsy in Chapter 12.

A number of studies have examined the use of Internet and social media platforms with regard to epilepsy. Researchers from Toronto, Canada conducted a study of Facebook and Twitter accounts that related to epilepsy.[225] They noted that Twitter had around 313 million users worldwide in 2016, and confined their study to accounts between June and August 2016 that were dedicated specifically to clinical epilepsy in humans, using the search terms 'epilepsy', 'epilepsies', 'epileptic', and 'seizure'. They estimated population data from the numbers of 'likes' and 'feeds', and they reviewed 100 out of a total of 400 accounts, classifying each according to the following categories: non-profit organizations, businesses, support groups, medical institutions, education, and journals. From these accounts they extracted the most recent 50 posts and tweets, and then analysed each of them. A total of 840 pages about epilepsy were 'liked' by just over three million people, and 137 Twitter pages were followed by 325,000 followers. The authors noted that this was an increase of 100 per

---

224 Scanfeld D, Scanfeld V and Larson EL (2010) Dissemination of health information through social networks: Twitter and antibiotics. *American Journal of Infection Control* 38, 182–188.
225 Meng Y, Elkaim L, Wang J et al. (2017) Social media in epilepsy: a quantitative and qualitative analysis. *Epilepsy & Behavior* 71, 79–84.

cent compared with data from an analysis conducted in 2012. The USA was the commonest source of Facebook pages, with 50 per cent originating from non-profit organizations and only 4 per cent from certified medical epilepsy centres. A similar result was obtained for the Twitter accounts. Dissemination of information about drug treatments and clarification of misconceptions were the commonest themes, followed by uplifting optimistic comments on living with epilepsy. There was also promotional information, especially from the USA, highlighting everything from Christmas cards to clothing and other accessories. Only 10 per cent of posts and tweets thanked medical staff, with a similar number seeking support groups or endeavouring to make policymakers, such as politicians, aware of epilepsy. Finally, and surprisingly, only 1 per cent of all posts related to epilepsy surgery.

The finding of an increase of 100 per cent in posts and Tweets between 2012 and 2016 highlights the potential for these platforms to increase knowledge and support and enable the sharing of experiences within the epilepsy community. The majority of pages belonged to epilepsy foundations and support groups, and a small number belonged to the medical epilepsy centres. Clearly this is a gap that healthcare professionals need to close. In the past a computer was essential for gaining access to information available on the Internet, but smartphones have now made such access available to many more people, irrespective of their educational background or socioeconomic status. Finally, the relative absence of posts on epilepsy surgery is noteworthy in view of the number of centres worldwide that offer this treatment option, and research evidence that it is underutilized. Clearly this is another issue that healthcare professionals need to address.

An earlier Canadian study from Dalhousie University in Nova Scotia focused on exploring how seizures were portrayed on Twitter, and the potential of the latter for disseminating information about treatment and care for people with epilepsy.[226] The authors used the search terms 'seizures' and 'seizure', with the hashtag symbol # added. Other keywords such as 'seize' were also investigated. Tweets from 31 March and 2 April 2011 were analysed. (Data from 1 April were excluded as it was felt that tweets sent on April Fool's Day would not be representative of the normal flow of messages.) A total of 1720 tweets were identified over the 48-hour period. The authors excluded 435 tweets that were not truly seizure-related, and classified the remainder as follows according to their interpretation of the content or source: 'metaphorical' (32 per cent of tweets); 'personal' (31 per cent); 'informative' (12 per cent); 'ridicule/joke' (9 per cent); 'miscellaneous' (8 per cent); 'opinion' (6 per cent); 'advice seeking' (2 per cent). The finding that just under 50 per cent of the tweets in this snapshot study either used the words metaphorically or in a joking, ridiculing manner was

---

226 McNeil K, Brna PM and Gordon KE (2012) Epilepsy in the Twitter era: a need to re-tweet the way we think about seizures. *Epilepsy & Behavior* 23, 127–130.

disappointing although unsurprising. The authors cited the following example of this kind of usage: 'What do you do if someone's having a seizure in the bath tub? Throw in a load of laundry.' This 'joke' was re-tweeted 77 times during the study period.

The finding that only 14 per cent of tweets were informative or came from those seeking advice or providing help indicates the extent of missed opportunities for using this platform in a more positive way. Twitter appears to have great potential for communication to and among the epilepsy community, staying abreast of treatment advances, communicating with healthcare professionals, and giving the general public a better understanding of the condition. The Dalhousie University researchers concluded that their study had 'demonstrated the prevalence of stigmatizing comments related to seizures', and that social media 'could be used productively to disseminate accurate information on seizures and epilepsy, but are currently propagating negative attitudes towards seizures with potential for fuelling stigma'.

The malicious potential of Twitter has been highlighted by the deliberate sending of animated videos and GIF (graphic interchange format) files to the accounts of individuals known to have epilepsy, with the aim of precipitating seizures. Although the form of photosensitive epilepsy that is targeted by such behaviour is relatively rare, this is a very harmful and potentially fatal form of cybercrime. A particularly high-profile case was recently profiled by Reis Thebault in the *Seattle Times*.[227] He described how Kurt Eichenwald, a prominent Dallas-based journalist with epilepsy, had posted a tweet that was highly critical of President Trump. Soon afterwards, Eichenwald received a GIF that caused a strobe light image to flash violently across his computer screen behind the message 'YOU DESERVE A SEIZURE FOR YOUR POSTS'. Within seconds he did indeed experience a seizure. The FBI subsequently arrested the sender, a criminal prosecution ensued, and the accused pleaded guilty to aggravated assault. Eichenwald's attorney stated that 'this electronic message was no different than a bomb being sent in the mail or anthrax sent in an envelope'.[228]

The reporting of the case resulted in an onslaught of 'copycat' flashing GIFs that were sent to people with photo-sensitive epilepsy. In the USA, in November 2019 the Twitter feed of the Epilepsy Foundation was subject to a cyberattack in which epilepsy-related hashtags were targeted by videos and GIFs of strobing and flashing lights. This attack was deliberately planned to coincide with National Epilepsy Awareness Month.[229] In the UK, the Epilepsy Society has urged the Government to ensure that such attacks fall within the law, by including them in the Online Harms Bill. This would exert pressure on social media companies, who so far, according to the Chief Executive of the society, Clare Pelham, have

---

[227] www.seattletimes.com/nation-world/nation/a-tweet-gave-a-journalist-a-seizure-his-case-brings-new-meaning-to-the-idea-of-online-assault/
[228] www.nytimes.com/2017/03/17/technology/social-media-attack-that-set-off-a-seizure-leads-to-an-arrest.html
[229] www.edition.cnn.com/2019/12/17/tech/epilepsy-strobe-twitter-attack-trnd/index.html

responded with a 'deafening silence' when requested to take immediate action to eradicate this dangerous behaviour.[230]

YouTube is the world's largest video-sharing platform, second largest search engine, and the third most visited site after Google and Facebook. It attracts 30 million visitors per day, with 5 billion videos watched and 300 hours uploaded every minute. It is difficult to censor, and its impact on the beliefs and behaviours of people cannot be measured easily, so its influence on public perception of illness in general will inevitably remain an unknown quantity. Depictions of seizures on YouTube have had mixed effects on the public perception of epilepsy. A search of the keyword 'epilepsy' on YouTube UK produces over 160,000 results that range from inappropriate Victorian freak shows to highly educational and valuable material. The latter covers a wide range of topics, from safety of medication in pregnancy to the classification of seizures and lists of 'things not to say to people with epilepsy'. The American Academy of Neurology has published a helpful guide for patients and their families, the Red Cross has produced a practical guide to first aid, and the University of California has published a history of 'epilepsy: the sacred disease'. These are all examples of how YouTube's positive educational potential, when professionally harnessed, can be viewed alongside the many moving accounts of people living with the condition and overcoming obstacles to achieving their goals. However, few studies have evaluated YouTube's accuracy and its impact on people with epilepsy.

The authors of a study of social media and epilepsy conducted at Dalhousie University in Halifax, Canada[231] commented that, at the time of writing (in 2010), public education initiatives in relation to epilepsy had not achieved the progress made in relation to diabetes and breast cancer, and they speculated as to why this was so, given the rapid expansion and wide availability of the Internet. They searched YouTube using the terms 'epilepsy' and 'seizures', and identified the top ten videos on the basis of the number of 'hits' that they obtained. These consisted of eight amateur and two professional videos with titles such as 'graphic epileptic seizure footage' and 'real seizure captured in crowded mall'. When they had assessed the number of 'hits' that each video had obtained they reviewed the comments left by viewers and reassessed these again 1 month and 6 months later. The ten videos were visited 1.5 million times, were cumulatively accessed 3200 times a day, and attracted a total of 8803 comments, confirming the power of YouTube to reach and attract comments from vast numbers of people. The number of hits per video ranged from 62,313 to 521,657. Interestingly, the amateur videos attracted six times as many comments as the professional ones, and generated more discussion, despite generally being poorly lit and not filmed with

---

[230] www.telegraph.co.uk/technology/2019/12/20/deafening-silence-social-media-companies-epilepsy-cyber-attacks/
[231] Lo AS, Esser MJ and Gordon KE (2010) YouTube: a gauge of public perception and awareness surrounding epilepsy. *Epilepsy & Behavior* 17, 541–545.

a steady camera. The comments ranged from the derogatory to the empathetic, with most providing an opinion rather than seeking information and further knowledge. Of most concern was the finding that some of the comments indicated that the viewer found seizures comical, with posts such as 'LOL' (laugh out loud) and 'ROFL' (roll on the floor laughing). However, the majority of the videos elicited more sympathetic than unsympathetic comments, with only two, due to the nature of their content, attracting the majority of negative opinions. The 'real seizure in a crowded mall' was interesting in that the seizure was faked and it focused on the reactions of bystanders, most of whom walked straight past and ignored the event. A video showing a person having a seizure while playing a video game was also faked and used for comic effect. The authors concluded that their study showed that misinformation about and stigmatization of epilepsy are prevalent among YouTube users. However, they also pointed out that as healthcare professionals and epilepsy charities can post videos too, the platform provides an opportunity for educating the public, reducing stigma, dispelling myths, and allaying fears.

In a more recent study, Victoria Wong and her collaborators from Portland, Oregon widened their research to include 100 YouTube videos.[232] Unlike the previously mentioned study from Dalhousie University, this study classified the videos on the basis of their content rather than the comments that they evoked, and the authors used a similar classification to that adopted in the Dalhousie study of the portrayal of seizures on Twitter. During April 2012 they located their subject matter by using the search terms 'seizures' and 'epilepsy', and then identified their top 100 videos. For each clip identified, they noted the origin, view count, and whether it was a professional production or a poorly lit, shaky amateur one. Two reviewers then independently assigned the videos to a category and rated them according to five-point scales with regard to accuracy and positive (sympathetic) or negative (derogatory) content. A total of 36 videos (44 per cent) were categorized as personal or anecdotal, 31 (38 per cent) as educational, and the remainder comprised advice seeking, advertising, and opinion. There were 54 amateur videos and the remainder were professional, with 28 videos actually showing a seizure taking place (in 22 videos the seizures were in humans, and in 6 they were in animals). In total, 85 per cent of the videos were considered to be sympathetic to people with seizures, 9 per cent were judged to be neutral, and only 6 per cent were regarded as derogatory. In terms of accuracy, 51 per cent were considered to be accurate and only 9 per cent were considered to be completely misleading. This study clearly yielded positive findings, and the authors concluded that YouTube has the potential to significantly reduce the stigmatization of people with epilepsy. However, the writer of this book, who has

---

232 Wong VS, Stevenson M and Selwa L (2013) The presentation of seizures and epilepsy in YouTube videos. *Epilepsy & Behavior* 27, 247–250.

not had the opportunity to analyse the comments made on the video clips, feels that the authors do not have quite such firm grounds for optimism. Nevertheless, their conclusion that YouTube appears to offer a more sympathetic and accurate portrayal of epilepsy than other social media platforms is noteworthy.

Paula Brna, also from Dalhousie University and working with the same team of research colleagues, took a different approach to investigating whether the seizures shown on YouTube were correctly diagnosed and classified.[233] In view of the educational potential of the YouTube platform, this important study aimed to assess the accuracy of the diagnosis of epilepsy and the information provided by the clip. A similar search using the keywords 'seizures' and 'epilepsy' was conducted on a single day in autumn 2011. A total of 13,425 'seizure videos' were identified, the vast majority of which were excluded from the study for a variety of reasons, including the presence of embedded text (which made independent analysis impossible), duplication, and animated film and videos from healthcare organizations (as it was assumed that these would be accurate). In total only 167 videos were suitable for review by four neurologists, and 80 per cent of these videos were of people under 18 years of age, including infants. Only 24 videos showed adults, and in 10 videos the age of the individual could not be determined. In fact, only one-third of the videos that purported to depict seizures were judged by the reviewers to do so, while nearly a third depicted what the experts regarded as non-epileptiform events. These results should be treated with caution, given the small number of adults in the study and the large number of exclusions. However, they do highlight the possibility that the indiscriminate use of video-sharing websites where the content is inaccurate and misleading could be harmful, especially to those who are seeking to diagnose their own children.

Conclusion

In this chapter we have covered a time period during which the whole face of the media has changed dramatically and irreversibly. The benefits of the Internet and social media platforms are self-evident, in that people with specific health conditions now have the opportunity to be better informed, to challenge orthodoxy, and to take control of their condition and its treatment. However, misleading or 'fake' information is also widespread and can have potentially harmful effects when knowledge is sought indiscriminately. The news media are most likely to project a negative image of seizures and of people with epilepsy. The YouTube

---

[233] Brna PM, Dooley JM, Esser MJ et al. (2013) Are YouTube seizure videos misleading? Neurologists do not always agree. *Epilepsy & Behavior* 29, 305–307.

platform is more positive, followed by the Facebook and Twitter platforms, although research studies on social media and epilepsy are sparse and have been conducted by only a handful of centres. Health-orientated information on the Internet can never be fully regulated, due to the vast size and global nature of this platform. Ensuring the accuracy of content that relates to epilepsy thus represents a challenge, but it also provides an opportunity. Accurate video representations of a seizure have much more impact than written or verbal descriptions, and have great potential to increase public knowledge about epilepsy and reduce the stigma associated with the condition. However, it seems likely that the majority of people who search for information about or comment on epilepsy are those who are themselves either directly or indirectly affected by the condition. Meanwhile many members of the non-affected public may continue to believe the myths and misleading information. The few studies that have been described in this chapter show that when words relating to epilepsy or seizures are used outside their true medical context, the resulting posts are usually flippant or derogatory. It is this misuse of the language of disability that is most stigmatizing of all, yet terms such as 'spastic' and 'epileptic' are still used by many in a pejorative manner as part of the lexicon of insults. So long as this continues to be the case, stigma will persist despite the best endeavours of educators and institutions.

Finally, the healthcare profession has been slow to grasp the opportunity to use the social media platforms to educate, communicate with, and support the community of people living with epilepsy. This situation needs to be addressed as a priority.

CHAPTER 9
Famous people with epilepsy

We have already mentioned many writers, poets, artists, musicians, and actors who are believed to have had epilepsy. Lists of 'famous people with epilepsy' can be found on numerous websites, including those of reputable epilepsy charities and other organizations that wish to demonstrate what can be achieved by individuals with the condition. However, careful examination of the evidence often casts doubt on its accuracy.

In this chapter we shall consider some famous people from the past whose epilepsy was known for certain, claimed, or disputed, before going on to discuss a number of present-day 'celebrities' with the condition.

At this point it is worth briefly mentioning some of the erroneous claims that have been made in the past. In 1902, a letter published in the *British Medical Journal* bearing the title 'Epilepsy and Genius' described a lecture by **Sir William Broadbent** (1835–1907). It quoted him as stating that it was 'an undoubted fact' that men of military, literary, and scientific genius had been 'epileptic'.[234] Broadbent was one of the most eminent physicians of his day (and was also physician to Queen Victoria), so his opinions carried much weight not only within the medical profession but also among the public. The author of the letter (identified only by the initials F.G.C.) castigated Broadbent for his lack of evidence and accuracy, and went to the opposite extreme, suggesting that such focusing of attention on genius had led hospital teaching to neglect 'the tendency of epileptics to become insane, and … the frequency with which hysteria and other morbid mental phases are manifest in those epileptics who are not actually lunatics or dements'.

---

234 www.bmj.com/content/1/2144/301.3

The constantly expanding lists of famous people with the condition include (among many others) Socrates, Alexander the Great, Julius Caesar, Napoleon Bonaparte, Peter the Great, Handel, Tchaikovsky, and Alfred Nobel. In fact most individuals with epilepsy would find it difficult to relate to such a roll call of high achievers, which could in turn reinforce feelings of underachievement and failure. These unsubstantiated 'famous names' are indeed far removed from the real-world problems that are faced on a daily basis by people with epilepsy.

In 2005, John Hughes, an American neurologist, published the findings of a detailed study of the medical histories of 43 famous historical figures, in which he reviewed the evidence to support claims that they had suffered from epilepsy. He reported that none of the 43 individuals had had epilepsy, and in each case he was able to provide an alternative diagnosis for their symptoms, the most frequent diagnoses being 'psychogenic attacks', 'attacks of anguish, nervousness, fear, agitation, or weakness', and 'alcohol withdrawal seizures'.[235]

He quoted Peter Fenwick, a London-based neuropsychiatrist, as saying 'It is likely that the earlier accounts of temporal lobe epilepsy and temporal lobe pathology and the relationship to mystic and religious states owe more to the enthusiasm of their authors than to the true scientific understanding of the nature of temporal lobe functioning.'[236] In fact, some of the names on Hughes' list of 'non-epileptics', such as Joan of Arc, can be disputed, and his dismissal of the French author Gustave Flaubert is inconsistent with the compelling evidence that was described in Chapter 4 of this book. However, Hughes has demonstrated how implausible it is that many of these historical figures had epilepsy, not least because of the limited information available and the lack of documented eye-witness accounts.

In this inevitably selective review of famous people from the past whose names have been linked with epilepsy, I shall begin with **Muhammad** (570–632), the prophet and founder of Islam. According to Owsei Temkin's comprehensive account of the history of epilepsy, the first reference to Muhammad's epileptic seizures was made by the eighth-century Byzantine historian Theophanes (*c.* 758–817), who wrote that Muhammad's wife 'was very much grieved that she, being of noble descent, was tied to such a man, who was not only poor but epileptic as well'.[237] Bearing in mind that Christian Byzantium was openly hostile to Islam, this account could well have been religious propaganda designed to discredit belief in Muhammad. Frank Freemon, an American physician and qualified historian, concluded that Muhammad may have had epilepsy, based on a study of two texts, one of which he quotes as stating that 'at the moment of inspiration, anxiety pressed the Prophet and his countenance

---

235 Hughes JR (2005) Did all these famous people really have epilepsy? *Epilepsy & Behavior* 6, 115–139.
236 Hughes JR (2005) A reappraisal of the possible seizures of Vincent van Gogh. *Epilepsy & Behavior* 6, 504–510.
237 Temkin O (1971) *The Falling Sickness: A History of Epilepsy from the Greeks to the Beginnings of Modern Neurology*, 2nd edition. Johns Hopkins University Press, Baltimore, MD. pp. 150–154.

was troubled. He fell to the ground like an inebriate or one overcome by sleep.'[238] He based his argument for epilepsy on the repetitive nature of the Prophet's visions, the hallucinatory imagery, and the loss of consciousness, while conceding that there was a lack of recognition of his epilepsy among his contemporaries, who had no doubt witnessed these 'attacks'. Freemon concluded that 'Although an unequivocal decision is not possible from existing knowledge, psychomotor or complex partial seizures of temporal lobe epilepsy would be the most tenable diagnosis.'

Joan of Arc (1412–1431), also known as the 'Maid of Orléans', was a heroine of the Hundred Years War between the English and the French over the right to rule France. She was eventually canonized as a Catholic saint, and her life has been the subject of numerous plays, paintings, and films. At her trial at the age of 19, prior to her execution by burning at the stake on 30 May 1431, she stated that for over six years she had experienced visions of saints telling her to drive the English out of France. It has been widely suggested that her visions and hearing of voices may have been hallucinatory symptoms of temporal lobe epilepsy. However, the evidence is sparse and open to subjective interpretations.

Historical records of Joan of Arc's trial provide a detailed description of the episodes during which she heard voices (auditory hallucinations) and saw visions (visual hallucinations). Hallucinations occur when a person sees, hears, smells, tastes, or feels something that does not exist. They commonly occur in individuals with psychotic disorders such as schizophrenia, but can also occur in those with temporal lobe epilepsy. In Joan of Arc's case, the differential diagnosis for her hearing of voices includes schizophrenia, epilepsy, and genuine spiritual episodes.

Giuseppe d'Orsi and Paolo Tinuper, from the Epilepsy Centre at the University of Bari, Italy, studied the documentation of Joan of Arc's 'Trial of Condemnation' in order to investigate the nature and basis of her hallucinations.[239] They identified events during which the sound of voices was often, but not always, followed by a bright light and images of saints. The episodes were brief, and were sometimes triggered by the sound of bells, which suggests musicogenic epilepsy. The authors quote directly from Joan of Arc's account (given during her public examination) of her first attacks: 'I was thirteen when I had a Voice from God for my help and guidance. The first time that I heard this Voice, I was very much frightened; it was midday, in the summer, in my father's garden. ... I heard this Voice to my right, towards the Church; rarely do I hear it without its being accompanied also by a light. The light comes from the same side as the Voice. Generally it is a great light.' Whether she saw

---

238 Freemon FR (1976) A differential diagnosis of the inspirational spells of Muhammad the Prophet of Islam. *Epilepsia* 17, 423–427.

239 d'Orsi G and Tinuper P (2006) "I heard voices ...": from semiology, a historical review, and a new hypothesis on the presumed epilepsy of Joan of Arc. *Epilepsy & Behavior* 9, 152–157.

individual saints or attributed voices to them is unclear, although she did describe St Michael surrounded by all the Angels of Heaven, and said 'I wept, I should like to have been taken away with them.' What she actually saw is uncertain and inconsistent. Sometimes she gave the impression of seeing the very saints who were speaking to her, and on other occasions just a light or distorted imagery: 'I do not know if they had arms or other members.' Similarly, the voices were either clear – for example, saying 'Go into France! Go, raise the siege that is being made before the city of Orléans' – or they were indistinct, consisting of 'several words I could not readily understand'.

These episodes occurred many times a month, sometimes two or three times a day, and often upon waking from sleep. The diagnosis of epilepsy here comes purely from Joan of Arc's testimony at the time of her trial. There is no personal written account (as she was illiterate), no eye-witness description, and no medical assessment of her physical or mental state. A psychiatric explanation such as schizophrenia has been suggested by some authors, but the positive nature of the messages she heard, as well as the fact that the voices came from outside her and from the right, rather than being internalized, argues against such an explanation, as does the joy and ecstasy that she felt on receiving them. D'Orsi and Tinuper go even further down the epilepsy route by suggesting that she may have had the specific inherited seizure syndrome of autosomal dominant partial epilepsy with auditory features (ADPEAF), based on the features of the attacks documented at the trial as well as the suggestion that her father might have been prone to similar attacks. This rare and undescribed form of epilepsy could not possibly have been considered by the medical profession at that time. Genetic tests for ADPEAF are now available, but in Joan of Arc's case cannot be used, as she was burnt at the stake, after which two further burnings were ordered to destroy her body completely. It is widely believed that her ashes were raked into the River Seine, although this has not been confirmed.

Tsar **Peter the Great** (1672–1725), who ruled the Russian Empire from the age of 10, is best known for modernizing Russia and transforming it into a major power, and for founding the city of St Petersburg. He never enjoyed good health, and he died as a result of kidney failure following bladder surgery. From an early age he was described as nervous and prone to attacks of twitching and agoraphobia, which resulted in him avoiding places that induced panic. The writer Alex De Jonge describes how he developed a twitch that 'in later years distorted his face to the point of a convulsion',[240] and attributes this to his having witnessed the horrific hacking to death by rebels of two men who were confidants and friends of his family. Some authors have interpreted the close relationship between this traumatic event and the onset of his twitching episodes as evidence that his 'attacks' were psychogenic

---

240 De Jonge A (1980) *Fire and Water: A Life of Peter the Great.* Coward, McCann and Geoghegan, New York.

seizures. Others have suggested that they were alcohol withdrawal seizures related to his habitual excessive consumption of alcohol. The latter view is supported by a record of him having a convulsion after attending a particularly heavy drinking party.

The evidence that Peter the Great had epilepsy comes mainly from the American historian Robert Massie's Pulitzer Prize-winning biography of the Russian ruler, which states that, following an attack of measles at the age of 22, he experienced episodes in which 'his face sometimes began to twitch uncontrollably. This disorder, usually troubling on the left side of his face, was no more than a facial tic lasting only a second or two. At other times, there would be a genuine convulsion, beginning with a contraction of the muscles on the left side of his neck, followed by a spasm involving the entire left side of his face, the rolling up of his eyes until the whites could be seen.'[241] Massie comments that such attacks then progressed to a state of unconsciousness, with recovery occurring one to two hours later. This appears to be a clear description of focal onset epilepsy becoming generalized, with the initial focal component closely resembling the type of epilepsy that was subsequently described by John Hughlings Jackson.

There can therefore be little doubt that Peter the Great had epilepsy, and Massie also provides information about some of the ways in which the condition affected him. For example, he preferred not to sleep alone due to fear of having a seizure. The Queen of Prussia witnessed one of his seizures and was so alarmed by it that she fled for assistance. Another onlooker, Cardinal Kollonitsch (the Primate of Hungary), remained with him and later described continuous shaking of the left arm and leg, and an absent fixed stare. Epilepsy clearly did not affect Peter the Great's status at court or among his subjects, nor did it inhibit his ability to transform Russia from a remote, backward country into a world power. The American neurologist John Hughes (whose study of 43 famous historical figures was discussed earlier in this chapter) has evaluated Peter the Great's epilepsy and its possible cause, and concluded that he developed severe encephalitis (inflammation of the brain) as a neurological complication of a measles virus infection contracted in his twenties. He suggests that focal left-sided and generalized epilepsy developed as a complication of the resulting brain damage, and that over time it resulted in progressive weakness of the Tsar's left arm and leg.[242] However, if this had indeed been the case, it is likely that additional cognitive problems would have developed as a result of the encephalitis. In fact there is no evidence of this, and indeed his considerable achievements argue strongly against such a hypothesis.

Clearly Peter the Great's status as an all-powerful Tsar protected him from stigmatization and discrimination, and thus his epilepsy was no obstacle to achieving his ambitions for

---

241 Massie RK (1980) *Peter the Great: His Life and World*. Alfred A. Knopf, New York.
242 Hughes JR (2007) The seizures of Peter Alexeevich = Peter the Great, father of modern Russia. *Epilepsy & Behavior* 10, 179–182.

himself and his people. The fact that his epilepsy has been airbrushed out of most accounts of his life may well reflect his chroniclers' belief that any reference to the condition would detract from his perceived greatness.

Napoleon Bonaparte (1769–1821) might seem to be a perfect example of the link between military genius and epilepsy that was proposed by Sir William Broadbent (see page 205). Throughout his life Napoleon experienced episodes during which his face would become distorted; he would lose consciousness, and he would end up rolling on the ground. According to Cesare Lombroso (1835–1909), an Italian physician and criminologist, Napoleon was prone to outbursts of extreme temper, and any blackout associated with this was fabricated for the purpose of manipulating situations.[243] Many experts concur with the view that Napoleon had 'fits' of some kind, but also agree with Lombroso that the rages that ended with him throwing his body about were contrived to manipulate others. For example, David Chandler, one of the foremost Napoleonic historians, described the attacks as 'hysterical epilepsy' and coined the term 'Conqueror's syndrome' to refer to the controlling context in which they were deployed.[244]

Evidence to support the view that Napoleon had epilepsy comes from a number of sources. In 1896, Edmund Andrews, a surgeon at the Mercy Hospital of Chicago, wrote an article about Napoleon's 'alleged epilepsy'.[245] Far more recently, a biography by the British historian Frank McLynn included a description of a seizure that occurred while Napoleon was in bed with Mademoiselle George, who subsequently spread news of the event far and wide in order to humiliate him.[246] Alan Schom, an American historian and biographer of the great military leader, cites an episode that took place in 1805, on an occasion when Napoleon was in the company of the Empress Josephine. After dining with the Empress, and while holding her in his arms, he collapsed in 'a prolonged epileptic convulsion, foaming at the mouth, and vomiting on recovery'.[247] Josephine must have witnessed many of his attacks, as McLynn commented that others were alarmed when these occurred, but she was not. Charles-Maurice Talleyrand, Napoleon's chief diplomat, had heard rumours about the seizures, but was nevertheless terrified when he first witnessed a prolonged attack, which lasted for around 15 minutes. On recovering from these episodes, Napoleon always demanded complete silence from those who had witnessed them.

Eye-witness accounts of Napoleon's fits suggest that, if they were epileptic, they were generalized seizures, and, as far as can be ascertained, he was never given any of the limited

---

243 Lombroso C (1891) *The Man of Genius*. Walter Scott, London.
244 Chandler DG (1973) *Napoleon*. Saturday Review Press, New York.
245 Andrews E (1896) Napoleon's alleged epilepsy. *Journal of the American Medical Association* 16, 655–656.
246 McLynn F (1997) *Napoleon: A Biography*. Jonathan Cape Ltd, London.
247 Schom A (1997) *Napoleon Bonaparte: A Biography*. HarperCollins Publishers, New York.

treatments that were available at that time. In a detailed study of the 'attacks' experienced by Napoleon, the American neurologist John Hughes (mentioned several times earlier in this chapter) speculated about the possible causes of the condition, rather than whether or not it was epilepsy. He concluded that the Emperor experienced a combination of genuine epileptic seizures and what he termed 'psychogenic attacks'. He commented on the post-mortem finding of a scar on Napoleon's forehead, but rather than attributing the epileptic seizures to a head injury, he suggested that they were caused by chronic uraemia that had developed as a complication of gonorrhoea. However, in the absence of information about Napoleon's age at the onset of his epilepsy, and the frequency of his attacks thereafter, any theory of causation can never be more than conjecture.[248]

The Swedish chemist and engineer **Alfred Nobel** (1833–1896) is best known for inventing dynamite and founding the Nobel Prizes. The American neurophysiologists William and Margaret Lennox stated that Nobel 'was subject to migraine and convulsions from infancy'.[249] The only evidence to support their view was a poem entitled 'You say I am a riddle', assumed to be autobiographical, which was written by Nobel when he was 18 years old:

> *My cradle looked a deathbed, and for years*
> *a mother watched with ever anxious care,*
> *so little chance to save the flickering light,*
> *I scarce could muster strength to drain the breast,*
> *and the convulsions followed, till I gasped*
> *upon the brink of nothingness – my frame*
> *a school for agony with death for goal.*

If he had indeed had a convulsion while breastfeeding, it is possible that he could have learned about the event from his mother, who had already witnessed the death of five of his eight brothers. It is possible that he had a febrile convulsion (a seizure caused by a fever). However, only a small proportion of such cases go on to develop epilepsy. Moreover, a definitive account of Nobel's life, including his health, written by the Swedish physician Erik Jorpes, makes no mention of either infantile convulsions or adult epilepsy.[250] Thus, although his name is frequently included in lists of famous people with epilepsy, there appears to be little, if any, evidence that he had the condition.

---

248 Hughes JR (2003) Emperor Napoleon Bonaparte: did he have seizures? Psychogenic or epileptic or both? *Epilepsy & Behavior* 4, 793–796.
249 Lennox WG with Lennox MA (1960) *Epilepsy and Related Disorders*. Little, Brown & Company, Boston, MA.
250 Jorpes JE (1959) Alfred Nobel. *British Medical Journal*, 1, 1–6.

Another famous historical figure whose name is frequently linked to epilepsy is **Theodore Roosevelt** (1858–1919), the 26th President of the USA. Several websites, including the Epilepsy Foundation's 'Epilepsy Hall of Fame'[251] and Healthline's '12 Famous Faces of Epilepsy',[252] include his name on their lists. Moreover, the website of the Montgomery County Board of Developmental Disabilities clearly states that 'Throughout his life, Roosevelt suffered from epilepsy, prone to epileptic seizures, but that didn't stop him from his convictions.'[253] Neither Nathan Miller in his biography[254] nor Roosevelt himself in his own autobiography[255] make any reference to epilepsy, but instead they focus on his poor health due to debilitating asthma. In childhood, Roosevelt experienced severe night-time episodes of breathlessness, during which he feared he would die. His doctors had no remedy for the condition, and he would often sleep sitting up. When he was fighting for breath his father would carry him round the family home. As he grew older, on the advice of his father he subjected himself to bouts of extreme physical activity, such as rowing, boxing, and alpine walking, and eventually successfully overcame his asthma. Clearly in Roosevelt's case, inaccurate reporting and misinformation led his wheezing symptoms to be confused with epileptic seizures, and this myth has been perpetuated by the tendency of websites to copy information rather than seek out the source evidence.

William Morris (1834–1896) was an English textile designer, poet, novelist, and social activist who became the major force in the Arts and Crafts Movement. Although some websites include him in their lists of famous people with epilepsy, it was his eldest daughter Jenny who was diagnosed with the condition at the age of 15, and who thereafter suffered greatly from the enormous stigma that surrounded the disease in Victorian England. The attitudes of the time and their lasting impact on William and Jane Morris and the art that they developed were described by Leslie Forbes, who herself had epilepsy.[256]

Jenny excelled at school, but her life changed after she had a generalized convulsion (which was attributed to a boating accident in an attempt to render it more respectable) and was diagnosed with epilepsy at the age of 15. Eminent neurologists were consulted and potassium bromide was prescribed, despite its severe side effects. This was at a time when epilepsy was not mentioned in the social circles in which the Morris family moved. Jenny and her sister May were both taken out of school because of concerns that the epilepsy was hereditary, and from then on Jenny was cared for at home by her mother Jane, and was rarely left on her own.

---

251 www.epilepsy.com/connect/forums/epilepsy-friends-com-general-discussion/epilepsy-hall-fame
252 www.healthline.com/health/celebrities-epilepsy#1
253 www.mcbdds.org/329/Theodore-Roosevelt
254 Miller N (1992) *Theodore Roosevelt: A Life*. William Morrow & Company, Inc., New York.
255 Roosevelt T (1913) *Theodore Roosevelt: An Autobiography*. The Macmillan Company, New York.
256 Forbes L (2016) *Embroidered Minds of the Morris Women. Part One: Don't Remember*. Forbes & Thomas, London.

Jenny was never placed in an institution, but the burden of care placed on her family took its toll. In 1892 her mother wrote to the poet Wilfred Blunt, expressing her feelings about her daughter's seizures: 'It is not that Jenny is getting worse, but my nerves have given way under the great pressure of being continually in the house with her.'[257] In 1901 she wrote that 'Jenny is so much slower in speaking and apparently in thinking than she was a year ago.' The extent to which her slowness of thought and speech was due to the bromide treatment rather than the epilepsy itself is unclear. She subsequently required the care of two nurses, became delusional, and attempted suicide by trying to throw herself out of a window. After her parents died, a legacy provided for her care in a series of nursing homes until her death at the age of 74.

The epilepsy itself and especially the shame and stigma surrounding it had a huge effect both on Jenny and on the rest of her family. Wendy Parkins from the University of Otago has made a detailed study of the health of Jenny's mother, Jane Morris.[258] At the age of 29 she had become a chronic invalid, her condition being non-specific and possibly psychosomatic in nature. She certainly suffered from depression and melancholia, which could account for her almost constant ill health. Rosalind Howard, a family friend, described witnessing an attack, and commented on how Jenny's epilepsy had affected the female members of the family: 'I have never seen anything of the sort before and was horrified. What a horrifying thing it is and how hard it must be for her sister and delicate mother to bear such shocks.'[259] Jane, writing to Wilfred Blunt in 1885, expressed her own emotions as follows: 'It has been a dreadful grief for us all, worse for me, as I have to be constantly with her. I never get used to it. … Every time the thing occurs it is as if a dagger were thrust into me.'[260]

The reaction of Jenny's father, William Morris, to her epilepsy has been documented by Fiona MacCarthy in her biography.[261] She comments on the close relationship that eventually developed between father and daughter, and quotes Jenny as stating after his death that she had lost 'not just her father but her main companion and last real link with the outside world'. Although he had always left Jenny's care to others, his frequent letters to her convey deep affection despite the shame and guilt that he felt about her severe epilepsy. He steadfastly refused to allow her to be placed in an asylum or institution. In May 2018 the 'Embroidered Minds Epilepsy Garden' was created for the Epilepsy Society at the RHS Chelsea Flower Show in London. It aimed both to raise awareness of epilepsy and to celebrate the lives of Jenny Morris and Leslie Forbes, the journalist and broadcaster who up until her death in 2016 had done so much to bring the Morris family's story to public attention.

257 Sharp FC and Marsh J (eds.) (2012) *The Collected Letters of Jane Morris*. The Boydell Press, Woodbridge.
258 Parkins W (2008) Jane Morris's invalidism reconsidered. *Nineteenth-Century Gender Studies* 4.2 (summer issue).
259 Kelvin N (ed.) (1984) *The Collected Letters of William Morris*. Princeton University Press, Princeton, NJ.
260 Parkins W (2013) *Jane Morris: The Burden of History*. Edinburgh University Press, Edinburgh. p. 157.
261 MacCarthy F (1994) *William Morris: A Life for our Time*. Faber & Faber, London.

The American comedian **Bud Abbott** (1895–1974), who is listed on the Epilepsy Foundation's 'Epilepsy Hall of Fame' website, appeared with his stage partner Lou Costello in films, radio, television, and comic strips, becoming perhaps the most popular comedy act of the 1940s and 1950s. In their biography, Steven Cox and John Lofflin have documented the complex relationship that existed between the two performers.[262] At the age of 30, Abbott developed frequent sudden-onset epileptic seizures, and in order to keep the stage act going would incorporate them into the performance, with Lou simply carrying his partner off stage as though nothing was amiss. The manner in which Lou managed the situation without blame or embarrassment created a bond between the two men that was to last for the rest of their lives. Abbott's stage persona was that of the self-assured, confident 'straight man'. However, in real life he was insecure and extremely anxious about having seizures during a performance. He started drinking to calm his nerves, and this led to a long-term battle with alcoholism. He once told a friend that his anxieties about having seizures in public would cause him to wake up in the night screaming. He eventually withdrew from showbusiness and lived quietly in retirement until his death at the age of 77. During their working career, the supportive Costello insisted that Abbott be paid more than him, commenting that 'Comics are a dime a dozen. Good straight men are hard to find.' Abbott's epilepsy was concealed from his adoring public, and Costello's actions ensured that it remained a secret.

We shall end this inevitably selective review of famous historical figures who may or may not have had epilepsy by considering seizures caused by alcohol and drugs. As mentioned when we discussed the composer Modest Mussorgsky and the actor Richard Burton in Chapter 7, the distinction between drug- or alcohol-induced seizures and true epilepsy is by no means clear cut. Alcohol withdrawal seizures have commonly been called 'rum fits' because they were recognized in sailors who, once they were at sea, rapidly consumed their ration of rum, and then, following alcohol withdrawal, would have convulsions. Without treatment this state often progressed to delirium tremens with a rapid pulse rate, high temperature, acute confusion, and a significant risk of death. Convulsive seizures typically started within 12–48 hours of cessation of drinking, during which time the alcohol blood level dropped rapidly.

The American poet, short story writer, and critic **Edgar Allan Poe** (1809–1849) has found his way into the pantheon of famous people with epilepsy as a result of his delirium tremens and memory blanks. He was one of three children who, deserted by their father and following the early death of their mother, were each taken into the care of a different family. Edgar constantly argued with his foster father, and at a young age became prone to binge drinking and blackouts or memory blanks. With mounting gambling debts from his time in the army and then at

---

262 Cox S and Lofflin J (1997) *The Abbott & Costello Story: Sixty Years of "Who's on First?"* Cumberland House Publishing, Nashville, TN.

university, Poe started to write and sell his short stories and poems, and eventually became one of America's most accomplished writers. Alcohol misuse had a destructive effect on all of his relationships except that with his adored cousin Virginia Clemm, whom he married when she was just 13 years old. After her early death from tuberculosis, Poe's drinking worsened. There is no evidence of epileptic seizures occurring, but his frequent episodes of memory loss and delirium tremens have been well documented.[263]

In 1848, Poe was found semiconscious outside an Irish pub in Baltimore, wearing ragged clothes that were not his own. He was admitted to Washington College Hospital, by which time he was showing features of delirium tremens, with twitching, sweating, and hallucinations. He lapsed into unconsciousness and within three days had died, at the age of 40. Although it seems likely that Poe did experience alcohol withdrawal seizures, there is insufficient evidence to support the widespread claim that he should be included in the pantheon of writers with epilepsy. Some have even gone so far as to attribute his argumentative character and unreliability to him having the 'epileptic personality'. (For further information about the evidence for such a personality type, see Chapter 11.)

The English poet and critic **Algernon Swinburne** (1837–1909) has been included in the lists of famous people with epilepsy as a result of his alcohol withdrawal fits. The little information that we have about his health comes from a biography written by Edmund Gosse a few years after Swinburne's death.[264] It suggests that he was a curious combination of frailty and strength, with an addictive personality. At a young age he was apparently hyperactive, and as an adult displayed extremely uninhibited behaviour. The entry on Swinburne in encyclopedia.com describes him as 'living a dissolute life of heavy drinking and masochistic sexual practices. His dissipation had brought on a number of attacks similar to epileptic fits, but his amazing energy had enabled him to return each time to his frenzied style of life.'[265] This quote echoes the Victorian belief that sexual excess can cause seizures, and that people with epilepsy engage in abnormal sexual practices. Swinburne occasionally had seizures in public, usually a short time after he had drunk himself into a state of unconsciousness. Throughout the 1860s and 1870s this cycle of heavy drinking, collapse, and 'drying out' occurred repeatedly. Eventually his friend and legal adviser, Theodore Watts-Dunn, took him into his own home, where he forcibly imprisoned him in order to break the pattern of destructive behaviour. Swinburne eventually died not of alcohol-related causes, but from pneumonia. There is no suggestion that he ever experienced an unprovoked seizure, and therefore he cannot be said to have had epilepsy.

---

263 Silverman K (1992) *Edgar A. Poe: Mournful and Never-Ending Remembrance.* HarperPerennial, New York.
264 Gosse E (1917) *The Life of Algernon Charles Swinburne.* Macmillan and Company, London.
265 www.encyclopedia.com/people/literature-and-arts/english-literature-19th-cent-biographies/algernon-charles-swinburne

The American novelist, short story writer, playwright, and actor **Truman Capote** (1924–1984) has earned his place amongst the famous with epilepsy as a result of his alcohol withdrawal fits. He had a very traumatic childhood, witnessing the collapse of his parents' marriage when he was only four years old. Thereafter he was cared for by distant elderly relatives. He soon became dependent on alcohol and drugs, and in 1981 according to his biographer Gerald Clarke, he experienced a seizure that resulted in six days of hospitalization. His doctors attributed the seizure to alcohol misuse, but Capote apparently 'pointedly disregarded the admonitions of his doctors'.[266] Clarke describes how one of Capote's doctors met him later on, when he was once again in the early stages of alcohol withdrawal, and bought him a pint of vodka to try to prevent the inevitability of further withdrawal seizures.

The authors of Capote's obituary in the *Los Angeles Times* (published on 26 August 1984) raise questions about his seizures and epilepsy, stating that 'Capote was hospitalized in April, 1983, in Montgomery, Alabama, after test showed a "toxic level" of dilantin and phenobarbital in his system. Doctors said he had a "bad reaction" to the drugs, which are used to control epileptic-type seizures.'[267] These drugs are used to treat epilepsy, and would not normally be prescribed in a situation where the seizures were caused by an avoidable trigger such as alcohol. It is possible that the seizures, which had initially been caused by alcohol withdrawal after heavy drinking sessions, were now persisting despite his abstinence, in which case Capote could then be regarded as having epilepsy. The website of the Edmonton Epilepsy Association of Northern Alberta includes Capote in its list of 'Famous People with Epilepsy',[268] but one should bear in mind that this list also includes Alfred Nobel, Lenin, Leo Tolstoy, Leonardo da Vinci, and the asthmatic Theodore Roosevelt, so should perhaps be treated with caution.

It is significant that the comprehensive review by the neurologist John Hughes of the myths surrounding famous people and epilepsy does not mention anyone who lived beyond the early 1980s.[269] The relative lack of public awareness of present-day 'celebrities' with epilepsy suggests that most of those individuals would prefer to remain silent about their condition. Perhaps they have been advised by publicists and managers that admitting to their epilepsy could harm the public image that they wish to project. Alternatively, their reticence about the condition may reflect the fact that epilepsy is more commonly concealed than are other long-term conditions. (We shall discuss the issue of concealment in more detail in Chapter 12.) The few who have been open about their condition have often been seizure-free for some time, or only have seizures very infrequently, or have sustained some type of brain

---

266 Clarke G (1988) *Capote: A Biography*. Simon & Schuster, New York.
267 www.latimes.com/local/obituaries/archives/la-me-truman-capote-19840826-story.html
268 www.edmontonepilepsy.org/epilepsy/living/famous.html
269 Hughes JR (2005) Did all those famous people really have epilepsy? *Epilepsy & Behavior* 6, 115–139.

injury which, because this was beyond their control, makes their seizures more acceptable to the public. This silence and reticence is regrettable to the extent that people in the public eye who have epilepsy can be powerful role models for others with the condition. Stories from all walks of public life have led to positive changes in the public's perception of and empathy towards people with mental health problems. Famous individuals with mental illness are increasingly becoming champions for their condition, and, for example, growing numbers of sports players are admitting to seeking support for mental health problems, but so far this is not the case for epilepsy.

A prevalence study conducted in the USA showed the lifetime risk of developing epilepsy to be approximately 1 in 60,[270] representing a significant proportion of the population. During 2017 and 2018 there were 791 footballers registered to play for the 20 clubs in the English Premier League, and 650 Members of Parliament in the House of Commons at Westminster. However, at the time of writing I am not aware of any Premier League footballer who has admitted to having epilepsy, and to my knowledge only two Members of Parliament have done so. Perhaps this reflects a fear in the sports and political arenas that the opposition would view epilepsy as a sign of vulnerability. In 2010 the Conservative **Paul Maynard** (1975–) became the first British Member of Parliament to admit to having epilepsy, and he has subsequently become vice-chairman of the UK epilepsy charity Epilepsy Action. Soon afterwards, a fellow Conservative Member of Parliament, **Laura Sandys** (1964–), declared her epilepsy, adding that she had been seizure-free for around seven years. One of the most prominent political advocates for people with epilepsy was the Irish politician and former Lord Mayor of Dublin **Joe Doyle** (1939–2009). Doyle never concealed the fact that he had had epilepsy from the age of 16, and for many years he was an active supporter of the Irish Epilepsy Association. In the USA the former Governor of Hawaii **Neil Abercrombie** (1937–) and the US Congressman **Tony Coelho** (1942–) have both been publicly open about their epilepsy, and have campaigned for increased research funding and improved disability rights. In their book on high-profile Americans with disabilities, Brian McMahon and Linda Shaw of Virginia Commonwealth University relate how Coelho's neurologist explained to him that he had epilepsy and told him that 'The good news is that you don't have to serve in Vietnam, but the bad news is that you won't be able to become a Catholic priest – more specifically, a Jesuit.'[271] At that time the Roman Catholic Church still regarded epilepsy as being somehow related to demonic possession, and therefore viewed people with the condition as unsuitable for ordination.

---

270 Kobau RH, Zahran H, Thurman DJ et al. (2005) Epilepsy surveillance among adults. *Morbidity and Mortality Weekly Report. Surveillance Summaries* 57, 1–20.
271 McMahon BT and Shaw LR (eds.) (1999) *Enabling Lives: Biographies of Six Prominent Americans with Disabilities.* CRC Press, Boca Raton, FL.

There can be few greater influences on the young and their developing views and perceptions than the celebrity culture associated with popular music, social media, and sport. We have already mentioned a number of popular musicians who have been open about their epilepsy (see Chapter 7). Other more contemporary names include **Lindsey Buckingham** (1949–), the lead guitarist and vocalist in the group Fleetwood Mac, who at the age of 29 experienced a seizure while touring with the band. This may have been an isolated event, and it was successfully controlled with anti-epileptic drugs, but rumours of ongoing minor epilepsy lingered thereafter.[272] **Lil Wayne** (1982–), the American rapper, was forced to go public about his epilepsy in 2013 after an MTV news feature announced that he had been rushed to a Los Angeles hospital 'again' because of seizures. From the punk rock era, **Adam Horovitz** (1966–) of the Beastie Boys and **Richard Jobson** (1960–), Scottish singer-songwriter of the Skids, have both been open about their epilepsy.

Horovitz has given many interviews about his condition, in which he has described what seems to be photosensitive epilepsy, as he has experienced seizures on a photoshoot and while watching television. To this day he avoids flash photography and wears a medical alert bracelet on his wrist. He has also incorporated his epilepsy into the lyrics of the band's songs: 'Well I'm an epileptic, a skept-o-leptic check it. I'm cutting up the beats from the bear I clept it.'[273] Jobson recounts in his autobiography an incident that occurred when he was 15 that left him 'suffering with epilepsy',[274] and in an article published in *The Scottish Sun* (13 January 2018) he commented that 'Throughout my life I've had epilepsy and there was a period where the amount of seizures I was having was so intense it was making me incredibly ill.'[275] He has gone on to become a successful filmmaker, television presenter, and writer.

Turning now to influential figures in sport, the American track and field athlete **Florence Griffith Joyner** (1959–1998), also known as Flo Jo, was regarded as the fastest woman athlete of all time, and her 100-metre and 200-metre world records still stand today. After winning three gold medals at the 1988 Olympics she retired from athletics, but her involvement in fashion design and acting kept her in the public eye until her death at the age of 38 from suffocation during a severe sleep-related seizure. She had been diagnosed with epilepsy eight years earlier, and had initially taken her prescribed anti-epileptic drug treatment regularly. However, at the time of her death no such drugs were found in her bloodstream. Joyner was a global role model in terms of her athletic and subsequent achievements. However, her sudden death, which might well have been preventable, also publicly highlighted the importance of taking anti-epileptic medication regularly in order to control the condition.

---

272 Brunning B (2004) *The Fleetwood Mac Story: Rumours and Lies*. Omnibus Press, London.
273 'The Skills to Pay the Bills' lyrics © Universal Music Publishing Group 1992.
274 Jobson R (2018) *Into the Valley*. Wymer Publishing, Bedford.
275 www.thescottishsun.co.uk/news/2088923/band-richard-jobson-stuart-adamson-the-skids/

The famous cricketer and former England captain **Tony Greig** (1946–2012) found his epilepsy in the public spotlight when a story in the Australian newspaper *The Sydney Morning Herald* (12 September 1978) highlighted the question raised by many, given his condition, about his ability to make captaining decisions. Grieg had decided to break away from the English cricket establishment to join and recruit fellow players to a new league set up by the Australian television mogul Kerry Packer. When commentators used his epilepsy to question his judgement, Greig took legal action and won his court case. After this involuntary 'outing' of his epilepsy he admitted to having experienced seizures since the age of 14, which were partially controlled by drugs and by sleeping before matches. When his seizures, which were preceded by an aura, occurred on the field during play, they were explained as heat stroke by sympathetic team managers. During one match a convulsive episode led to him being physically restrained in front of thousands of spectators. Throughout his playing days the press focused on his vulnerability as a person with epilepsy, rather than highlighting his courage in continuing to play the sport on the public stage, and the strictly regulated lifestyle that he had to maintain in order to minimize his attacks. After the end of his sporting career, Greig went on to champion the cause of epilepsy, speaking regularly to the media about his experiences, and becoming epilepsy ambassador for the charity Epilepsy Action Australia.

Jonathan (Jonty) Rhodes (1967–), a former South African international cricketer, was regarded as the greatest fieldsman of his time, renowned for his phenomenal catches, stops, and throws. Throughout his international cricket career, which spanned a decade, it was common knowledge that he had epilepsy. He had an unusual form of the condition, and despite the fact that his symptoms first appeared when he was 6 years old, it was some time before the diagnosis was finally made. He described his seizures as 'mild'. They were only brought on by a bang to the head and concussion, so by avoiding contact sports such as rugby football (very popular in South Africa) and taking other safety precautions he was able to control the condition without taking medication, and to continue to drive. Rhodes has done much to destigmatize epilepsy in South Africa. He acknowledges that his own condition is mild and that he can take practical measures to avoid seizures, whereas others with epilepsy face discrimination both socially and in the workplace, and cannot drive. He is a tireless ambassador for Epilepsy South Africa, hosting events, fundraising, and raising awareness of the condition. His story raises the thorny question (which will be discussed in Chapter 12) of whether people with epilepsy should play contact sports in which minor head injuries are likely to occur.

The story of the outstanding American-born cycling champion **Marion Clignet** (1964) highlights the stigma that surrounded epilepsy in the late 1980s, leading to silence or reticence about the condition among people who suffered from it. After being diagnosed with generalized tonic–clonic epilepsy at the age of 22, she lost her driving licence and then took up cycling simply as a means of getting from one place to another. This soon developed into a sporting passion, and before long she was performing competitively at the highest level. Despite her impressive track record she was not picked for the 1990 US World Championship team, as her epilepsy was considered to pose a risk to the rest of the team. The precise nature of the risk was never specified, although it seems most likely that there was concern that she might have a seizure when cycling at speed, and then collide with other athletes. The French authorities did not share this concern, so instead of giving up her sport she applied for dual nationality. She went on to win Olympic silver medals in 1996 and 2000, as well as six world titles, all under the flag of her adopted country of France, and she became an ambassador for epilepsy. She is quoted as saying 'I'm really not sure how far I would have pushed myself if I didn't have epilepsy' (*Irish Mirror*, 12 February 2015),[276] indicating how much she felt the need to prove herself. After her retirement she helped to design bikes that would be safe for cyclists who experienced frequent and sudden seizures. If anything, the discrimination that she experienced early in her career only fuelled her motivation to succeed and to become a role model for others with epilepsy in similar situations.

The European and world champion 400-metre hurdler **Dai Greene** (1986–), who was diagnosed with epilepsy at the age of 17, has become a powerful advocate for the role of lifestyle factors in seizure control. In newspaper interviews he has explained how his condition had been worsened by alcohol and lack of sleep, and that it was only after switching to a healthy lifestyle, in combination with anti-epileptic drug therapy, that he was able to achieve much better control of his condition. After winning the World Championship in South Korea he began to speak openly about his epilepsy, explaining how his focus on athletics had helped him to get to university, and how the avoidance of late nights and heavy drinking had helped him to control his condition, rather than vice versa. His openness about epilepsy, his advice on the need to avoid triggers and remain fit, and his status as a world champion provides an inspiring role model. He has also become an ambassador for the UK charity Young Epilepsy.

Another high-profile sportsperson with epilepsy is the Chicago White Sox baseball player **Greg Walker** (1959–), who was reported in the *New York Times* (1 August 1988) to have 'suffered a second seizure this morning, but was stabilized without further complication'.[277] After he had been admitted to a local community hospital for tests and treatment, his team doctor was forced to admit that Walker had experienced another seizure a few days earlier while fielding balls during a training session. At the age of 29, now that his epilepsy was public knowledge, Walker admitted to having had the condition from the age of 4. Little

---

276 www.irishmirror.ie/news/irish-news/health-news/irelands-rugby-coach-joe-schmidt-5148914
277 www.nytimes.com/1988/08/01/sports/walker-suffers-second-seizure.html

mention was made of his epilepsy thereafter, and his fans did not seem disconcerted by the news. He returned to the baseball field eight months later, playing against the California Angels. He had now undergone full medical investigations and was on drug treatment. An article published in *Sports Illustrated* (17 April 1989) covered his return, and it concluded (notwithstanding the unfortunate use of the term 'epileptics') that 'For epileptics, he is a source of inspiration. Greg had one of the most public seizures it is possible to have in America, and if he had failed in his comeback, epileptics may have doubted themselves. That didn't happen because Greg didn't let it happen.'[278]

The British boxer **Terry Marsh** (1958–) remains an enigma in terms of whether or not he has epilepsy. Marsh had already become the British, European, and International Boxing Federation light welterweight world champion when he started to experience dizzy spells. He consulted a Harley Street neurologist, and the resulting diagnosis of epilepsy ended his boxing career in 1987 at the age of 29. He was a fireman to trade, and not surprisingly was no longer able to pursue that occupation either. He tried unsuccessfully to regain his boxing licence on the basis of new medical evidence, claiming that his attacks had been caused by consuming an excessive number of chocolate bars. Subsequently he was unsuccessfully sued for libel by the boxing promotor Frank Warren, who claimed that Marsh had allowed him to sign a contract for a fight while knowing he was suffering from epilepsy. Marsh's own self-published biography[279] offers no clear evidence about the epilepsy question. If he did indeed experience epileptic seizures, the possibility that repeated head injuries sustained during his 200 or so bouts were a causal factor cannot be ruled out. Due to the high risk of head injury, boxing is not recommended for people with epilepsy, and none of the world boxing authorities will grant a licence to a person with a diagnosis of epilepsy.

In the game of rugby union, the fact that no protective headgear is worn is causing increasing concern about the long-term consequences of repeated head injury. This has led to the introduction of stringent rules for removing injured players from the field of play after such an injury for an immediate assessment and an estimate of the length of time for which they should be rested. One might not expect a person with epilepsy to be engaged in this particular sport at its highest level, but the Scottish international rugby player **Tom Smith** (1971–) has proved to be the exception, and an inspiration to those with epilepsy who wish to play the game. Smith's epilepsy started in his late teens, with the seizures occurring at night while he was asleep. He played as a prop forward, one of the most physically demanding positions in the team, and went on to represent the British and Irish Lions on tours of South Africa and Australia. In an article in the *Telegraph* newspaper (27 October 2000)

---

278 www.si.com/vault/1989/04/17/119751/just-happy-to-be-here-opening-day-1989-was-special-for-white-sox-first-baseman-greg-walker-eight-months-ago-he-thought-he-had-died
279 Marsh T (2005) *Undefeated: My Story*. Terry Marsh Publishing.

he commented that 'Everyone thinks that when you have epilepsy you cannot take part in physical sports, and you don't get more physical than rugby, but that's not the case. I was told I could still play, as long as I took care of myself.'[280] In the same week, in an interview with the *Scotsman* newspaper (24 October 2000), he was quoted as saying 'I have been fortunate that my epilepsy hasn't been too serious – on a scale of one to ten of how serious it could be, I'd rate myself just a one – but of course you do think about what could happen sometimes and how it could affect you.'[281] Nearly a decade later, at the age of 37, in an interview with the *Independent* newspaper (25 April 2009), Smith said 'I've been suffering from epileptic seizures – Grand Mals, they call them – since I was 18. Until three years ago, the attacks always happened in my sleep. Then, three years ago, I had a waking attack, which meant I had to forfeit my driving licence for 12 months. Three weeks after getting it back, I had another one. Another year off the road.'[282] In the same interview he described his daytime attacks and highlighted the transient short-term memory problems that followed them: 'I've had to be careful not to return to rugby too quickly after an attack, because the short-term memory loss can be very acute. I played a Calcutta Cup match against England after having a seizure on the day of the game, and believe me, it wasn't the best idea I ever had. ... But I consider myself fortunate to have had such a long career in professional sport in spite of my problem, and I talk of it openly because I want other sufferers to know that epilepsy doesn't have to be a barrier to achievement.' He remains one of the most articulate sports players with epilepsy, and is continuing to raise awareness of the condition both through the epilepsy charity Epilepsy Scotland in his native Scotland, and in New Zealand.

The American NFL football players **Tiki Barber** (1975–), his twin brother **Ronde Barber** (1975–), and **Jason Snelling** (1983–) played with the New York Giants, Tampa Bay Buccaneers, and Atlanta Falcons, respectively. They have all spoken publicly about their epilepsy and demonstrated that, even in this toughest of sports, high levels of achievement are possible for people with the condition. The Barber twins experienced seizures from early childhood, but both went on to have successful NFL careers, Tiki spending ten seasons in the league before becoming a media sports pundit, and Ronde leading his team to the 2002 Super Bowl victory. Jason Snelling was affected by seizures from his mid-teens, but subsequently became a running back; he retired from his Atlanta team in 2014 after a 5-year career as an NFL player. In an interview early in his career he described the relief he felt when he was diagnosed and finally found out what was wrong, but also his dismay at needing to take drug treatment. Initially he kept his epilepsy a secret, but when he eventually started to

---

280 www.telegraph.co.uk/sport/rugbyunion/4774560/About-Rugby-Smiths-epilepsy-burden.html
281 www.scotsman.com/sport/rugby-union-2-14915/smith-tries-to-put-illness-in-perspective-1-639541
282 www.independent.co.uk/sport/rugby/rugby-union/club-rugby/tom-smith-i-played-right-after-one-seizure-ndash-not-a-good-idea-1673944.html

speak about it he found people much more supportive than he had expected. Snelling had no concerns about seizures occurring while he was playing, as exertion had never been a trigger. His seizures eventually responded to medication, abstention from alcohol, and a healthy lifestyle. He became involved with the Epilepsy Foundation, and through various awareness-raising activities he campaigns to reduce the stigma associated with epilepsy.

It is disappointing that few in the world of soccer have spoken so candidly about their seizures. One exception is the Port Vale captain **Leon Legge** (1985–), who was first diagnosed at the age of 16, following a seizure on the training ground. He has reported being seizure-free on medication for two years, and has become an ambassador for the charity Young Epilepsy. In an article published in the *Evening Standard* (9 December 2010) he commented that 'At first it was something that got to me, but you learn to deal with it. Once you're on the right medication you can get on with things and lead a normal life. Luckily, I had a mild case.'[283]

It was mentioned earlier how very few current film, television, and social media celebrities have admitted to having epilepsy. It seems likely that one of the main reasons for this is the increasing importance of image. Reality television and social media have produced a new type of celebrity who is basically 'famous for being famous'. For example, **Katie Hopkins** (1975–) is a British media celebrity who started out as a contestant in the television programme 'The Apprentice', and has subsequently become an outspoken broadcaster and contributor to national newspapers. Her forthright views expressed on Twitter have been very controversial, and she has been accused of insensitive and even racist comments. She has been equally outspoken about the fact that she has epilepsy. She first experienced 'blank spells' during her teens. The side effects of her initial treatment with carbamazepine led her to stop taking the drug, and she lost confidence in her physicians. After university she concealed her epilepsy in order to gain a place at the Royal Military Academy at Sandhurst. There her epilepsy worsened, she experienced major tonic–clonic seizures, and when her past medical records came to light she was not allowed to graduate and take up a commission in the army. She then embarked on a business career, continued to conceal her epilepsy, and became a contestant on two reality TV shows. During National Epilepsy Week in May 2009 she finally spoke at length about her experience of living with the condition, in an interview with the *Daily Mail* newspaper.[284] Subsequently, in response to criticism that she was using her epilepsy for self-promotion, she commented that many people with epilepsy want to see more public figures 'coming out' and being honest about living with the condition, thereby reducing the stigma associated with it. In an article in the *Mail on Sunday* (4 March 2017) she shared her experiences of undergoing

---

[283] www.standard.co.uk/sport/football/epilepsy-has-not-stopped-leon-legge-achieving-his-goal-6545183.html
[284] www.dailymail.co.uk/health/article-1179775/Apprentice-star-Katie-Hopkins-Why-I-kept-Sandhurst-dark-epilepsy.html

epilepsy surgery.[285] At the time of writing, the extent to which this surgery has improved her symptoms is unclear. However, Hopkins has done much to bring the reality of epilepsy to a wider audience. Her concerns are shared by many people who are living with the condition, and she has been a powerful voice speaking on their behalf.

Conclusion

The lists of 'famous people with epilepsy' that can be found on numerous websites are inaccurate and make claims that cannot be substantiated. The problem with diagnosing historical figures is that the evidence is anecdotal, medical records are often non-existent, and of course the individuals concerned are no longer available to be questioned. The margins of error in over- and under-reporting epilepsy are immense. These famous names from the past are cited by charities and other epilepsy organizations to promote the message that people with epilepsy can be high achievers in a wide range of fields. However, this motivational approach is so far removed from the real-world problems that are faced on a daily basis by the average person with epilepsy that it runs the risk of reinforcing feelings of failure. The idea that epilepsy and genius go hand in hand might be an attractive one, but the population with epilepsy is fairly similar to the general population in terms of IQ range, albeit skewed slightly by the increased incidence of epilepsy in people with learning disabilities and acquired brain injury. In contrast to historical figures, present-day 'celebrities' with epilepsy will have their condition better documented, eye-witness accounts are available, and the individual is available to give a personal account of their condition. Yet we continue to place the main emphasis on people from the past, no matter how inaccurate their diagnosis might be, because of the general reluctance of present-day celebrities to step forward and admit to having epilepsy, to act as role models and advocates for those who have the condition, and to challenge public perceptions of the disorder.

Sports players are more likely to be open about having epilepsy, and this may reflect the need for drug testing, which requires them to declare all the medications that they are taking. These individuals are potentially powerful role models, but in some areas of sport, such as Premier League football in the UK, no one has stepped forward so far. A similar lack of role models can be found in other fields, notably theatre, film, and popular music. The various reasons for the silence or reticence of well-known or influential individuals who could potentially dispel myths, reduce discrimination and stigmatization, and educate the wider public about epilepsy will be discussed in more detail in Chapter 12.

---

285 www.dailymail.co.uk/debate/article-4281498/KATIE-HOPKINS-Surgery-end.html

PART IV

Epilepsy in society

CHAPTER 10
Epilepsy, laws, and officialdom

In this chapter we shall look at the law in relation to the normal daily activities and experiences of people with epilepsy, wherever possible viewing such legislation from a global perspective.

Most aspects of our lives are governed by rules and regulations designed to protect ourselves and others. Disabled people can be advantaged or disadvantaged by legislation, and in general the lawmakers' understanding of health-related issues lags some way behind that of informed healthcare professionals. Consequently, many of the laws and regulations that people with epilepsy have to comply with today reflect outdated misunderstandings or ill-informed prejudice.

The eugenics movement

In developing countries, legislation or the lack of legal protection can be partly ascribed to the firmly held and inaccurate perception of the causes of epilepsy, along with the prevailing belief that it is an untreatable condition. In the Western world, many of the laws from the late nineteenth century onward reflected the influence of the powerful and persuasive eugenics movement on politicians and policymakers. These laws were based on the doctrine that those with disabilities were inferior and a burden to the state, and therefore should not be given the same rights as the able-bodied.

Eugenics is defined as the practice or support of controlled selective breeding of human populations to 'improve' the population's genetic composition – for example, by compulsory or voluntary sterilization. In Chapter 2 we provided a brief description of the role played by **Francis Galton** (1822–1911), a cousin of Charles Darwin, in the emergence of the eugenics movement.

Galton was one of the founder members of the Eugenics Society, the original aim of which was to promote public awareness of hereditary disease and to encourage 'social responsibility' by using controlled breeding to prevent the transmission of such disease from parents to offspring. The Society used its journal, *The Eugenics Review*, to promote ideas and publish research relating to eugenics. Prominent scientists and sociologists regularly expressed their views in its articles and letters, in particular Galton, Julian Huxley (1887–1975), and Leonard Darwin (1850–1943) (Charles Darwin's fourth son). The latter, despite his lack of formal scientific training, became a leading eugenicist and, as Chairman and then President of the British Eugenics Society, carried the mantle of the movement well into the twentieth century.

A number of prominent literary figures, including H.G. Wells (1866–1946) and George Bernard Shaw (1856–1950), fiercely defended those eugenicists who discouraged people with genetic defects or inheritable 'undesirable traits' from having children. We can assume that epilepsy would have fallen into both of these categories.

Across the Atlantic, in 1903 the American Breeders Association (ABA) was founded by agricultural scientists to promote eugenic research. The prominent American biologist Charles Davenport (1866–1942) played a key role in shifting the emphasis of the ABA from agricultural to human heredity. He founded the Eugenics Record Office in 1910, established links with Nazi Germany, and edited their eugenics journals both before and during the Second World War. In his book *Heredity in Relation to Eugenics* (1911), which became a standard text for medical students despite its flawed scientific reasoning, he stated that 'It is a reproach to our intelligence that we as a people, proud in other respects of our control of nature, should have to support about half a million insane, feeble-minded, epileptic, blind and deaf, 80,000 prisoners and 100,000 paupers at a cost of over 100 million dollars per year.'[286]

In the early twentieth century, eugenics began to identify itself as an emerging science, and four international eugenics conferences were held between 1911 and 1932. The first of these, euphemistically called the International Hygiene Exhibition, took place in Dresden. It was widely reported in the British press, and was featured in the *British Medical Journal* and in *Hansard*, the official record of the proceedings of British Parliament, thus attracting the attention of politicians and policymakers.

Criticisms were occasionally levelled at the eugenicists, most vocally by the English writer G.K. Chesterton (1874–1936) in his book *Eugenics and Other Evils* (1922), in which he predicted that genetics would be misused to engineer a society in which the poor and the

---

286 Davenport C (1911) *Heredity in Relation to Eugenics*. Holt & Company, New York.

ill were suppressed. Nevertheless, increasing numbers of countries established their own eugenics societies and incorporated compulsory sterilization into their legal code.

Theodore Roosevelt Jr (1858–1919), the 26th President of the USA, stated his strong desire that 'the wrong people could be prevented entirely from breeding', and created the Heredity Commission with a view to achieving this aim in America. As a consequence of this initiative the Eugenics Record Office (ERO) was established in Cold Spring Harbour, New York, generously funded by some of America's leading philanthropists. In 1914 the founders of the ERO passed their sterilization law, which advocated compulsory sterilization for the 'feebleminded, insane, and dependent', including the 'socially inadequate' and 'epileptics'.

The Virginia statute that allowed the compulsory sterilization of people who were considered to be 'genetically unfit' was upheld by the United States Supreme Court in the case of Buck v Bell (1927). The decision of the court was delivered by Oliver Wendell Holmes Jr. (1841–1935), Associate Justice of the Supreme Court of the United States. The plaintiff, Carrie Buck, was an 18-year-old girl with epilepsy who had been committed to the Virginia State Colony for Epileptics and Feebleminded, along with her mother. Both were considered to be 'feebleminded', and Carrie's 7-month-old illegitimate child was reported to show 'backwardness'. John Bell was the superintendent at the Colony responsible for the sterilization, which the Supreme Court ruled was lawful on the grounds that 'three generations of imbeciles are enough'. This case gave the green light for laws on eugenic sterilization to be passed in 30 states, and the Supreme Court's ruling has never been overturned.

Throughout the 1930s, further support for the campaign to reduce society's burden of disabled and 'degenerate' people was provided by such powerful politicians as Woodrow Wilson (1856–1924), the 28th President of the USA, and Winston Churchill (1874–1965), the future British Prime Minister. By 1938, a total of 29 states in the USA had passed laws permitting compulsory sterilization for people with presumed genetic conditions such as epilepsy. In the late 1930s, links became established between the eugenics movements in America and Britain and that in Nazi Germany. Leon Whitney, a prominent member of the American Eugenics Society, praised Hitler for introducing compulsory sterilization in 1933 via the Law for the Prevention of Hereditarily Diseased Offspring, which defined feeblemindedness as conditions affecting the nervous system, including epilepsy. In his book *The Case for Sterilization*,[287] a copy of which was requested by Hitler, Whitney stated that '400,000 known defectives in Germany', of whom around 60,000 had epilepsy, were subject to the new law. This involved collaboration between neurologists, psychiatrists, and the Nazi party, thus giving academic respectability to the concept of racial hygiene. Anti-Semitism employed the same 'cleansing' procedures during the Holocaust.

---

287 Whitney LF (1934) *The Case for Sterilization*. Frederick A. Stokes Co., New York.

In Germany the physicians who had been complicit in the compulsory sterilization and extermination of disabled people, including those with epilepsy, were eventually convicted in 1946 at the Doctors Trial in Nuremberg. At an international level, the eugenics movement became less visible after the Second World War. Many of the compulsory sterilization laws were subsequently repealed, and in 1978 the US Federal Sterilization Regulations were introduced to prevent coercive sterilization. However, to this day the movement's legacy continues to contribute to the burden that many people with epilepsy experience, both in terms of prejudiced attitudes towards the disabled, and in the resurgence of eugenics ideology as a tool of the political far right.

Rules and regulations

Today, in many developed countries, epilepsy is a recognized disability and people with the condition are protected by disability legislation and regulations. However, they can still be subject to some laws and regulations – for example, with regard to employment or holding or reapplying for a driving licence – that appear to be unjust or discriminatory. The misperception that people with epilepsy are a danger to others has resulted in excessively restrictive regulations that only add to the subjective burden of illness, by generating feelings of anger and frustration. Such regulations often reflect deep-seated fears and prejudices that border on the superstitious. Of course there is a logical rationale for some specific regulations, such as those relating to uncontrolled epilepsy and fitness to drive. However, others have a less rational basis, such as being denied the right to co-pilot a plane after several decades of freedom from seizures. There are also inconsistencies between one country and another – for example, with regard to driving restrictions, which range from lifelong driving bans to the requirement to have been free from seizures for more than 12 months, and vary in terms of the type of vehicle that can be driven (private, public, or heavy goods vehicles).

The **right to marry** – a fundamental right – requires legal regulation by the state as it establishes a contract that involves inheritance and the ownership of property. The false claim that the eugenicists made about epilepsy was that it was predominantly an inherited disease and was always associated with 'feeblemindedness' and mental illness. For these reasons they viewed compulsory or voluntary sterilization as a means of eradicating the condition. The legal prevention of marriage (assuming that most children were born in wedlock) offered an alternative solution. By the mid-1950s a total of 17 states in the USA had prohibited the marriage of people with epilepsy, and it was a crime not just for the 'epileptic' to marry, but also for a person without epilepsy to knowingly marry a person with the condition.

Earlier in the twentieth century, the New England state of Connecticut introduced a statute prohibiting men who were 'epileptic, imbecile, or feeble-minded' from marrying women under 45 years of age, which at that time was assumed to be the upper limit of the reproductive age span for women. Similarly, women under 45 years of age who were 'epileptic, imbecile, or feeble-minded' were prohibited from marrying men of any age.[288] The Connecticut courts declared such a marriage a criminal act, commenting 'that epilepsy is a disease of a peculiarly serious and revolting character, tending to weaken mental force, and often descending from parent to child, or entailing upon the offspring of the sufferer some other grave form of nervous malady, is a matter of common knowledge, of which courts will take judicial notice. ... One mode of guarding against the perpetuation of epilepsy obviously is to forbid sexual intercourse with those afflicted by it, and to preclude such opportunities for sexual intercourse as marriage furnishes. To impose such a restriction upon the right to contract marriage ... is no invasion of the equality of all men before the law, if it applies equally to all, under the same circumstances, who belong to a certain class of persons.' The same flimsy logic underpinned the sterilization laws (mentioned earlier in this chapter) that had been passed in 29 US states by 1938, without either defining epilepsy or noting how commonly it was inherited.

In 1905 the Connecticut courts ruled that concealment of epilepsy would result in entitlement to divorce on the grounds of fraudulent contract. The state of New Jersey was slightly more liberal, allowing people with epilepsy to marry if they could provide a certificate of approval from 'two regular physicians' (the definition of 'regular' was not provided). In Ohio, a marriage licence would not be granted if either of the applicants was 'a habitual drunkard, epileptic, imbecile or insane, or who at the time of making an application for said licence is under the influence of any intoxicating liquor or drug'. These now outdated laws reflected profound misunderstandings about the diverse causes and manifestations of epilepsy, and over time it became apparent that they could no longer be justified scientifically. In 1955 the state of North Carolina changed its law so as to allow marriage of individuals whose seizures were under control, reflecting a move away from the inheritance-dominated legislation, and by 1980 the last US state had repealed the legislation that prevented people with epilepsy from marrying.

In Britain there were no laws preventing an individual with epilepsy from marrying, although until about 50 years ago there was legislation that would allow such a marriage to become null and void. The Matrimonial Causes Act (1937) stated that a marriage had grounds for annulment if 'either party to the marriage was at the time of the marriage

---

288 Dike SM (1913) State laws regulating marriage of the unfit. *Journal of the American Institute of Criminal Law and Criminology* 4, 423–425.

subject to recurrent fits of insanity or epilepsy.' The then-Archbishop of Canterbury, Cosmo Lang, argued against the inclusion of epilepsy in this act, commenting that 'It would not be suggested in such a case that that incurable disease [epilepsy] was a ground on which the man could get rid of his wife and send her to an institution and marry someone else.' However, it was not until 34 years later that the Nullity of Marriage Act (1971) finally acknowledged this and removed epilepsy as a grounds for declaring a marriage void.

In some parts of the world, including India and China, epilepsy continued to be regarded as a legal reason for annulling or prohibiting marriage. The Hindu Marriage Act (1958) stated that a marriage could only be solemnized if neither party had ever suffered from epilepsy or insanity. In 1976 the Indian Government replaced this with the Marriage Law Amendment Act (1976), which stated that any person who experienced recurrent attacks of epilepsy or insanity could not have a legally valid marriage, and that any such marriage that had taken place would be made void by divorce. In 1996 the Indian Epilepsy Association challenged the legal validity of the Act, and the Government removed the legislation in 1999. Today in India the marriage of a person with epilepsy is legally valid and the condition is no longer regarded as acceptable grounds for divorce. Despite these changes, prejudiced attitudes persist, and in India it is still common practice for people with epilepsy to conceal this fact prior to marriage. The authors of a very recent appraisal of the specific issue of epilepsy and arranged marriage[289] noted that divorce rates were considerably higher in people with epilepsy who had entered an arranged marriage. They commented that 'marital plans and aspirations should be discussed with the family of the person with epilepsy in a timely and proactive manner. The benefits of disclosing epilepsy during marital negotiations should be underscored.' They do not tell us what effect such disclosure might have on the perceived eligibility of a potential partner. However, it is perhaps unsurprising that, worldwide, people with epilepsy have a lower likelihood of being married or in a long-term relationship than the general population. As part of a collaborative study of epilepsy-related stigma, a research group from Peking University in China reported that only public servants with epilepsy have their health costs reimbursed, but it did not provide pointers to any legislation.[290] Detailed information on the law and marriage in China is scarce, but anecdotal accounts indicate that epilepsy remains a major hurdle to obtaining a marriage licence. The UK Foreign and Commonwealth Office guidance (published in 2019) advises that it is no longer possible to marry in China unless one of the couple is Chinese, but again makes no reference to any regulations relating to disability, including epilepsy.

---

289 Singh G, Pauranik A, Menon B et al. (2016) The dilemma of arranged marriages in people with epilepsy. An expert group appraisal. *Epilepsy & Behavior* 61, 242–247.
290 Yang R, Wang W, Snape D et al. (2011) Stigma of people with epilepsy in China: views of health professionals, teachers, employers and community leaders. *Epilepsy & Behavior* 21, 261–266.

The human right to freedom of movement is a fundamental one. However, in the USA, until the 1970s it was legal to deny people with seizures access to restaurants, theatres, recreational centres, and other public buildings. From then on the Americans with Disabilities Act (1973) offered protection, much of which was qualified, only accepting an individual if any reasonable accommodations deemed to be necessary were made. For example, if a person with epilepsy wanted to join a swimming club, membership might be conditional on the use of a floatation device while in the pool. This stipulation could be made irrespective of whether or not the person's seizures were controlled, and on account of its unreasonable nature could be seen as prejudiced against those with epilepsy. Sadly, 'reasonable accommodations' can be deployed to subtly discriminate against the individual by making the adjustment demeaning (as in this example). Recreational facilities such as gyms and health clubs can thus exclude people with epilepsy by suggesting unacceptable accommodations, and in doing so they obey the letter but not the spirit of the law. However, the Americans with Disabilities Act does prevent a restaurant manager from asking an individual with epilepsy to leave or to sit in another area due to concern about other customers' reactions. It also prevents hoteliers from declining overnight bookings for similar reasons.

Movement from one country to another is a major issue that often involves the need to consider healthcare costs and employment prospects. People with long-term health problems incur considerable financial costs, and their entry to another country can be perceived as a societal burden. Until 2002, immigration laws in Canada could prohibit the entry of people with epilepsy whose healthcare costs might be regarded as excessive. The Canadian Immigration Act (1976) stated that people with disabilities, including epilepsy, were prohibited from becoming permanent residents if they might be reasonably expected to be a burden on health and social service systems. The key phrase here was 'reasonably expected', giving unlimited power to the legal decision maker, and little opportunity for those turned down to make a successful appeal. The Immigration and Refugee Protection Act (2002) replaced this legislation, allowing residency for those with disabilities if they could be sponsored by a partner or parent or were granted refugee status, regardless of the potential impact on health or social care systems. A subsequent Supreme Court ruling instructed immigration authorities, when making decisions, to assess the family members of disabled children in order to identify whether they had sufficient financial and other resources to provide support without posing an 'excessive burden on social services'. It therefore seems that the degree of severity of a person's epilepsy remains a bar to Canadian residency if their immediate family are unable to provide financial support.[291]

---

291 MacNaughton H (2011) *Epilepsy and the Law: What are the Legal Rights of a Person with Epilepsy in British Columbia?* Victoria Epilepsy and Parkinson's Centre, Victoria, BC.

Tuberculosis is the only specific health condition that automatically rules out immigration to Australia. However, individuals must declare any pre-existing condition, and are assessed on a case-by-case basis, so prevention of entry on other health grounds is certainly not ruled out. Conditions such as HIV, cancer, and heart disease are frequently cited, but there have also been cases of applicants with mental illness and epilepsy who have been denied a visa. Health grounds are second only to security concerns in determining whether Australian visa applications will be rejected. In 2009 the Australian Parliament Joint Standing Committee on Migration conducted an inquiry into the treatment of people with a disability who were seeking citizenship. Complex partial seizures and poorly controlled epilepsy were deemed to impose significant healthcare demands and costs. The committee recommended formal medical examination of all individuals with significant health problems, and stated that 'a visa applicant will be found not to meet the health requirement if they result in significant costs to the Australian community'. In 2012 the threshold placed on medical costs to Australia visa applicants was increased for the first time in a decade in an attempt to reduce perceived Government discrimination against people with a disability.

In the USA the first federal immigration law was introduced in 1882. It prohibited entry to any 'lunatic, idiot, or person unable to take care of himself or herself without becoming a public charge'. Such a broad definition of unsuitability was open to wide interpretation. The subsequent Immigration Act of 1903, also known as the Anarchist Exclusion Act, was more precisely framed and defined four inadmissible groups, namely anarchists, people with epilepsy, beggars, and prostitutes. The impetus behind these moves to prevent 'undesirables' from entering the USA was the assassination of President William McKinley in 1901 by the anarchist son of Polish immigrants. The Immigration Act of 1907 again highlighted the undesirability of those with epilepsy, barring entry to 'all idiots, imbeciles, feebleminded persons, epileptics, insane persons, and persons who have been insane within five years previous'. In 1965 a series of amendments were made to the Immigration and Nationality Act of 1952, and epilepsy was no longer considered an absolute ground for exclusion, although it was still regarded as a mental condition.[292] People with epilepsy are now allowed to enter the USA, but they still have to face the hurdle of obtaining healthcare insurance and being eligible to access appropriate and often expensive treatments. Interestingly, a recent US study showed epilepsy to be less prevalent among the recent immigrant population than in the non-immigrant population. There are two possible reasons for this. The first is the so-called 'healthy immigrant effect', whereby, due to their ability to travel, a newly arrived immigrant community might be healthier than the general population at their destination. The second

---

292 Moore JE (1970) Mental illness exclusions in United States immigration procedures. *Case Western Reserve Journal of International Law* 3, 71–87.

reason is that healthcare costs may deter people with epilepsy from making the journey in the first place. The Trump administration's promise to deport large numbers of illegal immigrants came into sharp focus when a recent story highlighted the plight of a Mexican couple whose 8-year-old daughter, born in the USA, has severe epilepsy. The parents explained that if they had to return to Mexico with their daughter she would have a very short life expectancy.[293]

In the UK, immigration law never appears to have restricted the right to residency of people with epilepsy, although in recent years, in the context of a healthcare system that is free at the point of delivery, there have been concerns about the additional costs that any long-term illness might incur. This has been offset to some extent by the introduction of the Immigration Health Surcharge (IHS), which is paid for when making a visa application. This surcharge entitles migrants to use the National Health Service (NHS) within the UK without additional charge. It was introduced under the Immigration Act 2014 to cover non-European Economic Area (EEA) nationals seeking to reside in the UK for longer than six months. The surcharge is the same fixed amount irrespective of whether the individual is healthy or has a long-term condition such as epilepsy, and was designed to ensure that all such migrants made an adequate contribution to the cost of NHS care.

In developed countries the **right to drive a vehicle** is widely regarded as a fundamental requirement for undertaking normal daily activities, and the ability to drive is often essential for employment. Any condition that transiently deprives people of their awareness makes driving a car, lorry, bus or train, or piloting an aeroplane, a hazardous activity. Epilepsy is just one of many conditions in which loss of awareness or consciousness can occur while the affected person is in control, yet it tends to attract the most media attention when tragic accidents occur. There is no question that a person who experiences blackouts must not drive. However, there is controversy about two central questions relating to driving and epilepsy. When can a person who no longer has seizures and whose epilepsy is considered to be under control be regarded as safe to drive again? And what type of vehicle are they planning to drive? Another controversial issue is that of confidentiality, when a healthcare professional has to consider whether they have a responsibility to report a person with ongoing seizures whom they know is continuing to drive illegally. The final issue concerns how to monitor people with controlled epilepsy who are now legally allowed to drive, and how frequently to review their driving status without infringing their human rights. Legislation should be unambiguous and designed to protect all road users, including those with epilepsy. The term 'controlled epilepsy' frequently appears in the laws that define a person's safeness to drive, but the actual definition of this term is unclear (for example, whether the warning or aura

---

293 Wiener J (2017) The deportation fears of immigrants with disabled children. *The Atlantic*, 19 May 2017. www.theatlantic.com/health/archive/2017/05/deportation-disability/526986/

of an attack alone without loss of awareness, or the persistence of nocturnal attacks when the individual is asleep safe in their bed at night, should be regarded as criteria for restricting driving).

Let us begin by considering an example of what can happen when a person with uncontrolled epilepsy continues to drive. In November 2011 a BBC News item described how a driver with a history of epilepsy had caused the death of a woman by playing what the police described as 'Russian roulette' with his condition. The driver was jailed for six years after crashing into four cars while having an epileptic seizure. This accident resulted in an elderly woman being fatally injured and three other people, including a 2-year-old child, being seriously hurt. In court the driver admitted causing death by dangerous driving, and also pleaded guilty to three charges of causing grievous bodily harm. After the trial a police spokesperson commented that 'the driver had a serious medical condition but was self-employed and felt he needed to drive. He will have to live with the consequences of his actions for the rest of his life.' The driver had apparently not disclosed the full extent of his condition to the Driver & Vehicle Licensing Agency (DVLA). A spokeswoman for Epilepsy Action, an epilepsy charity, stated that there were strict rules for drivers who had been diagnosed with epilepsy: 'It is against the law for people with epilepsy who have seizures to drive unless their seizures occur only during sleep. All drivers with a diagnosis of epilepsy must inform the DVLA. People with epilepsy who have been seizure free for one year can drive. However, all drivers have a legal obligation to inform the DVLA if they have a seizure, and they must stop driving. They can apply or reapply for a driving licence as long as they have been completely free from seizures for one year.'[294]

This type of tragic story is repeated regularly in the press, highlighting the collective responsibility that we all have to others, the fact that the need to drive to earn a living can be misplaced (as in this example of a self-employed driver), and the civic duty to self-report to the authorities.

In the UK the DVLA has produced guidelines to enable medical practitioners to advise their patients on their medical fitness to drive; these can also be freely accessed online.[295]

Many UK epilepsy charities provide excellent information sheets and online information to help both the healthcare professional and the patient to navigate the regulations. The DVLA Guide states that an individual can apply for a driving licence after they have been seizure-free (irrespective of whether they are on medication) for 1 year. People with ongoing sleep-related seizures who then have a single daytime seizure must wait until they have been

---

294 Quoted on BBC News, 18 November 2011.
295 Driver & Vehicle Licensing Agency (2019) *Assessing Fitness to Drive: A Guide for Medical Professionals*. assets.publishing.service.gov.uk/government/uploads/system/uploads/attachment_data/file/834504/assessing-fitness-to-drive-a-guide-for-medical-professionals.pdf

free of daytime seizures for 3 years before they can be granted a licence. If an individual does not have epilepsy but experiences a solitary seizure, they must stop driving for 6 months while specialist assessments and investigations are undertaken to identify any cause (e.g. brain tumour) that might necessitate a further delay before the patient can resume driving. Finally, any person with epilepsy who is seizure-free and has been granted a driving licence will only be granted a permanent licence when it can be demonstrated that they have been seizure-free for at least 5 years.

The DVLA guidelines recognize two classes of drivers. Group 1 includes private vehicles such as cars and motorcycles, and Group 2 includes heavy goods vehicles and buses. Due to the higher risk of severe injury or death caused by accidents involving Group 2 vehicles, the law states that drivers of buses and lorries must have remained seizure-free, while off medication, for at least 10 years before licensing may be reconsidered. The guidelines also address fitness to drive in those who have not had epilepsy but are deemed to be at risk of developing the condition (e.g. after brain surgery, head injury, or brain haemorrhage).

Under Canadian legislation, doctors are responsible for reporting patients with epilepsy to the driving authorities. For example, in British Columbia, all qualified medical practitioners are required to report any patient over 16 years of age who has a medical condition that may make it hazardous for them to operate a motor vehicle. The Canadian Medical Association's guidelines state that people with epilepsy may drive a private vehicle if they have been seizure-free on medication for over 6 months, provided that their treatment does not affect their coordination or alertness. People who continue to have sleep-related seizures can drive if they have been free from daytime attacks for at least 5 years. If a patient has been seizure-free for such a long period that they are taken off medication, they are not allowed to drive for the first 3 months after stopping treatment. People who stop medication of their own accord should not drive, and those with simple partial seizures can continue to drive if their alertness is not affected. The stricter regulations for drivers of commercial vehicles such as lorries and buses require the individual to have been seizure-free for at least 5 years, whether or not they are taking anticonvulsive medication, before they can resume driving.

In contrast, in the UK it is the individual with epilepsy who is responsible for reporting their condition to the driving authorities. Implicit in this is the protection of doctor and patient confidentiality. In some jurisdictions the reporting of patients with epilepsy is mandatory, and the doctor is at fault and legally liable if he or she fails to disclose the patient's condition. In other jurisdictions the doctor is not compelled to report patients with epilepsy, but doing so protects him or her from legal action for breach of confidentiality, because the doctor has acted in the public interest. Mandatory reporting is perceived by many doctors as compromising the bond of trust that is central to the unique relationship between doctor and patient. An important Canadian study of the impact of mandatory reporting by doctors concluded that although it was clearly hazardous for people with ongoing seizures to drive, there was no evidence that such reporting of patients by their doctors reduced the risk of an accident occurring. The study compared a group of patients from Ontario, where physician reporting was a legal requirement, with a group of patients from Alberta, where it was not. The researchers found that concerns about the impact of epilepsy compared with other medical risk factors (e.g. drug and alcohol misuse) on driving was disproportional, as the lifetime accident rate among licensed drivers was 58 per cent for people with epilepsy and 60 per cent for those without the condition, and in both groups the accident rate in the preceding 12 months was 9 per cent. Moreover, there was no difference in accident rates between individuals with epilepsy who had been reported to the driving authority by their physicians and those who had self-reported their condition.[296] This study suggests that people with epilepsy tend to be socially responsible with regard to reporting seizures to the vehicle licensing authorities.

Another important issue, not without controversy, concerns how much time should elapse following the last seizure before the authorities allow an individual to resume driving. Remission of epilepsy, manifested as freedom from seizures, is the primary aim of medical treatment. Although it can be induced by drug treatment, it may also occur spontaneously. The longer the duration of remission, the lower the likelihood of further seizures, and thus the safer it is to resume driving of a car or public service vehicle. In 2001 the consistency of epilepsy-related driving restrictions across the USA was studied by reviewing legislation from 50 states and the District of Columbia.[297] It was found that 28 states had laws requiring people with epilepsy to be free of seizures for a fixed period of time (ranging from 3 to 12 months), while the remaining states had what were termed 'flexible restrictions'. The duration of the seizure-free period that was required before resumption of driving varied widely from one state to another, raising questions about the need for a much more evidence-based decision-making process. There is considerable interest in the possibility that investigations such as the EEG could be used to identify whether people with epilepsy are safe to drive, and indeed the results of a recent study suggest that the reaction-time EEG could be used as a routine method of assessing driving ability.[298]

It is unclear how many people with poorly controlled epilepsy continue to drive despite having active seizures, so there are no firm data on the impact of this behaviour on the risk

---

[296] McLachlan RS, Starreveld E and Lee MA (2007) Impact of mandatory physician reporting on accident risk in epilepsy. *Epilepsia* 48, 1500–1505.

[297] Krauss GL, Ampaw L and Krumholz A (2001) Individual state driving restrictions for people with epilepsy in the US. *Neurology* 57, 1780–1785.

[298] Krestel HE, Nirkko A, von Allmen A et al. (2011) Spike-triggered reaction-time EEG as a possible assessment tool for driving ability. *Epilepsia* 52, 126–129.

of injury and death due to road traffic accidents. However, it has been suggested that up to 20 per cent of people with poorly controlled epilepsy continue to drive for domestic or employment purposes. There is no clear evidence that road traffic accidents are more common among drivers with epilepsy than among those without the condition, or that shorter restriction periods before resuming driving have a more detrimental effect than longer restrictions. One US study showed no increase in accidents when a 12-month restriction was subsequently reduced to 3 months.[299] Another study reviewed the incidence of car fatalities in the USA and found no difference between the 3-, 6-, and 12-month driving restrictions and the incidence of accidents.[300] These researchers also studied the death certificates of drivers who had died in car crashes, and found that only 0.2 per cent of them listed epilepsy as a contributory factor. Alcohol caused 156 times more deaths, and young age (16–24 years) caused 123 times more deaths, than epilepsy. This study also showed that the fatality rate for drivers in the general population was 2.6 times higher than that for drivers with epilepsy.

In a study conducted in the UK, a large sample of drivers with a previous history of epilepsy who had been seizure-free for at least 1 year answered a self-completion questionnaire and were compared with a sample of non-epileptic drivers. There was no overall increase in the risk of accidents among drivers with epilepsy who were driving legally, but there was a higher risk that accidents involving drivers with epilepsy would be more severe than those involving non-epileptic drivers.[301]

An Australian study found that the number of fatal accidents involving young drivers was 120 times higher than the number of epilepsy-related accidents.[302] The relative risk of a driver with epilepsy having an accident is lower than for young drivers, older drivers, driving while sleep deprived, or driving after consuming alcohol within the legal limit. A recent systematic review of 67 studies worldwide to examine the risk of people with epilepsy being involved in road traffic accidents showed a sevenfold increase. The prevalence of driving (i.e. holding a driving licence) ranged from 3 per cent to 90 per cent of people with epilepsy . The authors concluded that the differences in legal restrictions among the different jurisdictions accounted for this wide variation.[303]

---

299 Drazkowski JE, Fisher RS, Sirven JI et al. (2003) Seizure-related motor vehicle accidents in Arizona before and after reducing the driving restriction from 12 to 3 months. *Mayo Clinic Proceedings* 78, 819–825.
300 Sheth SG, Krauss G, Krumholz A et al. (2004) Mortality in epilepsy: driving fatalities vs other causes of death in patients with epilepsy. *Neurology* 63, 1002–1007.
301 Taylor J, Chadwick D and Johnson T (1996) Risk of accidents in drivers with epilepsy. *Journal of Neurology, Neurosurgery, and Psychiatry* 60, 621–627.
302 Black AB and Lai NY (1997) Epilepsy and driving in South Australia – an assessment of compulsory notification. *Medicine and Law* 16, 253–267.
303 Xu Y, Shanthosh J, Zhou Z et al. (2019) Prevalence of driving and traffic accidents among people with seizures: a systemic review. *Neuroepidemiology* 53, 1–12.

A neurological study of the features of epilepsy-associated vehicle accidents was recently conducted in Australia.[304] It identified only 62 seizure-related traffic accidents, compared with 137,000 non-seizure-related ones, providing evidence that seizure-related events occur relatively infrequently.

Another important factor to bear in mind is that people with epilepsy who are on medication are less likely either to misuse alcohol or to drink and drive. The Epilepsy Society of Australia, in conjunction with the National Roads Commission, developed national guidelines for driving with epilepsy. The responsibility for reporting epilepsy lies with the individual, and there is a legal requirement to notify the Driving Licence Authority in the specific state or territory. Healthcare professionals only have a public duty to report a patient with epilepsy if they consider that by continuing to drive he or she is posing a serious risk to the public and to him- or herself. Australian regulations require a minimum seizure-free period of 12 months, after which a conditional licence can be issued.

Ultimately the evidence as to whether or not a driver's epilepsy is controlled will be based on the reporting of seizures by a family member, work colleague, or other third party to healthcare professionals or driving authorities. It is important to note that the driver's self-reporting of freedom from seizures may be influenced by, for example, the need to drive in order to earn a living and support a family. Only a very small number of people with epilepsy are involved in road traffic accidents as a direct consequence of their condition, but the driving regulations with regard to epilepsy vary widely from one country to another. Perhaps greater involvement of epilepsy societies and of individuals with epilepsy in the drafting of guidelines and application forms is the way forward.

With regard to flying, federal regulations in the USA prevent anyone who has been diagnosed with epilepsy or who has experienced a 'disturbance of consciousness without a satisfactory medical explanation of the cause' from obtaining any type of pilot's licence. In order to obtain a pilot's licence for commercial or private transport purposes, the applicant is assessed by a Federal Aviation Administration-approved physician, and no certificate can be granted if there is a diagnosis of epilepsy or impaired consciousness. There are no federal laws restricting people with epilepsy from obtaining employment in other airline-related occupations (e.g. flight attendant, baggage handler, maintenance crew). In the UK, the Civil Aviation Authority's 'Neurological Guidance' indicates that a diagnosis of epilepsy disqualifies the affected individual from obtaining a pilot's licence 'unless there is unequivocal evidence of a syndrome of benign childhood epilepsy associated with a very low risk of recurrence, and unless the applicant has been free of recurrence and off treatment for more than 10 years.'

---

304 Neal A, Carne R, Odell M et al. (2018) Characteristics of motor vehicle crashes associated with seizures. *Neurology* 91, 1102–1111.

The occurrence of one or more seizure-related episodes after the age of 5 years is regarded as grounds for disqualification.

Thus in the UK the only epilepsy patients who may be issued with a pilot's licence are those who have had seizures during childhood, but have been seizure-free ever since, and have a normal electroencephalogram (EEG). This is a much stricter criterion than for road driving, based on the much higher numbers of injuries and fatalities that would be involved in the event of an accident. For the same reasons, UK guidelines on the eligibility of people with epilepsy to become train drivers appear to follow the Civil Aviation Authority's recommendations, and a history of blackouts and epilepsy after the age of 5 years would prevent them from obtaining a licence to drive trains. However, there appears to be no formal legislation, and suitability for training and employment as a driver is assessed by an occupational health specialist.

The **right to work** is fundamental to self-esteem and the ability to earn a living. The rates of unemployment and low income among people with epilepsy are double those in the general population. This may reflect prejudice, lack of opportunities, associated illnesses, or lack of availability of suitable employment. Undoubtedly there are certain occupations in which sudden loss of consciousness could be hazardous to others, but there are other occupations (e.g. policing, military service, firefighting) where a complete ban on entry seems disproportionate, reflecting a risk-adverse culture. In 1958, writing in the *Cleveland State Law Review*, the eminent American psychiatrist, educator, and lawyer Irwin Perr (1928–2018) stated that 'the problem of the epileptic at work is minimized because of one simple fact – it's almost impossible for an epileptic to obtain or keep employment. The usual story is that after one seizure at work the employee is fired. … Practically speaking, it is true that epilepsy presents a menace in certain occupational situations, and for the protection of the epileptic and others, he should not work at heights, driving, or with moving machinery – unless the epilepsy is completely under control.'[305] Perr goes on to quote the safety director of the Ford Motor Company: 'accidents are so low among epileptics that it would not convey any data worth looking at. Out of 165 epileptics, over a period of many years, we do not have one accident case worth mentioning.' He also draws attention to a case where a seizure-related work injury involved a person known to have pre-existing epilepsy falling into an ash pit and being fatally burned. This resulted in the employers being found liable because the injury, not epilepsy, was the cause of death.[306] The publicity of such a case could only serve to worsen the prospects of finding employment at a time when there was no legislation to protect people with epilepsy, and when the only cases coming to court were those in which epilepsy had been caused by a workplace accident.

---

305 Perr IN (1958) Epilepsy and the law. *Cleveland State Law Review* 208.
306 Rockford Hotel Co. v. Industrial Commission, 132 N. E. 759.

Let us now consider how people with epilepsy are currently protected against loss of employment opportunity, and against dismissal. We shall begin with a contemporary story involving the nursing profession in the UK. From the ages of 7 to 18 years, Jane, now 32, had seizures that could not initially be controlled by drug treatment. She then became seizure-free for a period of 5 years and her medication was stopped. During that time she attended university, gained an honours degree in science, and began to work in a laboratory. When her seizures recurred she was told that it was unsafe for her to work with others in a laboratory environment, especially as her work involved handling expensive and fragile equipment. Jane did not challenge this decision, and she left her job. Her seizures were now much milder than before, and with re-introduction of drug treatment settled to an infrequent sensation of a rising feeling in her stomach, with no loss of awareness. She interpreted this feeling as an aura of a seizure which never developed into a full-blown event. She was subsequently accepted to train as a nurse following a positive assessment by an occupational health physician. She was deemed a suitable candidate to pursue a nursing career, and no restrictions were imposed or adjustments suggested during any of her clinical placements or course work. However, after she had graduated and was seeking full-time employment, her history of epilepsy seemed to disadvantage her, despite the fact that no problems had occurred during the 3 years of her nursing training. She eventually found employment in a residential home, in a post well below her expectations in terms of promotional prospects and salary. Jane then applied for a post at her local hospital. This involved supervising nursing assistants and handing out drug treatment, both of which were tasks for which she had already been responsible in the nursing home. Jane did not declare her epilepsy at the time of applying for this post, which she felt would finally put her on the career ladder. She was interviewed and appointed and sent for her pre-employment medical check-up to the same occupational health service that had deemed her fit to embark on nursing training some years earlier. On the basis of their report the offer of the post was withdrawn, and Jane was left feeling guilty about the fact that she had not mentioned her epilepsy on her initial application form. She appealed the decision, but by that stage the post had been offered to someone else. Jane consulted a lawyer and with the aid of current legislation (Equality Act 2010) obtained an apology from her local hospital. The latter also informed her that as they had already filled the post for which she had applied, they would bear her in mind for any positions that might arise in the future.

This story highlights many of the problems that confront people with epilepsy as they enter the job market, in particular the implied lack of honesty in not declaring the condition at the outset, the over-reaction to the existence of the condition and the risk it might carry, and a failure to consider making any adjustments to the post in order to accommodate the successful applicant. The law does offer some protection, but this requires the person with epilepsy to seek legal advice and then embark upon a protracted, confrontational, emotionally upsetting, and potentially expensive process that might 'mark their card' for future job applications and promotions. Jane's victory was a hollow one, as she could not be given the post for which she had originally applied because it had been offered to someone else. There was also a risk that she would be regarded as litigious and therefore as someone to be avoided if she applied for a post in the same hospital at a future date.

In the UK the Disability Discrimination Act 1995 was the key legislation introduced to protect the rights of disabled people. This has now been repealed and replaced by the Equality Act 2010, which defines disability as 'a physical or mental impairment that has a substantial and long-term negative effect upon the ability to carry out normal daily activities'.[307] The Equality Act covers discrimination not just in relation to disability, but also in relation to age, gender, race, religion, and sexual orientation. Similar legislation can be found in many other countries. Both the Americans with Disabilities Act (ADA) 1990 and the Australian Disability Discrimination Act 1992 make it illegal to discriminate in any area of public life, including the workplace, schools and colleges, transport services, and public and private places that are open to the public. In India, under the Rights of Persons with Disabilities Act 2016, epilepsy falls into the category of chronic neurological conditions, although it is not (unlike other conditions, such as multiple sclerosis) mentioned by name.

There are an estimated 83 million disabled people living in China. The Law of the People's Republic of China on the Protection of Disabled Persons (1990) was introduced to protect individuals' rights to employment opportunities, access to education, legal liability, and care. By 2003, official data revealed that over 80 per cent of all disabled people were in public or private employment, with employers being legally required to reserve no less than 1.5 per cent of all job opportunities for people with disabilities. In 2008, the Regulations on the Employment of People with Disabilities were introduced to provide further protection against discrimination during the employment process. Despite the impression given that the rights of disabled people were protected, in 2013 a report by Human Rights Watch found that 43 per cent of disabled Chinese children are illiterate, compared with 5 per cent of the general population, and they are thus denied an education. The Chinese Government makes it mandatory for all university applicants to undergo a medical test before they are offered a place, and allows rejection on the basis of unspecified physical and psychological 'defects'. People with disabilities such as hearing impairment are not allowed to take certain courses, such as law and foreign languages. Most recent evidence suggests that in China

---

307 Details of the act, including information for employers on what questions are unacceptable when discussing health and disability at interview or in the workplace, as well as guidance on positive action in recruitment and promotion, can be found at www.gov.uk/guidance/equality-act-2010-guidance

today, despite the Government's claims to have improved protection of their rights, disabled people continued to be stigmatized, marginalized, and abused.

In the UK, Linda Delany and Joanna Moody from the Manchester School of Law have examined whether national disability discrimination laws have improved matters for people with epilepsy.[308] They point out that the Disability Discrimination Act (DDA) 1995 defines disability as long term if it persists for 12 months or longer, and that in the case of epilepsy such a definition is problematic, particularly if the condition is controlled but still requires medication, or is manifested as brief partial seizures, or is solely sleep-related. None of these circumstances, which are unique to epilepsy, fulfil the criterion of showing 'a substantial and long-term effect on the ability to carry out day-to-day activities'. Delany and Moody suggest that epilepsy could only be unequivocally covered by the DDA if the definition of disability was broadened to include short-lived and 'mild' events. Very few people with epilepsy would be likely to use the term 'mild' to describe their attacks, but that is how brief partial seizures or sleep-related seizures might be perceived by an onlooker or assessor. The authors concluded that the DDA did not cover the majority of people with epilepsy, and they questioned 'why mildly disabled people should be left to fend for themselves when they fall victim to prejudice'.

If a person with epilepsy believes that they have been discriminated against, they are obliged to provide medical evidence, usually resulting in costs they can ill afford, to show that they meet the statutory criteria for disability. Any reports that are obtained are likely to be objective and to fail to take into account the subjective impact of the seizures, revealing a fundamental misunderstanding of the specific nature of the employment and possibly overestimating the potential risks that such events pose to others. Delany and Moody cite an example of how one expert medical opinion can be successfully overturned by another expert, to the detriment of the employee. In this particular case a neurologist provided a report stating that an employee was safe to return to work, but was successfully challenged by the employer's doctor, who stated that the neurologist had no understanding of the hazards of the workplace.

Notwithstanding the issue of whether people with epilepsy fulfil the criteria for the DDA definition of disability, the DDA was intended to ensure that during the selection process, protection was given to those applying for a post or promotion, and that successful applicants would be allowed 'reasonable adjustments' to accommodate their disability within the workplace. Many job descriptions specify that applicants must have a driving licence or be willing to undertake shift work. Clearly these requirements disadvantage people with

---

308 Delany L and Moody JE (1999) Epilepsy, employment and the Disability Discrimination Act. Does legislation make a difference? *Seizure* 8, 412–420.

epilepsy, but they can only be regarded as discriminatory if it can be demonstrated that the job could be undertaken without the need for a driving licence or shift work. Finally, the DDA does not apply to businesses with fewer than 15 employees, or to fire, military, or police services.

In the UK the Disability Rights Commission (DRC) was established in 1999, and was subsequently replaced by the Equality and Human Rights Commission (2007). The DRC's roles were to enforce DDA legislation as well as to advise employers on how to integrate disabled employees in the workplace. It is unclear how effective the DRC was in enforcing the DDA in relation to discrimination against people with epilepsy. In 2005 the Public Interest Research Unit (PIRU) published a report on the DDA. This concluded that although the Act had allowed thousands of people to get financial redress through employment tribunals, it had manifestly failed to address discrimination against people with disabilities, whose employment and wage levels remained well below those of the able-bodied. Far from occurring only in exceptional cases, it was noted that institutional discrimination and widespread, often extreme, prejudice were still commonplace. It was felt that employees were unlikely to make a claim due to their lack of awareness of what protection the Act could offer, and poor understanding of the Act among the trade union officials who represented and advised them. Obstacles to making a claim that were highlighted by the report included not knowing where to go for advice, the need to submit applications on time, fear of victimization, and low expectations of success. During the period 2004–2005, a total of 236 DDA employment claims were successful, whereas 4437 claims were dropped or failed at tribunal. The report concluded that many claimants had no professional legal help or representation, and that 'even those who meet the narrow definition of disabled, and so might gain some protection under the Act, seldom have the resources to enforce their rights at an employment tribunal'. It was felt that employers either did not believe that the Act applied to them, or else believed that the Disability Rights Commission had such limited enforcement powers as to be effectively 'toothless.'

After the Equality Act 2010 replaced the DDA, people with epilepsy were better covered even if their seizures were controlled or they did not consider themselves to be 'disabled' as such. However, the Equality Act has fared little better than its predecessor. In 2016 the UK Parliamentary Select Committee on Equality reported on the Act's impact on the disabled. First they noted that in 2012 the funding of the Equality and Human Rights Commission (EHRC), which had a duty to enforce the Act, had been cut by 75 per cent. The Select Committee also noted that many lawyers had commented how few firms of solicitors would take on discrimination cases, as it was simply not cost-effective (in terms of available funding and time involved) for them to take on such work. Baroness Deech, Chair of the Committee, commented that 'Over the course of our inquiry we have been struck by how disabled people are let down across the whole spectrum of life.' The Committee called for a government minister with responsibility for the disabled, which must be seen as a positive step forward, but clearly the Equality Act has not served its purpose of protecting the human rights of people with disabilities, including epilepsy.

Under the Freedom of Information Act, the author of this book asked the Scottish Commission how many people with epilepsy had approached the cash-strapped regulators of the Equality Act, namely the EHRC, in Scotland during the two-year period 2016–2017, to use their legal powers. Their response was that a mother who advised them that her child had epilepsy had contacted the legal team in the EHRC in Scotland with regard to reasonable adjustments in school. They also provided advice to another advisor in relation to someone they were helping who had epilepsy, with regard to reasonable adjustments in the workplace. Apparently there was no recorded outcome for either of these cases. Moreover, no employers were approached regarding the integration of people with epilepsy in the workplace.

These responses have to be viewed against a backdrop of 45,000–50,000 people with epilepsy in Scotland. Either there is a negligible problem with regard to equality and human rights within this sizeable population, which seems unlikely, or else people with epilepsy are unaware of the EHRC's role in regulating the Equality Act. If the Act is not being regulated, for whatever reason, its effectiveness cannot be demonstrated.

Conclusion

Based on a brief review of what is inevitably somewhat selective evidence from around the world, it would appear that much of the legislation that restricts people with epilepsy in relation to fundamental human rights (such as marriage, the right to drive, employment, and the right to movement) is based on historical prejudices and misconceptions, exacerbated by the eugenics movement and perpetuated by the tabloid press and certain elements of social media. The view that disabled people are a burden on the able-bodied in society underpins many of the regulations that persist to this day. This is particularly pertinent in criminal law (see Chapter 11).

Paradoxically, the laws that have been relatively recently introduced to prevent discrimination against people with disabilities, including epilepsy, are loosely framed and lack the funding (and possibly also the will) to regulate their implementation. Even the legal definition of disability is open to interpretation. Despite the disability discrimination legislation, the rights of many continue to be disregarded, and prejudiced attitudes are still widespread. As recently as 2017 the Scottish Human Rights Commission commented that a recent increase in court fees was raising concern that this would 'have a disproportionate effect on disabled people and a negative impact on their ability to access justice and an effective legal remedy'. To date the Equality Act 2010 has not delivered on the promise of equality for disabled people, including those with epilepsy. Far from the legislation protecting the rights of the vulnerable, it is disabled people themselves who have to pursue justice by making emotional and financial sacrifices without any guarantee of the successful outcomes that they so often deserve.

CHAPTER 11
Epilepsy, behaviour, violence, and criminal law

It is well recognized that people with epilepsy often feel confused and disorientated during the period immediately after a seizure. Attempts to restrain someone in this 'twilight' state can be met with physical resistance and struggling. Only rarely, in what is termed the post-ictal state, does this constitute what might be perceived as deliberately violent behaviour. However, there is a risk of misinterpreting as violent or antisocial behaviour the 'automatic pilot' state that some people experience during or after a seizure. This state differs from simple confusion in that the affected individual behaves in a bizarre manner, often performing complex acts over which they have no voluntary control. Such states, which are known as *automatisms*, most commonly occur when the epilepsy arises in the temporal lobe of the brain. Let us consider two real-life case examples that demonstrate the potential complexity of such automatisms.

J.W. was a plumber with a long history of temporal lobe epilepsy. He was called to a house to install a new bathroom sink. When he had completed this task he experienced a seizure, and following the seizure he disconnected the newly fitted sink, went through to the family bedroom, climbed into the house owners' bed and fell asleep. When the owners returned and went upstairs to inspect the work, they found the plumber, fully dressed, asleep in their bed.

S.W., a baker who had been free of temporal lobe seizures for many years, had just driven his van to deliver fresh bread to a local shop, and while parked outside he had a seizure. After the seizure he carefully removed his entire stock of rolls and loaves from inside the van and stacked them in a neat pile on the pavement. He then climbed into the back of his van and closed the doors behind him. A passer-by witnessed this, and on opening the van doors found the baker inside, looking vacant and having removed most of his clothing.

Neither of these two examples of automatisms resulted in violence or involvement of the police, but clearly there was the potential for that to have happened. We shall now consider what exactly automatisms are, the way that they are perceived as antisocial or criminal acts, and how the law deals with them. Automatisms can be defined as any sequence of brief unconscious behaviours that cannot be voluntarily suppressed or modified so as to make them appear normal and socially acceptable. They may range from simple gestures such as lip smacking, swallowing, grimacing, or chewing, to complex acts such as undressing, cooking, showering, or even shoplifting. Clearly even a simple gesture could lead to unfortunate and potentially violent scenarios (for example, the effect of lip smacking by a passenger when a young girl or child gets on to a bus). For those people who have been unfortunate enough to have had an automatism in a situation where such behaviour is likely to be perceived as inappropriate, resulting in a complaint or even arrest, the legal process swings into action. This is often protracted, with an outcome that is commonly unjust and occasionally tragic. The following two case examples were reported many years ago, but could still easily occur today.

J.S. was a 40-year-old man with a longstanding history of frequent temporal lobe seizures dating from early childhood. Despite this he had defied the expectations of many, and was married with two young daughters, was in full-time employment, and was a homeowner. In 2001, shortly before Christmas, he had walked his daughter to her dance class and had then caught a bus to visit his mother, who was in hospital. After visiting her he realized that it was almost time to pick up his daughter, so he hailed a taxi. While sitting in the back of the cab he experienced a seizure. After this, when the vehicle was stationary at traffic lights, he flung open the door and ran away, weaving his way through heavy traffic. The taxi driver, assuming that he was trying to avoid paying his fare, ran after him, pulled him to the ground, and a struggle ensued before the police arrived and handcuffed him. A body search revealed that he had a penknife in his pocket. He was charged with breach of the peace and carrying a knife, and was told that he could face a custodial sentence. His case took nine months to come to trial. During that time he lost his job, defaulted on his mortgage repayments, lost his home, and his mother died. He was eventually sentenced to community service. His lawyer did not suggest epilepsy as a defence, as he considered that, in view of the very deliberate way that J.S. had negotiated his way through dense traffic, it could not be offered as a possible mitigating circumstance. No expert medical opinion was sought.

A.S. was a retired builder and an elder in his local church. He had never married, primarily because of his embarrassment about having epilepsy and the remoteness that he had cultivated as a consequence of this. However, he took great pride in his involvement with and status within his local community. He had attended his brother's funeral and then travelled home by train. After getting off the train and walking down the platform, his next memory was of being bundled into a police car as someone yelled 'You old pervert.' He was informed that while walking down the station platform he had unfastened his trousers and exposed himself in front of other passengers, including schoolchildren. The story that this 'pillar of the local community' had been charged with gross indecency was reported by the local press. It was several months before his case came up in court and he could profess his innocence, but he did not want his epilepsy to become a matter of public knowledge, and by now he was unable to leave his house without hearing shouts of abuse. A.S. never sought advice from his doctor, nor was he aware that his lawyer might request a medical report. Unable to cope with the overwhelming feelings of shame and humiliation, he committed suicide.

These two tragic stories highlight the consequences of lack of awareness and understanding of epileptic automatisms by the judicial process. The challenges of achieving wider recognition of the involuntary behaviours that are caused by epilepsy should not be underestimated. These include the need to teach law enforcement officers to correctly identify automatisms and distinguish them from drug or alcohol intoxication, other medical conditions, and antisocial or challenging behaviour, as well as the need to address the lack of formal training of police officers in epilepsy awareness. To complicate matters further, some individuals (with or without epilepsy) may falsely claim to have experienced an automatism in an attempt to avoid punishment for a deliberate criminal act. Clear criteria for a genuine automatism need to be identified to ensure that this situation cannot occur, and it is important to determine how to prevent genuine cases from being subjected to a protracted and expensive legal process before (hopefully) they are either found not guilty or have their case dismissed. The effects on people with epilepsy who have had to endure the court process because of an automatism cannot be underestimated, and include lowering of their mood, erosion of their confidence, worsening of seizure control, and heightening of their sense of injustice.

Epilepsy and violent crime

The earliest suggestion of a link between epilepsy, criminal activity, and deviance dates back to **Abul Qasim** (936–1013 ce), an Arab physician and surgeon, who described the 'demonic' form of epilepsy as being linked to criminality.[309] Thereafter the concept of '*furor epilepticus*', a

---

309 Temkin O (1971) *The Falling Sickness: A History of Epilepsy from the Greeks to the Beginnings of Modern Neurology*, 2nd edition. Johns Hopkins University Press, Baltimore, MD. p. 106.

condition in which a person with epilepsy might, during a sudden outburst of anger, commit an unprovoked act of violence, became established. Centuries later, the Italian criminologist and physician **Cesare Lombroso** (1835–1909) proposed that criminal degenerates were 'born criminal', and that this state was manifested by certain physical characteristics and conditions, one of which was epilepsy. This belief, which dominated thinking about criminology well into the early twentieth century, was based on physiognomy (the supposed art of using a person's facial characteristics to determine their temperament and character) and the degeneration theory (the belief that the human species was undergoing a process of evolutionary decline, and that conditions such as epilepsy were contributing to this). The American criminologist Marvin E. Wolfgang has described how Lombroso 'came to designate the epileptic criminal, the insane criminal, and the born criminal as separate types, all stemming from an epileptoid base'.[310] On a more positive note, Lombroso believed that epilepsy could also be associated with genius, albeit combined with ruthlessness and moral weakness, and he cited Napoleon as one example among many others.[311] He continued to influence criminology for many years, and had a significant number of followers who shared his belief that crime had important biological causes, one of which was epilepsy.

The pioneering British psychiatrist **Henry Maudsley** (1835–1918) famously suggested that 'when a murder has been committed without apparent motive and the reason of it seems inexplicable, it may chance that the perpetrator is found on inquiry to be afflicted with epilepsy'.[312] Like Lombroso, Maudsley supported the theory of degeneration, and he had a similarly negative view of epilepsy and believed that it was linked to criminality. In *Responsibility in Mental Disease* he described what he termed ictal and inter-ictal violence and assaultive behaviour in his patients with temporal lobe epilepsy. The eminent British neurologist **Sir William Gowers** (1845–1915) had noted that violence was a brief episodic feature of what he called 'epileptic mania'. In addition, his colleague, the pioneering English neurologist **John Hughlings Jackson** (1835–1911), documented what he perceived as the violent acts that could occur during epileptic automatisms.[313]

Among the first to systematically investigate the relationship between epilepsy and violent crime was **Charles Buckman Goring** (1870–1919), a British criminologist, prison doctor, and author of *The English Convict: A Statistical Study*. This study, sponsored by the British government, investigated whether criminals had physical conditions or psychiatric

---

310 Wolfgang ME (1961) Pioneers In Criminology: Cesare Lombroso (1835–1909). *The Journal of Criminal Law, Criminology, and Police Science* 52, 361–391.
311 Temkin O (1971) *The Falling Sickness: A History of Epilepsy from the Greeks to the Beginnings of Modern Neurology*, 2nd edition. Johns Hopkins University Press, Baltimore, MD. p. 367.
312 Maudsley H (1874) *Responsibility in Mental Disease*. D. Appleton & Company, New York.
313 Jackson JH (1958) Temporary mental disorders after epileptic paroxysms. In: Taylor J (ed.) *Selected Writings of John Hughlings Jackson. Volume 1.* Basic Books, New York.

abnormalities that distinguished them from the non-criminal population as Lombroso had earlier claimed. Goring studied 96 traits, including the presence of epilepsy in 3000 inmates, and on the basis of his observations and measurements concluded that although there was no anthropological type of criminal per se, it was an 'indisputable fact that there is a physical, mental, and moral type of normal person who tends to be convicted of crime: that is to say, our evidence conclusively shows that, on the average, the criminal of English prisons is markedly differentiated by defective physique – as measured by stature and body weight; by defective mental capacity – as measured by general intelligence; and by an increased possession of wilful antisocial proclivities – as measured, apart from intelligence, by length of sentence to imprisonment.'[314] He went on to suggest that society might profitably 'regulate the reproduction of those degrees of constitutional qualities – feeble-mindedness, inebriety, epilepsy, deficient social instinct, etc. – which conduce to the committing of crimes.'[315] It was not until the 1930s that the widely held belief in a link between epilepsy and crime was finally refuted, when a study from the US state of Michigan found that the prevalence of epilepsy among the prison population was the same as that among the general population.[316]

Having established that people with epilepsy do not have an inherent propensity to violence, research was then directed towards determining whether there was any link between seizure activity and acts of violence or aggression. Antonio Delgado-Escueta and his colleagues from the University of California in Los Angeles (UCLA) noted over a 90-year period from 1889 onward that in only 15 cases presented to the US Appellate Courts (the court sitting below the Supreme Court) had epilepsy been put forward as a defence for homicide, manslaughter, or disorderly conduct.[317] Prior to their study there had been a surge in the number of academic papers linking epileptic automatisms to violent behaviour, giving credibility to the defence of 'diminished responsibility' or 'insanity', although in reality this had been pleaded in only five cases throughout the USA in 1979. The media interest generated by such cases had led the public to believe that a person experiencing confusion as a result of a seizure might well exhibit violent behaviour, and therefore it was dangerous to be in their vicinity.

Antonio Delgado-Escueta and his colleagues assembled a panel of international epilepsy specialists to review television recordings and brainwave traces of patients who were believed to have behaved in an aggressive manner while having seizures. These individuals were selected from 19 epilepsy centres worldwide, and a total of 5400 recordings were studied. However,

---

314 Goring CB (1913) *The English Convict: A Statistical Study*. HMSO, London. p. 370.
315 Goring CB (1913) *The English Convict: A Statistical Study*. HMSO, London. p. 373.
316 Anderson CL (1936) Epilepsy in the state of Michigan. *Mental Hygiene* 20, 441–462.
317 Delgado-Escueta AV, Mattson RH, King L et al. (1981) The nature of aggression during epileptic seizures. *New England Journal of Medicine* 305, 711–716.

only 19 patients were identified as having shown aggressive seizure-related behaviours, which clearly demonstrates that such an association is very rare. The abnormal behaviours that were observed in those individuals ranged from damaging nearby inanimate objects to shouting and spitting, screaming and kicking, raising a fist, and scratching. Among the 19 patients a total of 33 seizures were recorded on closed-circuit television and then reviewed by the panel of experts. The panel concluded that it would be virtually impossible to commit murder during a seizure, as this would require a sequence of ordered, deliberate, and sustained movements, and no such movements occurred in any of the recorded attacks. Clearly, then, although random acts such as pushing, flailing, shouting, and even throwing objects can occur during seizures, directed and coordinated acts of aggression do not occur. Having ruled out the possibility that murder or deliberate assault could take place during a seizure, the authors turned their attention to less violent acts and disorderly behaviour that might occur during the confusion caused by a seizure, and they suggested specific criteria to help to determine whether or not such aberrant behaviours were the result of an automatism. These criteria will be discussed later in this chapter.

In their book *Having Epilepsy*, published in 1983, the American sociologists Joseph Schneider and Peter Conrad described the notion that epilepsy causes aggression and crime as a myth that is 'an example of the medicalization of deviance, the creation of medical definitions and theories for deviant behaviour – epilepsy's stigmatized status and behavioural manifestations make it likely that the link between epilepsy and deviance will continue to be advanced'.[318] Nevertheless, such myths persisted. In 1997, during National Brain Awareness Week, the *Baltimore Sun* (16 March 1997) quoted a neuroscientist as stating that 'Up to half of all patients with temporal lobe epilepsy suffer sudden outbursts of aggression and violence.' Studies of the relative size of the prison population with epilepsy were still being undertaken, and yielded conflicting results that reflected variation in the methodology used. In those few studies of prison populations that suggest a higher prevalence of epilepsy among perpetrators of violent crime or among young offenders, this could be explained by the socioeconomic factors that accompany the condition, such as unemployment, low income, and social isolation, rather than being directly attributable to epilepsy.

Further confusion has been caused by the fact that some studies have regarded changes in brainwaves alone, without any outward manifestation of epilepsy, as an explanation for violence. The case of the serial killer Peter Manuel, which will be discussed later, is an important example. A change in brain activity, as manifested on the electroencephalogram (EEG), without any visible physical change in the affected individual led to the suggestion

---

318 Schneider JW and Conrad P (1983) *Having Epilepsy: The Experience and Control of Illness*. Temple University Press, Philadelphia, PA. p. 42.

that the 'epileptic equivalent' can explain deviant behaviour. All human activities are the result of chemical and electrical changes in brain activity, but there is no scientific basis for the suggestion that aberrant behaviour can be attributed to seizure activity in the absence of the outward and visible signs of an epileptic seizure. Such a theory would result in people with epilepsy being viewed as prime suspects for any given violent act, and would stigmatize the condition further. One supporter of the epileptic equivalent theory went so far as to suggest that many horrific and apparently inexplicable crimes could be attributed to people with epilepsy.[319] As a result, brainwave abnormalities were regularly sought in the EEGs of individuals who had committed particularly gruesome acts of violence, with a view to demonstrating that a frenzy or 'brainstorm' was responsible for their behaviour.

In 1995, Pamela Blake and her colleagues conducted neurological assessments, including EEG recordings, of 31 convicted murderers.[320] These individuals were all awaiting trial, sentencing, or appeal, and were seen between 1989 and 1993 at the request of their defence lawyers. The subjects were all male, with an average age of 32.7 years at the time of their offence, and they underwent a combination of clinical examination, EEG, brain imaging (MRI or CT scanning), and neuropsychological testing. The authors quoted a study from the 1940s that showed abnormal EEGs in 70 per cent of those who had been charged with a murder that appeared to have been motiveless, and who were therefore deemed 'insane'. These homicides had been variously attributed to temporal lobe epilepsy, epileptic equivalents, or an entity termed 'episodic dyscontrol syndrome' or 'impulse control disorder'. Blake and her colleagues found that two of the men had been diagnosed earlier with epilepsy, which appeared to be unrelated to their crimes. Eight of the 20 individuals who had EEGs showed minor 'abnormalities.' Non-specific changes were noted on MRI scanning in 9 of the 19 subjects who underwent imaging. Histories of learning disability, cerebral palsy, alcohol misuse, and sexual abuse were common among the study subjects. The authors concluded that psychiatric illness, minor brain injury, sexual and physical abuse, alcoholism, and paranoia 'interacted to form a matrix of violent behaviour'. They did not suggest epilepsy or epileptic equivalents as explanations for the homicides that had been committed, but they did note the high incidence of neurological and psychological abnormalities. If the hypothesis that epilepsy alone can lead to violent crimes was correct, one would have expected to find supportive evidence in the group of subjects studied by Blake and her colleagues, but in fact no such evidence was found.

---

319 Bennett AE (1965) Mental disorders associated with temporal lobe epilepsy. *Diseases of the Nervous System* 26, 275–280.
320 Blake PY, Pincus JH and Buckner C (1995) Neurologic abnormalities in murderers. *Neurology* 45, 1641–1647.

Famous homicide cases

The case of **David Montgomery** has been described in a contemporaneous and detailed account.[321] This major trial was heard in Monroe County in 1871 and again in the Supreme Court the following year. The accused was defended by Mr Martindale and the people were represented by Mr Peckham. Montgomery was a young religious cart driver with a history of epilepsy that had given him the nickname of 'daft Davy'. His wife, a former prostitute, had given birth to their baby but thereafter had stayed only infrequently with him. The trial records comment that Montgomery 'during his infancy had been subject to epileptic fits and that he had had them on several occasions subsequently. He had a disease of the brain also.' After a week of these frequent seizures he was described as being left in an excited and delusional state, with a witness adding that 'he talked and acted like an insane man, his face was flushed and his manner excited'. On the afternoon before the killing, in the company of his uncle, he visited his wife and persuaded her to return and live with him once more, together with their 9-month-old child. The following morning he got up before she awoke, found an axe in the room, took it in his hand, raised it and held it for five minutes before decapitating her. When arrested he said 'I stood with the axe for about five minutes looking at her and then seemed impelled to strike her though I did not want to. I had to strike the blow. My temper got the better of me.' His father and brother had then intervened to prevent Montgomery cutting his own throat with a razor. Later that morning he was taken to jail and immediately fell into a deep sleep, and on waking he had no recollection of what had happened.

At the trial, three physicians described as being 'of the largest experience and greatest intelligence' expressed the view that he was insane at the time when the crime was committed, while other equally well-qualified medical experts disagreed. In directing the jury, the judge E.D. Smith stated that 'a man is not responsible for an act when, by reason of involuntary insanity or delusion, he is at the time incapable of perceiving the act is either wrong or unlawful'. He commented that there was no doubt that the prisoner had epilepsy that had begun in infancy and persisted up until the time of the crime, and he noted the divergent views of the seven distinguished physicians who had been called to give evidence for the prisoner and the people. He stated that all of the medical experts had agreed that 'epilepsy was a disease that affected his [Montgomery's] brain', and they concurred that fits impaired the mind and that this was the natural effect of the disease. The judge concluded that Montgomery's actions were only 'excusable when he is not conscious that he is violating the

---

321 Martindale (1873) *The People against David Montgomery, for the Murder of Mary Montgomery.* Diossy & Company, New York.

laws of God and man'. The jury deliberated and returned a guilty verdict, and the defence moved a motion for retrial on the grounds that the verdict was against the weight of evidence, there were conflicting medical opinions, and there were procedural irregularities in relation to the conduct of the jury (one juror had separated from the others during the trial and was seen discussing the case with members of the public). When the case came to the Supreme Court, the judges decided that the guilty verdict was correct and should be affirmed. They commented that despite the fact that 'some days before the killing the prisoner was partially insane, and at some times during that time more so than at others, there is no evidence that he was not capable of distinguishing right and wrong between noon on Saturday and the commission of the crime'. The Supreme Court emphasized the fact that the 'greatest degree of care and caution must be exercised in determining the question of capacity to commit crime, yet we must hold a man responsible whose acts and declarations prove him to be so far sane as to know that the act which he commits is, by the laws of God and man, wrong'.

Despite the clear legal outcome, the medical profession continued (unsurprisingly) to argue Montgomery's state of mind for some time. Gonzalez Echeverria, the Chief Physician at the New York Hospital for Epileptics and Paralytics, had followed the case with great interest and subsequently expressed his views in the *American Journal of Insanity*.[322] He believed that Montgomery had had a seizure on the morning of the murder and remained in a seizure state until he awoke in prison with no memory of what had happened. He believed that 'epileptics', after having a seizure, lacked control over reflex responses and therefore could not inhibit an irresistible impulse, in contrast to people without epilepsy. In other words, he was suggesting that people with epilepsy could perform complex unconscious acts, and he highlighted what he regarded as the 'extremely violent and uncontrollable reactions peculiar to the disease.' Dr William Hammond, who had testified for the people at the trial, had a very different view, believing that 'deliberation takes away the idea of an insane act'.[323] In summary, Montgomery was a person with epilepsy who wilfully committed murder, and not someone in a form of epileptic trance who had no control over their actions. As might be expected, the widely reported trial reinforced the public perception that individuals with epilepsy were more violent than the rest of the population.

The case of **Charles Edward Canham** was discussed at the General Meeting of the Medico-Psychological Association in May 1901 and subsequently reported by Dr Percy Smith, a physician specializing in mental disorders at Charing Cross Hospital, London.[324]

---

322 Echeverria MG (1873) Criminal responsibility of epileptics, as illustrated by the case of David Montgomery. *American Journal of Insanity* 29, 341–425.

323 Hammond WA (1872) Medico-legal points in the case of David Montgomery. *Journal of Psychological Medicine* 6, 62–76.

324 Percy Smith R (1901) A case of epileptic homicide. *Journal of Mental Science* 47, 528–540.

On 4 March 1901, Canham was tried at Nottingham Assizes for the murder of his wife and infant child. During 1873 and 1874, while serving with the British Army on the African Gold Coast during the Anglo-Ashanti wars, he became unwell and subsequently developed epileptic seizures. Despite the fact that his fits were becoming more frequent, he married, had eight children and remained in army service until 1891, when he left with an impeccable military record. He then worked as an insurance salesman. He was continuing to experience seizures, and was now taking potassium bromide for treatment. He was described by acquaintances as a religious person (he regularly preached and conducted open-air services) and a loving husband and father. However, payments from his insurance customers were beginning to disappear into his personal bank account. On the night of 29 November 1900, Canham and his wife had gone to bed as usual in the room that they shared with their youngest child. The next morning their eldest daughter found her mother dead in bed with multiple head injuries. The youngest child, whose throat had been cut, had also died. Charles Canham was sitting in a chair with his eyes closed and his head bowed. A coal hammer and a carving knife were lying in the room. Canham was unresponsive, and there was an empty bottle that had contained chloroform and oil of cloves on the washstand in front of him. He had to be carried in a limp state to the police station. There he was examined by the duty police surgeon who described him as 'not totally unconscious' as he had resisted having his mouth opened or being turned, had kept his eyes very tightly closed, and had responded when pressure was applied to a nerve. Two hours later he appeared to have recovered and was then able to understand the charges that were being brought against him. He denied any knowledge of the murders, stating that he could remember nothing until after his arrest, and claiming that the police had treated him roughly. He maintained that the last thing he could remember from the previous night was taking the chloroform and oil of cloves to treat a headache. However, he had no recollection of going to the coal cellar to get the coal hammer, or to the kitchen to collect the carving knife.

When cautioned he denied having had any motive, stating that 'I had no reason to kill my wife, but a thousand reasons against it.' In the absence of any obvious motive, despite the fact that he had made no mitigating plea of insanity, the doctors were asked to assess him. At trial, witnesses testified about his epilepsy and in particular a previous seizure-related act of unprovoked violence directed at his brother. He was described as often sitting down and staring for long periods, and having no recollection of these episodes on recovery. Other witnesses described prolonged fainting attacks that could occur as often as five or six times a day. In none of these episodes did Canham bite his tongue or urinate. His army commanding officer provided an exemplary testimonial, describing him as 'a warrant officer of first-class rank. There was hardly an office he was not fit to hold.

The prosecution claimed that Canham was in financial difficulties and had deliberately planned to kill his wife and child, although it was difficult to identify what he would gain from such an action. They also claimed that he had feigned unconsciousness after the incident. The defence argued that he was guilty but insane as a consequence of epilepsy. The medical evidence was provided for the defence by Dr Percy Smith (mentioned earlier) and by Dr Evan Powell, from the Nottingham City Asylum. Powell maintained that, despite Canham's deliberate search for the hammer and knife, none of the evidence was inconsistent with the murders having been committed during an epileptic state, and that Canham's mood swings and religiosity confirmed that he was epileptic. A third medical expert, Dr Thomson from the Norfolk Asylum, concurred that it was not only possible that the crime was committed in an epileptic state, but that this was highly likely to have been the case. In the absence of any alternative explanation, and in view of the opinions expressed by the medical experts, the judge instructed the jury to decide whether Canham was suffering from epilepsy, and if so, whether the evidence was consistent with a crime having been committed during an episode of 'epileptic mania'. The judge's summing up was clearly in favour of Canham, given the weight of the medical evidence together with the army testimonial emphasizing the exemplary record of the accused. The jury returned a verdict of 'guilty but insane' on the basis that this was an epileptic homicide, and Canham escaped execution. Instead he was detained indefinitely, although it is unclear whether this was in an asylum or in prison.

Today we would not accept that an epileptic seizure or mania could explain such a deliberately planned and executed act of violence. Canham had to collect his murder weapons from the coal cellar and the kitchen and then inflict his wife's head injuries and his son's neck injuries in a targeted manner with the appropriate instrument. The medical experts were convinced that he had epilepsy, yet nowhere in Dr Percy Smith's account is there a description of the recurrent stereotypical attack that is the hallmark of the condition. The virtually catatonic state in which he was found at the time of his arrest does not occur after a seizure, and the police surgeon's initial observations suggest malingering. The notion that Canham had epilepsy at all is highly debatable. In fact it seems much more likely that he managed to deceive the doctors and so evade justice. This case highlights the unchallenged power of expert medical opinion, whether or not it is correct, when it is confidently presented to judge and jury. It is interesting to speculate whether the medical experts had read and been influenced by Henry Maudsley's contemporaneous book, *Responsibility in Mental Disease*, with its much quoted mantra that 'When a murder has been committed without apparent motive and the reason of it seems inexplicable, it may chance that the perpetrator is found on inquiry to be afflicted with epilepsy.'[325] The widely reported case of Canham certainly gave further support to the myth that there is a link between epilepsy and violent crimes.

In 1961, **Arthur Earl Walker** (1907–1995), a distinguished neurosurgeon at Johns Hopkins Hospital in Baltimore, published an account of a patient on whom he had performed surgery 10 years previously, a review of the literature on epilepsy and murder, and criteria that he suggested should be considered when attributing a violent crime to an epileptic state.[326] Since his mid-twenties the unnamed patient had had a history of episodes in which he would twist, make groping movements with his hands, utter weird sounds, stare straight ahead, and mumble. A violent episode resulted in a brief stay in a state mental hospital. He was married with two children, and although his neighbours described him as a kind and considerate husband and father, they had also witnessed frequent domestic quarrels. On 27 December 1946 the local residents called the police when they heard screams and the sound of someone falling. On entering the house the police found the patient covered in blood, and his wife was lying dead in the bedroom, with 30 stab wounds to her body. On arrival at the police station the patient suddenly stared into space and started pulling at his trousers. He was committed to a mental hospital, where he kept telling his fellow inmates that he could not have killed his wife because she was so dear to him. He claimed to have no memory of the events of that night apart from being confined in a police cell. The court psychiatrist expressed the view that the patient had killed his wife during a post-ictal automatism. The patient remained in the state mental hospital until Walker operated on him to remove his left temporal lobe around five years later. The patient's epilepsy improved thereafter, but he remained in the state institution until his death about eight years later. Walker speculated that if surgery had been performed several years earlier, the homicidal act would not have occurred. However, he did not mention whether court proceedings were ever underway, and he conveyed the impression that the defence of post-ictal automatism was accepted without being tested. The case allowed him to review the available literature, starting with patients described in 1854 by the French psychiatrist **Louis Jean Delasiauve** (1804–1893). Delasiauve regarded epilepsy as simply a neurotic condition, and in a book chapter on the legal responsibility of the 'epileptic' he described a young butcher who had shot his uncle in the belief that the latter was about to kill him, and another individual, with a propensity for young children, who mutilated an 11-year-old girl. The first case was found to be guilty. However, the second was deemed to be devoid of his senses, on the basis of the frequency of convulsions, his state of stupor immediately after the attack, the ferocity of the attack, and the fact that it took place in broad daylight.

---

325 Maudsley H (1874) *Responsibility in Mental Disease*. D. Appleton & Company, New York.
326 Walker AE (1961) Murder or epilepsy? *Journal of Nervous and Mental Disease* 133, 430–437.

Walker also cited a patient of the American psychiatrist **Abner Otis Kellogg** (1818–1888). This case was a 40-year-old man who had been experiencing convulsions at least once a month for the past 10 years. Very early one morning he had a seizure that required his mother and his two sisters to help him back to bed. He grabbed a coal shovel, attacked his sisters, overturned the stove and set fire to the house, and then cut the throat of one of the sisters with a razor. For the next 10 days he was described as having multiple seizures before he finally woke up with no apparent knowledge of what he had done. According to Walker, Kellogg provided this brief anecdote without giving any indication of the individual's name, whether or not the case came to trial, and what the outcome was for the patient and his sister. Walker conceded that the frequency of criminal acts among people with epilepsy was relatively low, but then went on to quote Henry Maudsley in full, writing that 'Whenever we meet with isolated acts of violence, outrages on persons, homicide, suicide, arson, which nothing seems to have instigated, and when, upon attentive examination and thorough enquiry, we find a loss of memory after the perpetration of the act with a periodicity in the recurrence of the same act, and a brief duration, we may diagnose "larval" epilepsy.'[327] Clearly influenced by Maudsley's words, he postulated criteria to guide the process of law when deciding whether to attribute a violent crime to 'an epileptic state'. These included a definite diagnosis of epilepsy, a seizure typical of the accused, epilepsy immediately prior to the violent act, loss of awareness or impaired consciousness at the time of the act, the absence of any motive or premeditation, and failure to attempt escape or avoid detection. These are very sensible guidelines, but they perpetuate the concept of an epileptic basis for homicide and the belief in the 'epileptic furor'.

A few years later the English court case of Mr A illustrated the unchallenged power of the medical expert and the introduction of the unfortunate term 'epileptic homicide.' In writing up the report, John Gunn, who at that time was director of the research unit at the Institute of Psychiatry, London, failed to provide the court details.[328] Mr A, who was a habitual offender, had as a teenager developed seizures that led to several hospital admissions. He described subjective episodes of loss of awareness during these events. He met and subsequently married a social worker, and all seemed well until June 1963, when he informed a neighbour that his wife had gone to visit her mother and would be away for some time. Two days later he attended his local police station and confessed that he had killed her. The police found her body on the bed with multiple injuries apparently caused by a claw hammer. When interviewed, Mr A said that he had taken the hammer up to the bedroom the night before to nail a clothes rack to the wall, and on waking in the morning had picked it up and hit his wife several times with it. He

---

327 Maudsley H (1874) *Responsibility in Mental Disease*. D. Appleton & Company, New York.
328 Gunn J (1978) Epileptic homicide: a case report. *British Journal of Psychiatry* 132, 510–513.

stated that he then went downstairs, lit the fire, made a cup of tea for his wife, and only when he took it up to her did he realize that she was dead.

At the trial a prison doctor stated that the logical sequence of Mr A's actions and the absence of confusion and memory loss ruled out the possibility that any epileptic condition was causal. However, as in the case of Charles Canham described earlier, there was no obvious motive for such a violent act, and once again Henry Maudsley's sage advice would have been in the minds of those medical experts who were called to give their opinions and guide the judge and jury. The two eminent experts involved in Mr A's case were Sir Denis Hill (1913–1982), Professor of Psychiatry at the University of London, and Professor George Fenton, from the Institute of Psychiatry, London. Both were eminent experts in the field of forensic psychiatry, and Sir Denis Hill was an expert on the applications of electroencephalography (EEG) in psychiatry. Crucial to the outcome of the trial were their evaluations of Mr A's EEG findings, which they described as showing 'a generalized abnormality', especially over the right side of the brain, with unequivocal evidence of epileptic activity. They cautiously commented that 'It is not, of course, possible to say how this relates to the crime with which he is charged.' We do not know how the judge instructed the jury, but they were clearly impressed by the experts' opinions, accepted that Mr A's epilepsy had played a significant part in his behaviour, and found him guilty of manslaughter rather than murder. While serving a sentence of life imprisonment he experienced frequent seizures, which were considered to be of temporal lobe origin. These seizures were often associated with prolonged episodes of memory loss, but never with any acts of violence. Although John Gunn describes Mr A's case as one of epileptic homicide, he stops short of offering an explanation for the precise relationship between the murder and Mr A's epilepsy, and instead speculates mainly about what the sentencing outcome would have been if a plea of diminished responsibility had been successful. He does not mention the inconsistency of Mr A being able to remember the act of killing his wife and then attempting to conceal it by telling neighbours that she had gone away. Nor does he address either the deliberate nature of the attack or the absence of any witnessed seizure prior to it. The scientific speculation of the experts clearly outranked the considered and probably correct opinion of the prison doctor, leading the jury away from a verdict of murder, despite the obvious premeditation, to one of manslaughter. Once again the widespread reporting of this case in the press perpetuated the erroneous belief that people with epilepsy pose a danger to the public.

The over-interpretation of EEG evidence was highlighted in the trial of **Peter Manuel,** a notorious Scottish serial killer who murdered at least seven people, and was hanged in 1958 at Glasgow's Barlinnie Prison.[329] Manuel's crimes were gratuitously violent and appeared to

---

329 Nicol AM (2016) *Peter Manuel: Portrait of a Serial Killer.* Black & White Publishing, Edinburgh.

have little motive, so a medical reason for his behaviour was sought. At the time, epilepsy seemed to be a plausible explanation for such inexplicable violence, and his defence team presented EEG evidence that suggested that he suffered from frontal lobe epilepsy. However, Manuel decided not to introduce this evidence when he took over the presentation of his defence from his own lawyers. There was never any suggestion that the murders were committed during some form of epileptic trance or automatism. However, the belief that Manuel's psychotic personality was due to his epilepsy persisted among the wider public for many years, and contributed further to the stigma associated with the condition. Relatively recently the question of whether Manuel might have had epilepsy was resurrected by Dr Richard Goldberg, a reader in law at Aberdeen University, who speculated that Manuel might have suffered from frontal lobe epilepsy, which could have resulted in a defence of diminished responsibility. In an article published in *The Scotsman* (20 April 2008), Goldberg commented that had the EEG evidence for epilepsy been revealed at the time, it 'could have been enough to justify a verdict of culpable homicide'.[330] This sensationalist speculation about a notorious murderer had the effect of reviving prejudiced attitudes towards people with epilepsy, and perpetuating the myth that there is a link between the condition and criminal behaviour.

The high-profile trial of **Jack Ruby** (1911–1967) has already been described in detail in the discussion of the portrayal of epilepsy by the media (see Chapter 8, pp. 183–4). The extensive worldwide reporting of this case by the media exacerbated public misconceptions and increased the stigmatization of people with epilepsy. After the trial, Samuel Livingston summed up the case by stating that 'The "average reader" who has recently been exposed to the many newspaper articles relative to the Jack Ruby murder trial can understandably get the impression that epilepsy, murder, and crimes of passion are related. Many of my epileptic patients and also many employers of persons with epilepsy have contacted me. They cannot help but wonder if some such frightful thing could be perpetrated by them—or upon them. Since I have spent a medical career dealing with epileptic patients, I feel a sincere responsibility to express my opinion on this subject. To my knowledge, there are no reports in the current medical literature which prove that there is a higher rate of criminal action among epileptics than among other individuals.'[331] Livingston noted that the link between epilepsy and murder that had been made throughout Ruby's trial had severely damaged public attitudes to epilepsy as a physical condition, and he concluded sagely that 'I certainly would not question the fact that an epileptic might kill, not because he has epilepsy, but because he is a human being'.

---

330 www.scotsman.com/news-2-15012/did-authorities-ignore-medical-evidence-to-ensure-serial-killer-manuel-was-hanged-1-1166215
331 Livingston S (1964) Epilepsy and murder. *Journal of the American Medical Association* 188, 172.

One year before the Ruby case, **Edward Podolsky** (1902–1965), an American physician and writer, cited several legal cases to support his claim that one of the many traits associated with epilepsy was 'a tendency to homicidal activity'. He then listed what he regarded as the typical features of 'murder committed by epileptics'.[332] However, all of the cases he described as examples of seizure-related murder involved premeditation and complex actions (for example, killing and then burying the victim, taking a hunting knife to rob a grocery stall and inflicting multiple stabbings, concealing the murder weapon, and stabbing three individuals over a protracted period of time while on a rampage). In none of these cases was there any mention of a previous diagnosis of epilepsy, although one individual was described as having an abnormal EEG. In all of the cases there was apparently a lack of memory of the incident, but this does not prove the presence of epilepsy. Podolsky describes the case of a young man, discharged from the army with a diagnosis of epilepsy, 'coming to' in his car to find his girlfriend dead beside him, along with a wrench covered in blood. The jury appears to have been unconvinced that his epilepsy was relevant, as their verdict was murder in the first degree. The author's premise, based on the cases that he cites, is that lack of memory of the murder along with its violent nature are the characteristic features of a seizure-related killing. However, he undermines his argument by quoting a study of 50 murderers that reported that a third of those individuals claimed to have no memory of their violent act. A profile of low intelligence, personality disorder, and psychosis, but not epilepsy, was found in the individuals with amnesia, and although EEG abnormalities were identified, their frequency was not significantly different between the groups who could and could not recall their crime.[333] Despite the absence of any evidence to support such a statement, Podolsky concluded that 'epilepsy in certain instances leads to a form of impulsive behavior sometimes culminating in homicide. The epileptic impulsive character is intolerant of tension or frustration. Whatever he needs he must have. He cannot postpone reactions; he generally acts instead of thinking and reflecting about his action.'[334]

It is clear that, historically, much of the discussion about possible links between epilepsy and violent crime has been based upon anecdote, biased attitudes, and erroneous ideas, such as those of Podolsky. More recently, the application of statistical methodology to well-designed studies has been used to address the issue. A Swedish study conducted by a large team of authors with collective expertise in psychiatry, epidemiology, biostatistics, crime prevention, and prison and probation services investigated whether epilepsy and traumatic brain injury are linked with violent criminal behaviour.[335] Swedish population registers for

---

332 Podolsky E (1962) The epileptic murderer. *Medico-Legal Journal* 30, 176–179.
333 O'Connell BA (1960) Amnesia and homicide. *British Journal of Delinquency* 10, 262–276.
334 Podolsky E (1962) The epileptic murderer. *Medico-Legal Journal* 30, 176–179.
335 Fazel S, Lichtenstein P, Grann M et al. (2011) Risk of violent crime in individuals with epilepsy and traumatic brain injury: a 35-year Swedish population study. *PLoS Medicine* 8, e1001150.

the period from 1973 to 2009 were studied in order to identify any association between epilepsy and violent crime (defined as convictions for homicide, assault, robbery, arson, any sexual offence, or illegal threats or intimidation), compared with age- and gender-matched controls from the general population, and with unaffected siblings. It was found that 973 (4.2 per cent) of a total of 22,947 individuals with epilepsy had committed a violent offence. However, when individuals with epilepsy were compared with their unaffected siblings, thereby removing confounding factors such as socioeconomic background, no association at all was found between epilepsy and violent crime. These findings, which suggest that there is no evidence to support a link between epilepsy and violent criminal behaviour, clearly have the potential to reduce the stigma and erroneous beliefs surrounding the condition.

Researchers from South Korea reviewed the medical and criminal records of all patients with epilepsy who, over a period of 12 months, had been admitted to the National Forensic Hospital (a hospital-based correction facility for convicted criminals with psychiatric neurological illnesses) because they had committed an act of violence.[336] During this period, only 17 (2.2 per cent) of a total of 761 admissions had a diagnosis of epilepsy, and none of those individuals had experienced a seizure at the time of their crime, although seven had symptoms of alcohol intoxication. This large study showed no temporal relationship between seizure onset and the violent act that had led to incarceration, and indicated that when a person with epilepsy committed a violent crime, the incident always occurred between seizures rather than during or immediately after one.

Neil Pandya and his colleagues from the University of Saskatchewan in Canada identified conflicting findings in their recent case report and literature review.[337] They described the case of a 40-year-old woman with worsening temporal lobe epilepsy and escalating aggression. As her epilepsy failed to respond to a number of different drugs she exhibited increasingly violent behaviour that often coincided with seizure onset, and was particularly severe during the first 5 to 10 minutes after a seizure. Her violent behaviour resulted in over 30 convictions, and around 6 months after she had declined surgery for her epilepsy she had a dispute with a fellow tenant that led to a fatal stabbing of the tenant. The patient could not remember the act, which was not witnessed by any third party, and it is not known whether it was preceded by a seizure. The woman was found guilty of second-degree murder and was given a prison sentence. While she was serving her sentence the question of epilepsy surgery was reconsidered, and after further investigations she underwent surgery to remove her right temporal lobe. Her behaviour subsequently improved, so she was transferred

---

336 Kim J-M, Chu K, Jung K-H et al. (2011) Characteristics of epilepsy patients who committed violent crimes: report from the National Forensic Hospital. *Journal of Epilepsy Research* 1, 13–18.
337 Pandya NS, Vrbancic M, Ladino D et al. (2013) Epilepsy and homicide. *Neuropsychiatric Disease and Treatment* 9, 667–673.

from a maximum-security facility to a psychiatric centre. Her seizures are now controlled on a single drug. Although this case report describes how a person with epilepsy stabbed another individual after a dispute, it does not provide any evidence that the violent incident was seizure-related. Details of the trial are not available and, as mentioned earlier, inability to remember perpetrating an act of violence is common, and does not in itself constitute evidence of epilepsy-induced amnesia.

This particular case report does not present sufficient evidence to demonstrate a link between epilepsy and murder. However, Pandya and his colleagues have provided a valuable literature review on the subject of epilepsy and homicide. By searching Medline, the Index Medicus, and biographies of reviews, 50 cases were identified between 1880 and 2013 in which epilepsy was cited in court as a defence for murder or manslaughter. In the majority of these cases the type of seizure was not specified, but when it was, temporal lobe epilepsy was the most common form. Of these cases, 39 (78 per cent) showed no direct relationship between the murder and the timing of seizures, while in 11 cases (22 per cent) there appeared to have been a seizure at or around the time of the act (in 9 cases after the attack, in 1 case during it, and in 1 case 'between attacks', which would suggest there was no link whatsoever with epilepsy). The authors highlight the extreme nature of what they regard as epilepsy-related violence. In terms of outcomes, 62 per cent of these cases were found guilty of homicide and 38 per cent were not considered to be criminally responsible for their actions on the basis of insanity, and were discharged to long-term or indefinite care in a psychiatric facility. The main drawbacks of this review are that a search was made of the medical literature rather than the legal literature, the case reports spanned a long time period, during which medical understanding of epilepsy was improving, the case details were brief, and the cases came from different jurisdictions. The latter factor is particularly relevant if the death penalty was possible, where a defence of guilty but insane, with resultant lifelong incarceration, would be preferable. However, the overall message is a positive one, as the authors concluded that the link between epilepsy and aggression had been 'disproportionally emphasized', with only 11 cases of possible seizure-related homicide being identified in the English-language medical literature over a period of 133 years. It is now clear that any link between epileptic seizures and life-threatening violence has been grossly exaggerated. Finally, the authors highlighted international recommendations drawn up to help to determine whether or not a violent crime was the consequence of a seizure. Their evidence suggests that such criteria would rarely be needed to adjudicate in cases of homicide.

Finally we shall consider an earlier UK-based study that reviewed epilepsy cases in which a verdict of 'not guilty by reason of insanity' (NGRI) had been reached.[338] Comprehensive

---

338 Reuber M and Mackay RD (2008) Epileptic automatisms in the criminal courts: 13 cases tried in England and Wales between 1975 and 2001. *Epilepsia* 49, 138–145.

data for England and Wales for the period from 1975 to 2001 were obtained from the Mental Health Unit at the Home Office. The data covered both medical and legal perspectives, so were unlikely to have overlooked any relevant cases. Over the 26-year period, 13 epilepsy-related cases were identified, representing 7.5 per cent of all NGRI verdicts. The charges that were brought consisted of assault (7 cases), abduction (3 cases), arson (2 cases), murder (1 case), attempted murder (1 case), and burglary (1 case). Nearly two-thirds of the crimes were committed in a state of alcohol intoxication, and around half while the perpetrator was exhibiting psychotic symptoms. Such premeditated acts as burglary or kidnapping are clearly not consistent with an epilepsy-related state, whereas the high frequency of neuropsychological and psychiatric impairment, unemployment, previous history of criminality, and alcohol misuse among the offenders suggests that these environmental factors are much more relevant than epilepsy to the criminal behaviour. The authors of the study concluded that around one-third of the offences occurred during a post-seizure state, but the court reports provided little or no medical evidence on which to base such a conclusion, and the authors conceded that the verdict of NGRI might be related to factors other than the presence of epilepsy alone. However, this study does yet again demonstrate that acts of violent criminal behaviour directly linked to seizures are extremely rare and should not constitute a concern for the general public.

The 'epileptic personality'

Mental health problems such as depression and anxiety are commonly encountered in people with epilepsy. It is unclear whether these are a consequence of societal reactions, or biologically related to the condition itself, or a combination of both. The notion of the 'epileptic personality', especially with regard to antisocial and petty criminal behaviour, has become widespread as a result of prejudiced attitudes towards individuals with epilepsy. The concept of a specific personality disorder in people with epilepsy dates back to a psychoanalytical study of Napoleon Bonaparte that was published in 1917 by **Leon Pierce Clark** (1870–1933), a highly influential American psychiatrist and psychoanalyst. Clark stated that 'First … there is invariably present an epileptic constitution or make-up in those individuals who later develop epilepsy. The nucleus of this personality defect is a temperament of extreme hypersensitiveness and egotism and all that these two main characteristics entail. This defect in character is not to be taken in any narrow or moralistic sense, but is to be considered as a temperamental defect in a broad, biologic view, a personality defect which makes its possessor incapable of social adaptation in its best setting and which, if it remains uncorrected, renders the individual entirely inadequate to make a normal adult life.'[339] Clark's negative attitude, which suggested that a particular type of 'personality defect' might predispose an individual to epilepsy, did incalculable damage by giving rise to the idea that people with epilepsy invariably have an antisocial personality disorder. This belief, based merely on one healthcare professional's personal opinion, persisted among a number of psychiatrists for years, even after a rigorous study was conducted in the 1960s that tested Clark's hypothesis and yielded unequivocally negative results.[340]

The relationship between psychopathology and epilepsy has been extensively studied, and it is widely accepted that people with epilepsy suffer from a high incidence of mood and anxiety disorders. Many healthcare professionals continue to use the term 'epileptic personality', and some cite it as an explanation when their relationship with a patient with epilepsy breaks down. Throughout the twentieth century many articles published in reputable psychiatric journals reinforced the view that people with epilepsy exhibit particularly challenging and unreasonable behaviours that make it difficult to engage with them rationally. The authors of these articles described an inter-ictal state (i.e. one that occurred between seizures) in which individuals were likely to exhibit impulsive, egocentric, and argumentative behaviour. Some suggested that these traits reflected the brain injury underlying the epilepsy, while others proposed that the behaviours resulted from ongoing electrical seizure activity. These unsubstantiated views led increasing numbers of more affluent patients with epilepsy to the consulting rooms of psychiatrists for psychoanalytical treatment, yielding a very lucrative practice for those professionals.

In 1974, Stephen Waxman and Norman Geschwind, two distinguished American neurologists, defined what they considered to be the behavioural characteristics of the 'inter-ictal personality disorder'.[341] They compiled a long list of specific personality characteristics that they believed were frequently seen in and were unique to patients with temporal lobe epilepsy. The list included a wide range of negative traits (ranging from being over-pedantic and rambling in conversation to being obsessed with and articulating wildly about subjects such as religion and politics) and challenging behaviours (such as deviant sexual behaviour). The specific combination of excessive verbal output, excessive writing (hypergraphia), altered sex drive (usually hyposexuality), and rigidity or 'stickiness' in cognition and social interactions became known as Geschwind's syndrome. The existence of such a syndrome is subject to debate. Many authors have sought evidence for the 'epileptic personality' in the works and personalities of famous artists and writers. For example, Vincent van Gogh's

---

339 Clark LP (1917) A further study of mental content in epilepsy. *Psychiatry Bulletin* 2, 483–536.
340 Guerrant J, Anderson WW, Fischer A et al. (1962) *Personality in Epilepsy*. Charles. C. Thomas Publisher, Springfield, IL.
341 Waxman SG and Geschwind N (1975) The interictal behavior syndrome of temporal lobe epilepsy. *Archives of General Psychiatry* 32, 1580–1586.

religiosity and the copious volumes of letters that he wrote to his brother Theo, and Fyodor Dostoevsky's ecstatic seizures and well-documented hypergraphia (Figure 18) are frequently cited as evidence for an abnormal pattern of behaviour in people with epilepsy.

A later study from the Behavioural Neurology Unit at Harvard Medical School claimed that it had identified a total of 18 abnormal behaviours arising from the temporal lobe of the brain in people with epilepsy.[342] These behaviours included mania, aggression, anger, hostility, dependency, a sense of personal destiny, humourlessness, excessive and convoluted writing, high moral opinions, and paranoia (see Table 3). The authors suggested that these characteristics originated from abnormal electrical activity deep in the temporal lobe (the limbic region), where emotional responses were believed to reside. They even defined differences in behaviour according to whether seizures arose from the right or left temporal lobe, with 'catastrophic overemphasis of dissocial behaviour' arising from the left lobe. They also produced a questionnaire to help to classify the proposed aberrant personality of people with temporal lobe epilepsy.[343] Subsequent researchers were unable to replicate these findings, and have questioned the manner in which the original study subjects were selected, and whether they were screened to exclude coexisting psychiatric conditions or disorders such as Asperger's syndrome and autism.

In summary, the concept of an 'inter-ictal personality' remains controversial, as there is little evidence of any link between specific personality traits and epilepsy. Many of these behaviours can be exhibited by any person with a long-term medical condition, and most of them probably reflect the challenges of living with a disability and having to cope with the reactions and prejudices of other people. Recent researchers have suggested that any personality traits that are identified might reflect the need to cope with recurrent seizures, rather than representing a form of psychopathology found in temporal lobe epilepsy.[344] Moreover, many of these traits can be observed in people who do not have any physical or mental health problems. Ultimately it seems that the full range of behavioural features of the 'inter-ictal personality' or 'epileptic personality' are very rarely seen in a single individual. It seems highly unlikely that there is a link between this syndrome and epilepsy, yet these terms continue to be bandied about, with very harmful consequences for many people with epilepsy. Today, the persistent belief in the idea of an 'epileptic personality' has resulted in both the general public and law enforcers continuing to regard people with epilepsy as

---

342 Bear DM and Fedio P (1977) Quantitative analysis of inter-ictal behavior in temporal lobe epilepsy. *Archives of Neurology* 34, 454–467.
343 Bear DM (1985) Temporal lobe epilepsy and the Bear-Fedio personality inventory. *Neurology* 35, 284–286.
344 Tremont G, Smith MM, Bauer L et al. (2012) Comparison of personality characteristics on the Bear-Fedio inventory between patients with epilepsy and those with non-epileptic seizures. *Journal of Neuropsychiatry and Clinical Neurosciences* 24, 47–52.

inherently more likely to display aggressive and hostile behaviour than individuals without the condition.

Automatisms

At the beginning of this chapter we provided some case examples of automatisms and discussed the persistent myth that they might lead to violent behaviour and crime. It is well known that before, during, or after a seizure the affected individual may behave in an abnormal manner, being confused about where they are and misinterpreting the actions, motives, and reactions of those around them. Their resultant actions can be perceived by onlookers as threatening, especially when the affected person perceives attempts to restrain or soothe them as an invasion of their space. What we are referring to here is an *automatism* in which a person with epilepsy can still perform some basic actions while having no recollection of and little control over them. Abnormal behaviour associated with an automatism is a frequent reason for people with epilepsy coming up against the justice system, often with catastrophic consequences.

T.W. was a 25-year-old man with a longstanding history of complex partial (temporal lobe) epilepsy who had travelled to New York to visit a relative for Christmas and New Year. He had been anxious about his outbound night-time flight, but was seizure-free throughout. Although he was not usually a heavy drinker, over the holiday period he had consumed an excessive amount of alcohol and had kept irregular hours. Normally as part of his epilepsy self-management he kept regular hours and never forgot to take his anti-epilepsy drug treatment. He arrived at the airport to fly home only to find that his flight was delayed by several hours and that all of his anti-epilepsy drugs were in his checked-in suitcase rather than his hand luggage. Anxious and bored by the long wait until boarding, he went to the bar in the departure lounge, where he consumed three large beers. When the flight was underway he experienced the early warning symptoms of a seizure and swiftly removed himself from his fellow passengers by going to the toilet and locking the door. The cabin crew noticed his lengthy absence and heard banging sounds coming from the toilet. They knocked on the door but heard no response. They managed to open the door and found the passenger crouching on the floor and refusing to move. When they tried to physically remove him he started to struggle and the crew, with the help of a passenger, then wrestled him to the ground. He was now mumbling incoherently, fighting everyone off, and smelling strongly of alcohol. Fellow passengers, including children, were alarmed by his behaviour and the flight was diverted to the nearest airport, where the passenger was removed from the plane, charged with breach of the peace caused by 'air rage', and taken into custody. T.W. had no memory of the events that had occurred up until the moment when he was arrested. He was upset, remorseful, and had no access to his anti-epilepsy medication, which was in his suitcase. Because of his potentially life-endangering behaviour towards others on the flight, as well as an apparent assault on the cabin staff, he was facing a custodial prison sentence. Several months later, when the case eventually came to trial, expert medical evidence was presented and it was accepted that T.W.'s behaviour had been caused by an automatism outwith his control and was therefore not deliberate. He was advised to ensure that whenever travelling in the future he always kept his drug treatment with him and avoided consuming alcohol or becoming sleep-deprived. The publicity surrounding the trial led to T.W. losing his job and any future prospects of employment, as well as a worsening of his epilepsy as a result of the stress of being brought to trial.

Over the years, widespread media reports of inexplicably aggressive and antisocial behaviour around the time of a witnessed seizure, whether inter-ictal (between attacks), ictal (during attacks), or post-ictal (after attacks), have become deeply ingrained in the minds of the public. Ictal aggressive behaviour is usually resistive and undirected, but is often exacerbated by attempts to restrain or control the person with epilepsy, ceasing immediately if the person is left alone. It is usually a reaction to an external stimulus, and rarely occurs spontaneously. It most commonly occurs after the seizure when the affected person, in a confused 'twilight' state, misinterprets any external intervention, such as restraint imposed by a first responder. Therefore first aiders must be aware of the need to handle patients with epilepsy gently during this phase, rather than to forcibly sit them down, stand them up, or attempt to move them against their will. When complex automatisms are not triggered by an external factor but occur spontaneously after a seizure they can easily be interpreted by the casual onlooker as suspicious and possibly criminal, or as the effects of drug or alcohol intoxication. This is especially likely if the automatism is manifested as a complex act (e.g. walking around to the back of a neighbour's house and trying to open a window, or opening the door of a random stationary car and attempting to sit in the passenger seat). Such behaviour typically occurs after complex partial (temporal and frontal lobe) seizures, and is often complex and seemingly deliberate while being performed without conscious awareness or memory. When the individual is later told how they behaved, they cannot contradict or account for what they have done, as they have no memory of the event or its circumstances. Thus to the casual onlooker who has not witnessed the preceding seizure, the person with epilepsy may appear alert and aware of what they are doing, whereas in fact the opposite is true. Simple automatisms, which were discussed at the beginning of this chapter, can also be problematic.

The legal classification of automatisms merely subdivides them into those that are insane and those that are sane or non-insane. Because epilepsy arises in the brain, which is considered to be 'out of control', its resultant automatisms are legally classified as insane. In contrast, a person with diabetes can experience a 'hypo' when their blood sugar levels are low, and can behave in a strange and uncontrollable manner, but because the cause of the condition arises in the pancreas, where insulin is produced, rather than in the brain, this can be classified as a sane automatism, subject to certain legal tests of probability and foreseeability being met. The facts of each individual case will determine whether the outcome of a diabetic defence is classified as an insane or sane (non-insane) automatism. The notion that sane (non-insane) automatisms arise from an external factor such as a blow to the head or the injection of a drug is a useful rule of thumb when trying to navigate this complex issue.

This nonsensical distinction reflects a legal rather than medical understanding of the relationship between the brain and the body. The unusual behaviour originates from the brain in both epilepsy and diabetes, and can be identical, but because in diabetes the trigger is elsewhere in the body the law does not see the resultant state as being the result of an abnormal brain, whereas in epilepsy it does. In other words, the law sees the diabetic 'hypo' as remediable through altering the dose of its treatment or balancing the diet, and so the situation can be prevented from recurring. The same could be said of epilepsy, with regard to adjusting the drug treatment accordingly, but the law takes a negative stance on this. Describing an epileptic automatism as 'insane' and a diabetic automatism as 'sane' behaviour tells us more about prejudice than about wisdom. Here the law is making epilepsy a mental disorder and is lumping the brain and the mind together, whereas science tells us that they are separate entities that share the same house. Leaving the nomenclature aside, the practical differences between sane and insane automatisms are reflected in the fact that establishing a sane automatism results in a complete defence with a finding of not guilty to any charge, whereas a finding of insane automatism results in a finding of not guilty by reason of insane automatism, and an order can thereafter be made.

Over the years I have encountered a range of circumstances in which individuals have been prosecuted for relatively minor offences related to epileptic automatisms. To name just a few, these include resisting paramedics on entering an ambulance, manhandling police, urinating in public, removing one's clothing in public, becoming aggressive in a shop, banging dustbin lids together in a lane in the middle of the night, sitting in a taxi while refusing to pay the fare, walking up and down the aisle of an aeroplane, refusing to fasten a seatbelt, and fire raising. Many of the cases that I have encountered have pled guilty to the minor misdemeanours due to the costs of their defence, the difficulty and costs entailed in obtaining an expert medical opinion, being overwhelmed by the legal process, or the advice of their defence lawyer. This may be well and good with the first offence, where a custodial sentence is unlikely, but is regrettable if a second automatism offence transpires. I have also observed the consequences of people with epilepsy facing a criminal charge. Typically, increasing anxiety results in worsening seizures, and the individual concerned feels that they have lost control of their situation and become unfairly criminalized, as if having epilepsy in itself was not challenging enough. Self-esteem is eroded and job prospects are immediately reduced with a pending court appearance, and family conflict and depression often ensue. A recent study from the USA showed that suicide rates were 22 per cent higher in people with epilepsy than in the general population.[345] Among those with temporal lobe epilepsy the risk of suicide is even higher, being 25 times greater than in age-matched controls.[346] The trauma of an unfair and often delayed court appearance could just be the tipping point.

The problem is that people with epilepsy can, just like anyone else, commit crimes, and the law has to decide whether or not such an act is the result of an automatism. We have already mentioned a high-profile case in which the defence erroneously invoked epilepsy as an excuse for a violent crime. Generally, in order to convict an individual of a wilful act, the law requires evidence that the alleged crime involves both a guilty act (*actus reus*) and a guilty mind (*mens rea*). An illegal act does not make a person guilty unless their mind is also guilty. A guilty act will generally be proved by objective evidence – for example, by eye-witnesses, closed-circuit television, or forensic evidence. Proving a guilty mind requires proof of the intention to commit a crime, or knowledge that an action or lack of action would cause a crime to be committed. To demonstrate intent it is necessary to show that the accused knowingly committed a criminal act while entirely aware of their action and its consequences. Here there is a requirement to show that the individual was aware that what they were doing was wrong, and lack of such awareness is an integral component of the automatism. As mentioned earlier, the guilty act is not culpable unless the mind is also guilty. Thus a person with epilepsy who, for example, commits a breach of the peace during an automatism cannot be judged as guilty. In these circumstances the court accepts the special defence of automatism, referred to under statute as insanity. Scots law draws a distinction between the statutory defence of insanity and the defence of automatism. If during an automatism a person with epilepsy pushes another individual to the ground, who then sustains a severe head injury, a similar verdict might be expected. The concept of being found not guilty by reason of insanity dates back to 1843 and is referred to as the M'Naghten Rules named after Daniel McNaughton, who attempted to assassinate the then-British Prime Minister Robert Peel. It is when these rules are satisfied that the accused is adjudged to be not guilty by reason of insanity. Such a defence is recognized in Australia, Canada, England and

---

345 Tian N, W Cui, M Zack et al. (2016) Suicide among people with epilepsy: a population-based analysis of data from the U.S. National Violent Death Reporting System, 17 states, 2003–2011. *Epilepsy & Behavior* 61, 210–217.
346 Christensen J, Vestergaard M, Mortensen PB et al. (2007) Epilepsy and risk of suicide: a population-based case–control study. *Lancet Neurology* 6, 693–698.

Wales, New Zealand, the Republic of Ireland, and most US states. International criteria have been drawn up by the neurologist Antonio Delgado-Escueta and his colleagues to help the courts to decide whether or not an offence can be regarded as the consequence of an epileptic automatism (see Table 4).[347] These criteria are heavily dependent on investigations (EEG and video recordings) and are not practicable when less serious, but nonetheless potentially life-changing, charges come before the court.

The very nature of epilepsy does leave the door open to the verdict of sane automatism if an external force or factor can be shown to have caused the seizure that led to the automatism that resulted in the offence. Although seizures are obviously internal, arising in the brain, they can be triggered by external factors such as sleep deprivation, physical exhaustion, hunger, and failure to take anti-epilepsy medication. If medical evidence can prove, for example, that failure to take anti-epilepsy medication was the cause of the seizure, this external factor allows a defence of sane automatisms to the accused, and if accepted will result in acquittal. All of this means that the law has difficulty in grasping the blurred line between sane and insane automatism, and it raises the question of what happens to those individuals who have been found not guilty by reason of insanity. After a verdict of guilty the placing, or disposal, of the individual is based on the medical opinion as to what treatments are required to prevent the offence in question from reoccurring. A case would be adjourned to obtain background medical reports, which could lead to placement in a secure hospital.

Reform in the law in relation to automatism-related minor offences is long overdue. Individuals should be spared the judicial process if there is substantial evidence that an event is automatism-related. The following criteria to confirm such a situation would seem sensible: that the individual is known to have epilepsy, is known to have automatisms, is seen to have had a seizure, any violent action perpetrated is poorly directed and simple rather than complex, and the incident is out of character. The questions then arise as to who makes the decision not to prosecute, and how the medical evidence is collected and evaluated. The steadily decreasing funding for law and order in the UK brings little hope of sparing people with epilepsy from the bruising legal process to which they are subjected.

Conclusion

There is no evidence to support the suggestion that people with epilepsy have a violent predisposition. This longstanding myth has been reinforced by the confused and conflicting

---

347 Delgado-Escueta AV, Mattson RH, King L et al. (2002) The nature of aggression during epileptic seizures. *Epilepsy & Behavior* 3, 550–556.

literature on the subject. People with epilepsy are no more likely to commit murder or other violent crimes than anyone else, and the replacement of the anecdotal medical literature based on selective case studies with rigorously designed and statistically based studies has done much to dispel this damaging belief. Another myth is that of the 'epileptic personality', which was promoted by early selective studies that failed to account for the social impact of the illness or to compare its characteristics with the effects of other long-term health conditions on the personality. Those early studies appeared to set out to confirm their authors' theories and personal prejudices, and failed to provide information about the mental health of their study group, or the incidence of conditions such as Asperger's syndrome among them. The majority of individuals with epilepsy are as law-abiding as anyone else, indeed probably more so, given the lifestyle adjustments that they have to make, such as avoiding alcohol and the use of recreational drugs. Finally, the binary legal concept of sane and insane automatisms needs to be addressed, as this outdated terminology stigmatizes epilepsy and regards it as a disorder of the mind rather than of the brain.

CHAPTER 12
Stigmatization, discrimination, and social isolation

Public perceptions, attitudes, and opinions are strongly influenced by the media, which now often have a significant effect not only in areas such as marketing and political elections, but also in virtually every other aspect of daily life. Health-related messages that are backed by substantial financial resources can be very effective in shifting public perceptions. For example, the harmful effects of smoking are now well known. However, the organizations and charities that represent people with epilepsy do not have such resources at their disposal, and instead their attempts to influence public opinion have depended largely upon tireless campaigning and awareness raising about the condition. Many researchers have used questionnaires to assess the views of the general public about epilepsy, although the percentage of respondents tends to be low and also disproportionately well educated. In addition, surveys have been used to elicit the views of people with epilepsy and their families, carers, healthcare professionals, employers, and teachers. However, there are significant knowledge gaps with regard to knowledge and views about epilepsy among social workers, housing and benefits officers, law enforcement officers, and even nurses, despite the fact that these groups are heavily involved in the decisions, challenges, and life choices that are faced by people with epilepsy who are in their care.

The question arises as to why the acceptance of a condition as common as epilepsy is so problematic. In her book *Illness as Metaphor*,[348] Susan Sontag comments that chronic illness

---

348 Sontag S (1978) *Illness as Metaphor*. Farrar, Straus and Giroux, New York.

is viewed as a bad and undesirable state that attracts pity, victimization, and even revulsion. Epilepsy must be one of the highest-scoring chronic illnesses in this context. The irregularity and unpredictability of epileptic seizures, together with the loss of control, perceived 'deviant' behaviour, and abnormal body movements, make the condition unique among chronic disorders. This, combined with fear generated among those who witness seizures, ignorance about the condition, and historical attitudes of rejection, helps to explain why epilepsy is so stigmatized. This continuing prejudice also goes some way towards explaining why healthcare planners and research funders persist in giving epilepsy a lower priority than it merits.

Observing the way in which people react to a seizure provides a window into their fears and misunderstandings. As I mentioned in Chapter 6, I first witnessed a seizure when I was 10 years old, in a cinema. It was a matinée performance, and most of the small audience was sitting in the middle of the front few rows. Suddenly a man who was sitting on his own immediately in front of us stiffened, shouted out, and started to shake uncontrollably. The audience members quickly moved to the sides of the auditorium in order to distance themselves from him. A few minutes later a cinema usher appeared and marched him out of the auditorium, while the rest of us carried on watching the film. I can still remember his confused, dishevelled appearance and his unsteady progress up the aisle towards the door.

The second episode that I witnessed in a public place occurred around 20 years later, when my wife and I were standing in the ticket office at Paddington Station. I was a young hospital doctor who had seen seizures in the setting of the Accident and Emergency Department but not in the street. A smartly dressed man carrying a briefcase was buying his train ticket and suddenly fell to the ground, where he started to have convulsions. The ticket clerk quickly closed his hatch and moved to open an adjacent one, while the people who had been standing behind the man stepped round him to join the newly created queue. It seemed that their main concern was that this inconvenient incident might cause them to miss their trains, and they had no time to provide assistance or even show concern. When I hailed the ticket office staff and asked them to phone for an ambulance I was accused of being abusive and overreacting. In fact, everyone seemed more concerned about my attitude than about the man with epilepsy. When he eventually recovered I flagged down a taxi to take him to hospital, but the taxi driver refused to have him as a passenger. My wife and I then sat with the man until he had recovered sufficiently to make his own way home. He had been incontinent during the seizure and there were urine stains on his trousers. He seemed apologetic and went on his way. I have never forgotten the lack of concern and support offered during this incident, and the reaction of other people to a situation that they did not understand and clearly feared.

The situation is well summarized by a comment made over 60 years ago by Howard Fabing, head of neuropsychiatry at Christ Hospital, Cincinnati, Ohio. He observed that 'the improved medical condition of these patients often has little bearing on their chance for improving their social or economic opportunities. The doctor who succeeds in bringing an epileptic's seizures under control often runs smack into the stone wall of centuries of prejudice when he attempts to lead his patient into the next – the most important and rewarding – phase of therapy, that of rehabilitation, into the world of his fellow men.'[349]

Stigma

In 1997 the Indian neurologist Rajendra Kale commented in an editorial that 'the history of epilepsy can be summarized as 4,000 years of ignorance, superstition and stigma, followed by 100 years of knowledge, superstition and stigma.'[350] He cited a recent German study that had shown that around 20 per cent of respondents still believed that epilepsy was a mental disorder, and that a similar proportion would not want their children to marry anyone with the condition. Kale highlighted the US states that up until 1956 had prohibited marriage of people with epilepsy, and up until the 1970s had denied them access to public places such as theatres and restaurants. He reported that discrimination in developing countries was even more punitive and widespread. For example, in India a female with epilepsy had little chance of getting married, and surveys from rural Turkey showed that 70 per cent of people still believed that epilepsy had supernatural causes. It is against the backdrop of what is now more than 4000 years of stigma that we shall review the history of discrimination and its consequences.

Stigma is a Greek word that historically referred to a type of mark or tattoo that was cut or burned into the skin of criminals, slaves, or traitors. It is now defined as a degrading and debasing attitude through which society discredits a person or group of people because of a particular physical attribute, such as an illness, or because of their racial origin, sexuality, nationality, or religion. It may be directed toward an individual who is perceived as different from the 'normal' majority, or toward the friends, family, or associates of that person. The sociology literature on stigma has its own complex terminology, but there are some alternative terms in use that are more accessible to the layperson. For example, the term *internalized stigma* refers to stigma that is experienced by the individual, but is perhaps more easily understood as *perceived stigma*, and the term *interpersonal stigma* refers to stigma

---

349 Fabing HD (1958) Epilepsy and the law. *Medical Clinics of North America* 42, 361–373.
350 Kale R (1997) Bringing epilepsy out of the shadows. *British Medical Journal* 315, 2.

created by the attitudes and behaviour of others, but is perhaps better understood as *enacted stigma*. The sociologist J.L. Dell defined stigma as the relationship 'between the differentness of an individual and the devaluation society places on that particular differentness.'[351] For stigmatization to be maximally effective the stigmatized person must, to some extent at least, share some of the beliefs of those who are devaluing them. This becomes a vicious circle as their tacit acceptance of the negative stereotype has the effect of disempowering them. Many academic studies have attempted to measure stigma by means of rating scales, the aim being to determine how common it is, how much it varies between different cultures and among different conditions, and whether it can be reduced by educational interventions.

Erving Goffman (1922–1982), the acclaimed Canadian-American sociologist, and the author of *Stigma: Notes on the Management of Spoiled Identity*, suggested that an individual's relationship to stigma can be divided into three categories. The 'victim' is stigmatized and bears the brunt of the stigma, the 'normal' do not carry the stigma, and the 'wise' are those among the normal who show understanding of and empathy with the condition of the stigmatized. Examples of the 'wise' would include informed members of the public, supportive family members, and healthcare professionals. Goffman based his book on case studies in which he analysed stigmatized individuals' feelings, their relationship to 'normal' people, and the strategies that they used to cope with perceived rejection. Goffman defined stigma as a process by which the reaction of others 'spoils' normal identity. The opening words of his landmark book are worth repeating here: 'The Greeks, who were apparently strong on visual aids, originated the term *stigma* to refer to bodily signs designed to expose something unusual and bad about the moral status of the signifier. The signs were cut or burnt into the body and advertised that the bearer was a slave, a criminal, or a traitor – a blemished person, ritually polluted, to be avoided, especially in public places. Later, in Christian times, two layers of metaphor were added to the term: the first referred to bodily signs of holy grace that took the form of eruptive blossoms on the skin; the second, a medical allusion to this religious allusion, referred to bodily signs of physical disorder.'[352] Goffman goes on to describe stigma as a process whereby the negative reactions of others 'serve to spoil one's own social identity'. Stigmatized individuals are typically ostracized, undervalued, rejected, ridiculed, shunned by 'normal' society, and as a result subjected to social isolation. Thus stigmatization, discrimination, and social isolation are inextricably linked.

In 1983 the distinguished US sociologists **Joseph Schneider** and **Peter Conrad** published a book on the meaning of having epilepsy, entitled *Having Epilepsy: the Experience and*

---

351 Dell JL (1986) Social dimensions of epilepsy: stigma and response. In: Whitman S and Hermann BP (eds.) *Psychopathology in Epilepsy: Social Dimensions*. Oxford University Press, New York. pp. 185–210.
352 Goffman E (1963) *Stigma: Notes on the Management of Spoiled Identity*. Penguin, London. p. 9.

Control of Illness.[353] Based on the experiences of patients with the condition, it addresses not only stigmatization but also many other aspects of seizures. This largely forgotten and rarely quoted work was based on in-depth interviews with 80 individuals with epilepsy. From the material obtained, the authors were able to construct a first-hand account of how people with epilepsy coped with and managed their illness. It should be pointed out that this study was conducted at a time when patients were still rarely given an opportunity to express their personal opinions. When considering the validity of the authors' conclusions with regard to the wide spectrum of patients with epilepsy, it is important to bear in mind that neither the selection criteria for the participants nor their demographic characteristics (such as gender, level of education, and socioeconomic status) were specified.

Some of the comments made by the interviewees about discrimination included the following: 'The fact of having epilepsy. It isn't the seizures. I think they are a very minor part of it.' 'Its implications are enormous. The historical implications of epilepsy are fantastic. I'm lucky to have been born when I was. If I had been born at the beginning of this century I would have been discarded … probably locked up somewhere.' One woman described the reaction of others by comparing her seizures to 'having your pants pulled down in public'. Another patient commented that 'It's dirty, falling down and frothing at the mouth and jerking and the bystanders not knowing what to do.' A woman who had lost her job as a teacher said 'I understand it now and I'm not afraid of it. But most people are unless they've experienced it, and so you just don't speak to other people about it and if you do, never use the word "epilepsy". The word itself, I mean job-ways, insurance-ways … anything, the hang-ups there are about it. There's just too much prejudice so the less said about it the better.' Many of Schneider and Conrad's subjects conveyed shame about their seizures, but it is unclear whether this emotion was directly experienced by them or reflected the attitudes of those who had witnessed their attacks.

For many people with epilepsy, the negative response of others results in a loss of opportunities due to experiences of disclosure, driving restrictions, limited employment opportunities, insurance problems, and many other limitations. Discrimination can be overt, hidden, indirect, or legal, and is defined as the treatment of any person or group differently and in a way that is inferior to the way that people are normally treated, or as the unjust and prejudicial treatment of different categories of people. The perceptions of 'normal' people will define the degree of stigmatization and discrimination inflicted, and no one with epilepsy will have escaped the burden of this experience. However, it is less widely realized that family members and friends can also be affected, either merely through

---

[353] Schneider JW and Conrad P (1983) *Having Epilepsy: the Experience and Control of Illness*. Temple University Press, Philadelphia, PA.

association, or as a result of myths about genetics or misplaced concerns about the damaging emotional effects of being a carer.

The detrimental effects of unemployment on health are well established. When discrimination removes the opportunity to work, it results in loss of a sense of purpose and self-esteem, social isolation, stress caused by the economic impact, deteriorating mental health, and worsening seizure control. This downward spiral of events needs to be understood by those who discriminate against people with epilepsy. The American sociologist Robert Merton (1910–2003) coined the term 'unintended consequences' to describe the unforeseen outcomes of deliberate actions, and the emotional fragility of those who are discriminated against should not be underestimated. Although prejudiced attitudes and discriminatory actions do not invariably go hand in hand, in general our thoughts do usually govern our actions. It is important to study the attitudes of Goffman's 'normals' to epilepsy in order to identify what strategies might encourage the development of more positive perceptions, and to ascertain whether stigmatization and discrimination are declining or increasing over time.

In the 1970s, Janet Ries, a social psychology researcher at Washington State University, undertook a study that primarily focused on alcoholism and whether or not the 'normals' regarded it as a disease.[354] She interviewed 306 individuals in a US Midwestern urban community, asking questions about alcoholics, people with epilepsy, and blind people, and she compared the responses given for these three groups. The vast majority of the respondents felt that alcoholics had unfavourable characteristics and were the least socially acceptable group. Blind people were perceived as the most socially acceptable group, and perceptions of people with epilepsy were midway between those of the other two groups. Ries' results for people with epilepsy were revealing. In total, 53 per cent of respondents stated they would not want their children to marry individuals with the condition, 26 per cent would not rent them a room, 11 per cent would not work with them, 8 per cent would not want them to join a club of which they were a member, and 5 per cent would not want them to live in their neighbourhood.

As in the study by Schneider and Conrad, this research was conducted at a time when the methodology for analysing public opinion was in its infancy. Major advances in that field were made possible by the work of George Gallup (1901–1984), the American inventor of the Gallup Poll, a method of sampling public opinion by eliciting views from small samples of individuals representative of all social levels and groups. In 1935, Gallup set up the American Institute of Public Opinion, which at 5-year intervals from 1949 to 1979 asked a representative sample of the adult population for their views on epilepsy. He published

---

[354] Ries JK (1977) Public acceptance of the disease concept of alcoholism. *Journal of Health and Social Behavior* 18, 338–344.

this work with William Caveness (1909–1981), a neurologist and Head of the National Institute of Neurological and Communicative Disorders at Bethesda's National Institute of Health.[355] The results of their studies were positive, showing a significant reduction in prejudiced attitudes at each 5-year interval over the 30-year time period. The most positive comments were made by the better educated, more securely employed, younger, and urban respondents. In total, 63 per cent of the respondents knew a person with epilepsy, and 59 per cent reported having witnessed a seizure at first hand. This surprising result suggests that despite Gallup's involvement in the study, the sample was not representative of the general population, thus casting doubt on the representativeness of the opinions obtained and conclusions drawn. Over the 30-year study period, the proportion of respondents who considered epilepsy to be a form of insanity decreased from 41 per cent to 8 per cent, and the proportion who stated that they would not allow their children to play with someone with epilepsy declined from 43 per cent to 11 per cent. In 1949, 55 per cent of respondents believed that people with epilepsy should not be in employment, compared with 21 per cent in 1979. In the mid-1970s in the USA, the national level of unemployment was 8.5 per cent, compared with 23 per cent among people with epilepsy. This is despite a Department of Labour study that showed better safety records and indicated that there were only a few jobs that were unsuitable for people with epilepsy, such as working at height. At the beginning of the 30-year study period the Southern States were the most negative about people with epilepsy, but this regional difference had disappeared by the end of the survey period. Caveness and Gallup concluded that the educational efforts of healthcare professionals and charities, better drugs that provided improved control of epilepsy, and increased post-war employment prospects with better legislation in the areas of immigration, marriage, and driving, had all helped to improve public perceptions. However, there are other possible explanations. For example, awareness was raised after the war in Vietnam had resulted in a population of head-injured patients who were considered to deserve empathy as they had acquired their epilepsy 'through no fault of their own'. In addition, in subsequent years people with epilepsy were beginning to be portrayed more realistically by the media, television, and cinema.

Disappointingly, later surveys that asked slightly different questions revealed a continuing lack of knowledge and understanding. Ten years after the publication of Caveness and Gallup's research, a study that used similar methodology showed that 50 per cent of those surveyed had no understanding of the causes of epilepsy, and 20 per cent still believed it to be a mental health disorder. Two-thirds of respondents believed that an object should be placed in the mouth of someone having a seizure, 30 per cent thought that people with epilepsy

---

355 Caveness WF and Gallup GH (1980) A survey of public attitudes towards epilepsy in 1979 with an indication of trends over the past thirty years. *Epilepsia* 21, 509–518.

and their families were 'inferior' human beings, and 18 per cent believed that a person with epilepsy could be identified by their facial characteristics alone.[356]

Similar studies that were conducted throughout the 1980s and 1990s showed only a very slow improvement in awareness and understanding. All of them concluded that more public education programmes were required, with a view to shaping the attitudes of young people before they became influenced and conditioned by the views of their elders. With a view to achieving this, at the beginning of the millennium the Epilepsy Foundation of America sent out questionnaires to around 20,000 high-school students. Nearly 50 per cent of the respondents either believed that epilepsy was a mental condition or were uncertain about this, and 50 per cent did not know whether people with epilepsy should drive, work, or have children. One-third of the respondents were unaware of the basic concepts of first aid, and admitted that they would not know what to do if they witnessed a seizure. Only 50 per cent were confident that epilepsy was not contagious. One-third would not date a person described as an 'epileptic', and the majority believed that it was possible to tell if someone had epilepsy just by looking at their facial features. In 2002, Rosemarie Kobau and Patricia Price, from the Division of Adult and Community Health in Atlanta, Georgia, USA, conducted a survey to assess perceptions and knowledge of epilepsy and seizures within a US population.[357] Out of 5500 individuals who were surveyed, just over 4000 responded. The authors concluded that 'in the United States, epilepsy remains a mystery to a large segment of the population', and that despite the fact that 50 per cent of the responders admitted to having witnessed a seizure in person or on TV, or to knowing someone with epilepsy, 'levels of knowledge about the disorder are far below what they should be'. The mantra that 'groups would benefit from educational campaigns to improve knowledge of the disorder' is one that has been expressed by many researchers both before and since. However, the form that these campaigns should take and the ways in which their effectiveness can be measured have yet to be addressed.

The attitudes of the public in the UK to epilepsy were examined in a study conducted by Ann Jacoby and her colleagues at the Department of Public Health and Policy at the University of Liverpool, in conjunction with the Office for National Statistics.[358] From 3000 selected addresses, approximately 1600 adults responded to a short questionnaire. The respondents matched the sociodemographic characteristics of the UK population and therefore the answers could safely be assumed to be representative of the views of the wider

---

356 LaMartina JM (1989) Uncovering public misconceptions about epilepsy. *Journal of Epilepsy* 2, 45–48.
357 Kobau R and Price P (2003) Knowledge of epilepsy and familiarity with this disorder in the U.S. population: results from the 2002 HealthStyles Survey. *Epilepsia* 44, 1449–1454.
358 Jacoby A, Gorry J, Gamble C et al. (2004) Public knowledge, private grief: a study of public attitudes to epilepsy in the United Kingdom and implications for stigma. *Epilepsia* 45, 1405–1415.

public. The questions covered exposure to and knowledge of epilepsy, as well as opinions on employment, intelligence, personality, lifestyle, empathy, and the causes of the condition. In total, 16 per cent of the respondents attributed epilepsy to stress, 14 per cent attributed it to alcohol and drug abuse, and 13 per cent viewed it as a mental illness rather than a physical one. Most of the respondents could identify symptoms of epilepsy, but felt that a fall to the ground and shaking were its defining features, with less than 20 per cent being aware that it could also take the form of blank spells or 'absences' alone. With regard to employment, 60 per cent of the respondents felt that people with epilepsy should not be employed in the armed services, and 50 per cent believed that they should not become police officers. Occupations as firemen and lorry drivers were also widely regarded as inappropriate, and 25 per cent of respondents believed that teaching and nursing were unsuitable careers. One-third of respondents felt that people with epilepsy should not be employed in factory work, whereas only 6 per cent thought that they should be barred from working as shop assistants. Most of the respondents thought that working as a solicitor was appropriate, but training to become a doctor was considered out of the question.

The questionnaire also asked the respondents to state reasons why people with epilepsy were treated differently. This elicited the following comments, among others: 'They're known as freaks and people are wary of them', 'They are identified as being out of the normal, labelled as being abnormal', 'They are a health risk to the public', and 'It can be hard to tell if a person in a seizure is drunk or on drugs, and people are afraid to get involved as a result'.

There were also many positive comments, including 'Most people with epilepsy are as intelligent as anyone else', and 'Children with epilepsy should be allowed to play with others'. However, more than 50 per cent of respondents believed that people with epilepsy were destined to be treated as different, adding that they could see the potential for them to have a normal life, but that the attitudes of society were holding them back. The authors of the study compared their conclusions with those of earlier studies, noting that there had been a decrease in prejudice and misunderstanding, but adding that 'Future in-depth studies are needed to explore the reasons behind perceivers' [respondents'] "negative" attitudes, in order to meaningfully inform public attitude campaigns and ensure they are properly targeted, and hence to maximize the likelihood of their success.' Here, as in so many studies before and after it, the questions were formulated by a team of sociologists, psychologists, and statisticians, and only rarely were people with epilepsy asked for their input at this stage.

With regard to the 'future in-depth studies' that Jacoby and her colleagues have called for, the few that have been conducted subsequently have generally produced the same answers to similar questions. A multi-authored text, published in 2012 and aimed at promoting health and understanding of epilepsy, contained the admission that 'a large-scale, population-based survey specific to epilepsy has not been conducted in the United States in many years, so gaps in knowledge about contemporary attitudes and beliefs may exist.'[359] These studies have certainly shown a small positive change over time in the attitudes of Goffman's 'normals' to people with epilepsy. However, the ability of such surveys to truly reflect public opinion is questionable when respondents are aware that the answers they give are being used to assess their own personal attitudes. Thus they will tend to provide what they believe to be the most socially acceptable or expected response, despite reassurances that their contribution will not be attributed to them. Also we have no way of knowing the attitudes of the non-responders to the surveys, although it might be surmised that these would be less positive than those of individuals who were sufficiently interested and motivated to respond.

Jacoby's respondents believed that people with epilepsy should have a more normal life, but it was society, of which they were representative, that was preventing progress. This brings us back to the disconnect between thought and action. Meanwhile the authors of studies continue to suggest that their research will help to enable the development and appropriate targeting of educational programmes. Yet instead of assuming that, due to their learned helplessness, people with epilepsy need Goffman's 'wise normal' caring academics to pose questions on their behalf, we should begin by asking them directly about their own views on stigma and public awareness and what ideas they might have for improving the situation. These so-called 'expert patients' have a wealth of knowledge and experience that has already been recognized through their role in self-management programmes. Sadly, however, their voice is often ignored when studies are being designed, improvement of services and attitudes is being addressed, and legislation is being drafted.

Angelia Paschal and her colleagues from the University of Kansas Medical School worked with seven people with epilepsy to design questions to take out to those attending their local epilepsy centre.[360] The researchers pointed out that the stigma surrounding epilepsy had always prevented the condition from gaining the public health attention it deserved, and that as a result it had become a condition that policy makers seemed to feel they could afford to ignore. Paschal noted that 'in the formulation of previous educational interventions the opinions of epilepsy patients have been overlooked'. At the time when they were planning their project there was no existing questionnaire designed to ask people with epilepsy how they felt about their own condition. The researchers, in collaboration with their epilepsy patients, drew up a list of questions, and also asked respondents to suggest solutions for increasing awareness and reducing stigma. The survey was mailed out to 484 individuals, of

---

359 Institute of Medicine (US) Committee on the Public Health Dimensions of the Epilepsies (2012) *Epilepsy across the Spectrum: Promoting Health and Understanding.* National Academies Press, Washington, DC.

360 Paschal AM, Hawley SR, St Romain T et al. (2007) Epilepsy patients' perceptions about stigma, education, and awareness: preliminary responses based on a community participatory approach. *Epilepsy & Behavior* 11, 329–337.

whom only 165 (34 per cent) returned a completed survey. The majority of the respondents were women (62 per cent), on low incomes (54 per cent), and unmarried (54 per cent), with only 42 per cent of the total respondents in employment. These figures are consistent with findings in other studies of employment and marital status in populations with epilepsy. The study group were all attending a hospital epilepsy clinic and were therefore likely to have more severe epilepsy.

In total, 42 per cent of the respondents believed that the general public had negative views of epilepsy and that this had a negative effect on their own image of themselves. Around 20 per cent stated that at some time in the past they had denied having epilepsy altogether. Despite attending a hospital epilepsy clinic, one-third of the respondents said that they did not know anyone else with the condition, indicating both secrecy about the condition and a lack of peer support. The respondents commented that members of the public did not know how to react to epilepsy, and 90 per cent believed that the public were ill informed. When asked to list what they considered to be the most common public misconceptions, they suggested the following examples: 'All seizures are severe', 'Epilepsy is a mental illness', and epilepsy 'is contagious and consequently those with it should be socially avoided'. When asked about the best strategies for educating the public, they suggested television advertisements, workplace education programmes, pamphlets, and radio announcements, and two-thirds of the respondents mentioned the need to provide the public with better information on first aid. The authors highlighted the low response rate and the tendency of respondents to give the most socially acceptable responses, but they nevertheless concluded that stigma can only be eliminated by meaningful public education programmes. The questions of funding for the programmes, identification of the target audience, and how to measure the effectiveness of the programmes remained unanswered. Realistically, in the current financial climate it seems unlikely that charities and other providers will be able to fund long-term sustainable public education programmes. Sadly, then, although people with epilepsy were involved in its design, the conclusions and recommendations of this study have not led to any further progress.

No account of epilepsy and stigma would be complete without considering two classic and sadly overlooked studies. The first is by Graham Scambler and Anthony Hopkins from the UK, and the second, mentioned earlier, is by the Americans Joseph Schneider and Peter Conrad. Both were the result of meticulously documented interviews with people with epilepsy. They captured not just stigma but also the myriad of other aspects of being diagnosed and living with the condition. They remain as relevant today as when they were first published, and should be compulsory reading for all involved in the care of people with epilepsy. It is interesting that three out of the four authors were sociologists (Hopkins was the only medic), as up until that time ill health had been viewed primarily in the context of medical diagnosis and treatment. Scambler was then a young research student working with Hopkins at St Bartholomew's Hospital, London. Unlike most neurologists of that era, Hopkins was as interested in the social aspects of disease as in the medical ones. The funding for their research project was provided by the British Epilepsy Association and was modest by today's standards.

They started their study by investigating the incidence of stigma.[361] They then conducted a small survey of 85 adults without epilepsy in order to test three assumptions about perceptions of public knowledge: first, that the general public viewed epilepsy solely in terms of grand mal (convulsive) seizures; second, that epilepsy was a mental health disorder; and third, that people with epilepsy had antisocial personalities. Interestingly, they found the public better informed than predicted, and much less prejudiced than earlier studies had suggested. They then addressed the perceptions of epilepsy and its impact on the lives of a large number of people with the condition drawn from general medical practices in the London area. Over the course of the study they interviewed 108 individuals, all of whom were over 16 years of age and had either experienced at least one seizure in the previous two years or were on anti-epileptic medications for seizures that had occurred at some time in the past. The use of these criteria ensured that the participants represented the whole spectrum of the condition covered by an epilepsy diagnosis.

The researchers examined the impact of first being diagnosed with epilepsy, and found that the participants' main reactions were anger and resentment (for example, 'I cried for two days' and 'It's not a very nice word, is it?'). Not surprisingly, such negative reactions to being given the diagnosis were universally reported. The positive aspects of finally being given an explanation for the symptoms and the possibility of experiencing an improvement through treatment were not mentioned. This was in contrast to Schneider and Conrad's earlier findings that some individuals experienced relief when they learned, often after a long delay, what was wrong and that something could now be done to treat it. Scambler and Hopkins found that some of their subjects had tried to re-negotiate the diagnosis with their doctor, drawing upon uncertainties such as the lack of a cause or normality of tests. They also noted that doctors would occasionally feign initial uncertainty as a ploy to allow them to gradually impart a diagnosis that they believed their patient did not want to hear. This breaking of bad news in stages could be used by the patient to dispute their condition. Around 75 per cent of those diagnosed reported that they were given no reason why they had epilepsy, thus adding to the uncertainty and leading to comments such as 'If he doesn't even know what causes seizures, how can he tell they are epileptic?'

---

[361] Scambler G and Hopkins A (1986) Being epileptic: coming to terms with stigma. *Sociology of Health and Illness* 8, 26–43.

Next the authors explored what 'being epileptic' meant to their interviewees. They began by defining the differences between *enacted stigma* and *felt stigma*. As mentioned earlier in this chapter, enacted stigma refers to the experience of the unfair attitudes and behaviour of others, which are based on a person's perceived unacceptability or inferiority. This is different from felt stigma, which refers to a person's feelings of shame and expectation that they will be discriminated against by the unfair attitudes and behaviour of others. Nearly all of the participants in the study had experienced felt stigma, but only a third reported having been the victim of enacted stigma. This level of enacted stigma is surprisingly low. Felt stigma often resulted in a strategy of concealment in an attempt to appear 'normal'. This strategy had a negative effect on the affected person's relationships at home and in the workplace. The authors of the study highlighted the possible role of parents as 'felt stigma coaches' if they conveyed to their children, no matter how subliminally, that epilepsy was something bad that they were reluctant to discuss. Implanting this belief during childhood could result in a lifetime of feeling disproportionally stigmatized. The authors quoted one interviewee as commenting that 'Mother wanted to keep it a big dark secret and not let anyone know.' The possibility that some parents may even feel ashamed of having a child with epilepsy cannot be excluded, and clearly there is the potential for lifelong damage to be caused by the child's awareness of their parents' sense of shame. Only 25 per cent of the interviewees with childhood-onset epilepsy had been told their diagnosis by their parents, and around 50 per cent of their siblings were unaware of their brother's or sister's condition.

All of the interviewees reported that they had only disclosed their epilepsy to someone outside the family when that person had gained the status of a close friend. It was also more difficult to tell a potential partner about their condition, although this was sometimes done pre-emptively to ensure that the other person would be more prepared in the event of a sudden seizure occurring that might jeopardize the relationship. In total, 61 per cent of the interviewees had not disclosed their condition to their partner, and of those who had, one-third experienced the breakdown of their relationship. In situations of impending marriage, a strategy of concealment was much less likely. One interviewee stated that 'the only person I'll ever tell of the opposite sex is the man that can accept me as I am now and will say "Will you marry me?" I won't say yes until he understands fully, until he's come to the GP and I've asked the doctor to explain it all to him.' A third of those who were getting married were completely open about their epilepsy, a third partially concealed it, and a third concealed it altogether. A significant number of those who had admitted to having epilepsy after they became engaged did not go on to marry. It is not known what happened to the long-term relationships of those who continued to conceal their epilepsy.

Only 25 per cent of the interviewees who were in full-time employment had informed their employer of their condition. Some had mentioned that they experienced blackouts without specifically referring to epilepsy. More than 50 per cent had not disclosed their condition, and said that they lived with the daily threat of exposure, confrontation with their supervisor, and the risk of losing their job. Those who had informed their employer that they had epilepsy nevertheless concealed any sickness leave or hospital appointments. Although all of the interviewees who were in work felt that they had been stigmatized because of their epilepsy, less than 25 per cent could cite an episode of enacted stigma. Not surprisingly, the highest numbers of episodes were experienced by those who had told their employers about their condition. This suggests that the higher the number of people who knew about the individual's epilepsy, the greater the risk of that individual becoming the target of prejudiced attitudes. It also raises the question of whether confidentiality had been maintained after their disclosure.

A number of conclusions can be drawn from this study. First, enacted stigma was not experienced as frequently as other research studies and anecdotal accounts in the media suggest. Second, felt stigma was commonly experienced by all of the interviewees, and seemed to precede rather than follow any specific incident of enacted stigma. In other words, people with epilepsy seemed to be 'primed' to feel this type of stigma from the beginning, and anticipated its exacerbation by actual events. Third, concealment of the condition was a frequently used strategy for overcoming the problem of felt stigma, and had a significant negative effect on the affected person's relationships at home and in the workplace. Finally, felt stigma appeared to be a consequence of the perceived shame linked to having epilepsy, reinforced by the reactions of family members and wider society, and, in the case of childhood-onset epilepsy, the negative attitudes of some parents to their child's seizures.

Let us consider a case example that may help to illustrate these points. John was 18 years old and had a history of childhood-onset epilepsy. His parents rarely spoke about his condition, and he did not even know that it was called epilepsy until he was in his early teens. At school he always felt different from others, but he did not know why. He had just started a relationship and decided not to tell his new girlfriend that he had epilepsy, due to fear that she would reject him and end the relationship. One evening they went to the cinema and he became confused, started smacking his lips, and his expression then became vacant. When he came round he did not know where he was and did not recognize his girlfriend, who panicked and ran out of the cinema. He phoned her the next day but she did not return his calls. When he subsequently met her parents in the street they walked past him without acknowledging him. John, through his concealment, appeared to have become the victim of enacted stigma. Yet one might ask whether he was in fact responsible for the reaction of his girlfriend, who as a result of his concealment had been placed in a situation for which she was completely unprepared. Also, he had simply assumed that their relationship would not survive the disclosure of his epilepsy, whereas if he had told her about his condition in advance, the outcome might have been very different. As it was, he became wary of future relationships and even more prone to concealment. John's coping strategy had created a situation that only served to exacerbate his felt stigma, and his girlfriend's response was not one of enacted stigma.

As mentioned earlier in this chapter, the findings of Joseph Schneider and Peter Conrad, described in their book *Having Epilepsy: the Experience and Control of Illness*,[362] were obtained from interviews with 80 people who had at some time in their life been given a diagnosis of epilepsy; 90 per cent of these individuals were still experiencing ongoing seizures. Their study population contained more women than men, was predominantly young, and was mostly drawn from middle-income groups. A third of the participants had attended college, and 8 per cent had university or professional qualifications. In an attempt to make their study sample more representative of the entire population of people with epilepsy, the researchers asked the participants to pass on a letter of introduction to friends with the condition. Although one would expect them to have become acquainted with other epilepsy patients at clinics, through charities or within support groups, and so form friendships, it was found that very few of them knew other people with the condition, and isolation was commonplace.

Schneider and Conrad focused on how the informing, translating, and shielding roles of parents influenced the strategies that their children would use for coping with their epilepsy in adolescence and adulthood. They found that parents were usually the first to give a name to their children's seizures, often using terminology such as 'funny turns' or 'feelings' to describe them. One female interviewee said that her parents refused to speak to her about her attacks, and as a result she had no knowledge or understanding of whether these were 'normal' experiences or not until she reached adulthood. Although many parents concealed the nature of the condition from their children, not all of them did so. One interviewee stated that her parents 'didn't beat around the bush, trying to make it really simple ... they said you have had a seizure and now you're fine'. Schneider and Conrad refer to these as 'closed' and 'open' parental approaches, respectively. The authors suggest that the closed approach may lead to disability and dependence, whereas the open approach would seem more likely to reduce felt stigma and have a positive influence on adjustment and coping.

Schneider and Conrad asked their study participants to describe what it was like to have a seizure. Many of the interviewees responded that they did not know because they had not

---

[362] Schneider JW and Conrad P (1983) *Having Epilepsy: the Experience and Control of Illness*. Temple University Press, Philadelphia, PA.

experienced their seizures in the same way that eye-witnesses had. They were able to describe the warning feelings and the recovery phase, but not the attack, of which they were completely unaware. The social consequences of and embarrassment caused by seizures, along with the involvement of emergency services, were cited by many of the interviewees. One participant described how witnesses seemed uncomfortable because 'they panic more than anything else like – I don't want to be around you … I don't know what to do'. The researchers then asked the interviewees to describe their feelings when they were first diagnosed with epilepsy. They found that in many cases, after a period of diagnostic uncertainty, finally finding out what was wrong brought a sense of relief and optimism that an effective treatment would be available. Many felt that simply being given the name 'epilepsy' helped them 'to get a handle on it'. Sometimes the terminology used by their physicians (for example, 'seizure disorder' rather than 'epilepsy') caused confusion. One respondent commented 'They never used the word epilepsy. They said I had a seizure disorder. They don't like using the word "epilepsy" to anyone.' By avoiding using the term 'epilepsy', the patient's own doctor can effectively become their patient's 'stigma coach', reinforcing their feelings of shame about their condition.

In drawing conclusions from their study, Schneider and Conrad highlighted the importance of 'owning epilepsy and realizing self' (what might today be called self-management). They stated that 'A brighter future for people with epilepsy depends on gaining ownership and control over their illness. This means first and foremost that they acknowledge their epilepsy as part of them and, having done so, deny it to others as grounds for devaluing definitions and treatment. This must be done by people with epilepsy for themselves without significant reliance on outsiders, especially professionals.' They emphasized that disclosure was the key to reducing felt stigma and thus minimizing enacted stigma, and they suggested that revealing the condition to others had therapeutic value. Finally, they commented that 'epilepsy, like sex and death, must be made speakable. … It is only then that we can begin to banish the ghosts that have for so long made it mysterious and threatening.'

The global problem

Much has been written about Western culture and the stigmatization of epilepsy. There are an estimated 50 million people worldwide with epilepsy, and in developing countries the incidence of epilepsy is higher than in the 'developed' world, due to inadequate antenatal and postnatal care, other effects of reduced healthcare delivery, and poor sanitation, which increases the risk of brain infections. Worldwide, nearly 80 per cent of people with epilepsy are living in low- or middle-income countries, and according to the World Health Organization (WHO), the Western Pacific Region has the highest global incidence and prevalence.[363] All cultures and religions share a long history of demonizing people with epilepsy. It has been difficult to address this by means of educational programmes in countries that have inadequate financial resources to fund such programmes, and where other public health issues are perceived as more urgent. In 2007 the Director General of the WHO estimated that 90 per cent of Africans with epilepsy were not receiving basic drug treatment, and pointed out that traditional beliefs had led to the perception that the condition was untreatable. The above-mentioned WHO report on epilepsy in the Western Pacific Region highlighted violations of the civil and human rights of people with epilepsy, for whom there was little or no legislative protection. Discrimination with regard to access to education was commonplace, as was lack of equal opportunities generally. A study of attitudes to epilepsy in Laos, conducted in 2007, indicated the size of the task of de-stigmatizing the condition.[364]

Laos is bordered by China, Burma, and Vietnam, and around 70 per cent of its population are Buddhists, while the remainder predominantly practise Satsana Phi, the Tai folk religion. Epilepsy was known locally as 'mad pig disease', and 20 per cent of those interviewed believed that it could be transmitted by eating pork. Two-thirds of the interviewees stated that they avoided contact or sharing meals with people with epilepsy. Around 40 per cent expressed the view that people with epilepsy should not marry, have children, or be employed, and a similar proportion believed that epilepsy was a supernatural condition. Surprisingly, about 50 per cent of those with epilepsy who were interviewed expressed the same views. A study conducted by the same authors in Benin (formerly Dahomey), the French-speaking West African nation that was the birthplace of 'voodoo',[365] found that 70 per cent of the interviewees with epilepsy felt stigmatized and socially isolated, had marital problems, or suffered from anxiety. Many other studies have revealed similarly high levels of stigma in developing countries around the world.

In 1997 the WHO launched its *Global Campaign Against Epilepsy: Out of the Shadows*, the stated aim of which was 'to improve acceptability, treatment, services and prevention of epilepsy worldwide'.[366] The campaign involved a collaborative study by the WHO, the International League Against Epilepsy (ILAE), and the International Bureau for Epilepsy (IBE). They conducted a survey of 160 countries in order to evaluate the resources available

---

363 World Health Organization (2004) *Epilepsy in the Western Pacific Region: A Call to Action: Global Campaign Against Epilepsy*. WHO Regional Office for the Western Pacific, Manila.
364 Tran D-S, Odermatt P, Singphuoangphet S et al. (2007) Epilepsy in Laos: knowledge, attitudes, and practices in the community. *Epilepsy & Behavior* 10, 565–570.
365 Rafael F, Houinato D, Nubukpo P et al. (2010) Sociocultural and psychological features of perceived stigma reported by people with epilepsy in Benin. *Epilepsia* 51, 1061–1068.
366 www.who.int/mental_health/management/en/GcaeBroEn.pdf?ua=1

for and attitudes toward people with epilepsy. They looked not only at diagnostic facilities, such as the availability of scanning and brainwave recording (EEG), but also access to drugs, drug monitoring, and psychology services. In addition, the questionnaire covered health insurance, disability benefits, and the problems encountered by people with epilepsy, such as discrimination. The results were published in an atlas of epilepsy care,[367] which predictably showed that, globally, such care was inadequate to meet patients' needs, with low-income countries faring the worst. Benefits entitlement was available in 50 per cent of the countries surveyed, ranging from 84 per cent of high-income countries to only 15 per cent of low-income countries.[368] Although 75 per cent of healthcare professionals who were surveyed felt that social support was adequate, only 25 per cent of patients with epilepsy held this view. When asked what they perceived to be their biggest problem, 80 per cent of people who experienced seizures cited the social burden of their condition, whereas healthcare professionals cited drug availability as their major difficulty. Patients and healthcare providers alike agreed that community knowledge of epilepsy and the existence of stigma were major issues. The 'wish list' of healthcare professionals, which consisted of more effective drugs, improved diagnostics, larger numbers of healthcare staff, and improved access to epilepsy surgery, contrasted with that of their patients, who were more concerned about addressing the social effects of epilepsy. This discrepancy in priorities between providers and recipients of healthcare highlights the risks involved in not consulting the latter group when developing so-called 'patient-centred' services. Finally, although both groups agreed that there was a lack of educational provision, somewhat surprisingly they gave it a low priority.

Overall, this WHO-led survey identified a significant lack of funding, especially in low-income economies, as well as reduced opportunities for people with epilepsy, and the continuing problem of stigma. It did not offer specific solutions, but concluded by stating that 'It is hoped that the availability of essential information will lead to greater awareness among policy-makers of the gaps in resources for epilepsy care.'

Reducing stigma

In 2010, Hanneke de Boer from the Epilepsy Institute of the Netherlands, and one of the authors of the above-mentioned survey, published an update on the global situation.[369] Although she outlined the definitions and history of stigma, she made no reference to possible

---

367 World Health Organization (2005) *Atlas of Epilepsy Care in the World 2005*. World Health Organization, Geneva.
368 Dua T, De Boer HM, Prilipko LL et al. (2005) Epilepsy care in the world: results of an ILAE/IBE/WHO Global Campaign against Epilepsy Survey. *Epilepsia* 47, 1225–1231.
369 De Boer HM (2010) Epilepsy stigma: moving from a global problem to global solutions. *Seizure* 19, 630–636.

solutions other than stating that 'if all parties and individuals working in the field of epilepsy worldwide, or having a personal interest in the disease, or having epilepsy, join forces to deal with the challenges, turning them into actions, we should then be able to bring about global solutions.' She concluded, with very guarded optimism in terms of the timescale quoted, 'I am convinced that through continuing to take action over the next 60 years, the situation with regard to epilepsy stigma will look very different by 2070.'

In 2012 in the USA, the Institute of Medicine (IOM) published a lengthy report entitled *Epilepsy Across the Spectrum: Promoting Health and Understanding*. One of the key messages stated in its preface was that 'the stigma associated with epilepsy has to be eliminated.'[370] In 2014 a paper by several members of the IOM reviewed public awareness and knowledge, concluding that 'the public is generally lacking in basic knowledge about seizures and epilepsy.' The authors recommended a public education programme designed to inform the media and engage the public, acknowledging that epilepsy care received less funding than any other long-term neurological condition.[371] The stated goal of such a programme was to increase knowledge and foster positive attitudes among members of the public towards people with epilepsy. In order to achieve this objective, the authors identified eight key messages of which the public should be aware, which can be summarized as follows:

1. Epilepsy is common and includes all ages and ethnicities.
2. It represents a spectrum of conditions of varying severity.
3. It can occasionally be life-threatening, have an impact upon quality of life, and carry the risk of personal injury.
4. Nearly two out of three people with epilepsy are controlled with either no seizures or a significantly reduced number of seizures while on medication.
5. There are specialized epilepsy centres that offer diagnosis, new treatments, support, and occasionally surgery to people with epilepsy.
6. Basic first aid that can be administered by anyone is important to the well-being of people who are experiencing or recovering from a seizure.
7. Many people with epilepsy are fully functioning members of society, raising families, and in employment.
8. Finally, and importantly, 'the stigma associated with epilepsy can cause serious harm to the physical, mental and social well-being of a person with epilepsy'.

---

370 Institute of Medicine (US) Committee on the Public Health Dimensions of the Epilepsies (2012) *Epilepsy across the Spectrum: Promoting Health and Understanding*. National Academies Press, Washington, DC.
371 England MJ, Austin JK, Beck V et al. (2014) Erasing epilepsy stigma: eight key messages. *Health Promotion Practice* 15, 313–318.

The IOM intended these key messages to be relayed to the public by the media, which they suggested could promote epilepsy research and human-interest stories through news outlets and advocate the use of social media and the Internet to disseminate accurate information. However, this would require some mandatory mechanism to ensure balance, accuracy, and lack of stigmatization in media representations of epilepsy. Moreover, the IOM recommendations on coordinating public awareness are not specific, so it is difficult to envisage them being acted upon. The authors of the IOM report nevertheless believe that it provides a roadmap for future action aimed at eradicating stigma. Only time will tell if this is the case.

In devising solutions to stigmatization, we need to be able to accurately measure changes in the level of the problem. Interventions can be targeted at two groups, namely the stigmatizing general public, and the people with epilepsy who experience or observe stigmatization. Although it may be possible to reduce the emotional and psychological impact of stigmatization on the latter group through support groups and counselling, the prevention of harm occurring in the first place is preferable to minimizing its impact. Therefore the general public must be the main if not sole focus of interventions. The main tools available for this are education and social marketing. Education may be effective but needs to be regularly repeated to target audiences if it is to have a sustained effect. Social marketing, which is increasingly being used for health promotion, utilizes marketing strategies along with other approaches to influence behaviours for the greater social good. The message that it should carry with regard to people with epilepsy must emphasize that they are no different to anyone else, even though there are some situations in which they need to be treated differently. Social marketing has the potential to monitor and challenge inaccuracies in the media, educate specific groups, and increase public awareness of and contact with people with epilepsy, although its effectiveness in eradicating stigma has yet to be proven. Potentially one of the most effective tools for reducing stigma is the 'coming out' of famous people and media 'celebrities' with epilepsy who are open about their condition and champion the cause of those who suffer from it, although sadly this occurs only rarely at present.

With regard to ways of assessing the effectiveness of any programme designed to reduce stigma, various scales and questionnaires have been suggested for measuring the presence and level of stigma. However, it should be borne in mind that respondents will tend to give responses that reflect what they perceive to be the desired or most appropriate answer, rather than what they actually feel. For people with epilepsy, factors such as employment, relationships, social networks, and quality of life should be measured against the same outcomes as those for the general public, and only when the results obtained are the same for both groups can stigma be said to have been eradicated.

Employment

It is well documented that there are consistently higher levels of unemployment among people with epilepsy, and that those with the condition who are employed are more likely to have unskilled manual jobs, or occupations for which they are overqualified in terms of their education and skills. The unemployment rate among people with epilepsy is approximately double that of the general population. To some extent this can be related to factors such as seizure frequency and severity, related learning difficulties, the side effects of drug treatment, and the safety requirements of certain occupations, but the prejudiced attitudes of employers and work colleagues may well also be implicated. In 1950 a letter published in the *British Medical Journal* described the plight of people with epilepsy, referring to the 'need for training and work in specialized factories, living either in their homes or hostels with facilities for transport', and commenting that 'epileptics are unwanted in our midst, living wretchedly unhappy lives'.[372] The view that only 'specialized factories' would provide an appropriate work environment harked back to the epilepsy colonies of the late nineteenth century, and suggested that the views of potential employers of people with epilepsy had changed little since that time.

In the late 1950s, the Research Committee of the Royal College of General Practitioners (RCGP) in the UK conducted a survey to assess the employment status of people living independently with epilepsy. Contrary to expectations, nearly 700 (74 per cent) of the 940 people questioned were found to be in full-time work, and were described as 'men and women who did normal work and to whom epilepsy was no handicap as far as employability was concerned'.[373] These positive findings have not been replicated, and the survey failed to address either the general level of unemployment or the type of work offered to people with epilepsy. In 1965, Graham Jones, a senior medical officer for a major iron, steel, and tinplate producer based in Wales, published an article in the *Lancet* in which he expressed scepticism about the findings of the RCGP's Research Committee, and suggested that many people with epilepsy did experience employment problems and were embarrassed by their condition.[374] He outlined his 12-year experience of providing healthcare for 39 employees and job candidates with epilepsy in an integrated steelworks with a workforce of 1400 people. He described how three employees were dismissed because of their epilepsy, and three potential employees were not taken on by the company because they had admitted to having epilepsy during a pre-employment medical examination. He noted that many individuals had concealed

---

372 Swanston CN (1950) Employment of epileptics. *British Medical Journal* 2, 1170.
373 Crombie DL, Cross KW, Fry RJ et al. (1960) A survey of the epilepsies in general practice: a report by the Research Committee of the Royal College of General Practitioners. *British Medical Journal* 2, 416–422.
374 Jones JG (1965) Employment of epileptics. *Lancet* 2, 486–489.

their epilepsy because 'it was well known locally that many organizations would not employ anyone admitting to a history of epilepsy and would dismiss any employee unfortunate enough to have his condition disclosed'. He commented that those with epilepsy who were employed were generally working in a restricted capacity in menial, uninteresting, and poorly paid occupations. Summarizing his audit, Jones stated that whereas 15 of his 39 subjects had apparently experienced no problems in gaining satisfactory employment, the other 24 individuals had been dismissed, refused employment, or forced to give up their normal work and accept a more menial and less well paid job within the steelworks. This study was far more detailed than many others of its time, and it also differed from them in its finding that two-thirds of workers with epilepsy had employment problems. Some of the contemporaneous studies went so far as to suggest that any problems with employment could be attributed to the individuals themselves, rather than to the employers or the occupation concerned. One such study quoted from unpublished data that 'the frequency of attacks bore no relation to poor work record, but personality and intelligence were the most important factors'.[375] In 1971 the Office of Health Economics in the UK published its report, *Epilepsy and Society*, which confirmed Graham Jones' assertion that up to two-thirds of people with epilepsy had experienced employment problems, which included working in mundane and low-paid jobs for which they were overqualified in terms of their education and vocational training.[376]

In 1985 the pharmaceutical company Labaz organized a conference on epilepsy and employment and identified three specific issues that appeared to restrict access to work, namely the genuine hazard to the individual and their work colleagues in the event of a seizure (for example, working at height), the perceived hazard (for example, the erroneous belief that time would be taken off work and therefore the individual would be less productive than their co-workers), and the anxiety and prejudiced attitudes of employers and co-workers. In fact, two decades earlier, in the 1960s, evidence had been obtained that refuted this, showing low accident and sickness rates among people with epilepsy.[377] However, as it was published in a specialist journal it escaped the attention of prospective employers. An editorial published in the *British Medical Journal* that covered the above-mentioned conference on epilepsy and employment noted that nearly 50 per cent of job applicants did not mention their epilepsy when applying for posts.[378] The recommendations that emerged from the conference were that future appointment processes should follow the UK Civil Service model, consisting of an application form and a medical declaration, with the latter not being viewed until the

---

375 Dominian J, Serafetinides EA and Dewhurst M (1963) A follow-up study of late-onset epilepsy. II. Psychiatric and social findings. *British Medical Journal* 1, 431–435.
376 Office of Health Economics (1971) *Epilepsy and Society*. Office of Health Economics, London.
377 Udel MM (1960) The work performance of epileptics in industry. *Archives of Environmental Health* 1, 257–264.
378 Gloag D (1985) Epilepsy and employment. *British Medical Journal* 291, 2–3.

candidate's merits had been assessed and an appointment made. The candidate could then be rejected only after a full medical assessment that took into account any genuine physical hazards that the job might entail. This process would prevent any prejudiced attitudes of the employer from influencing the appointment process, thus enabling the final decision to be based on the candidate's ability, not their disability.

In 1978 the findings of an American study that examined the attitudes of major companies in the San Francisco Bay Area over a 20-year period were published.[379] The authors sent out questionnaires in 1956 and 1966, and repeated the exercise again in the 1970s. Their results showed that over a 20-year period the number of companies that had employed an individual in the knowledge that he or she had epilepsy had risen from 7 per cent to 43 per cent, dismissal rates had decreased from 14 per cent to 0 per cent, and the number of posts that employers considered suitable for people with epilepsy had risen. Although this study seems to suggest that attitudes had improved, only 40 per cent of those who were sent a questionnaire responded, and the underlying concerns expressed about safety at work remained unaltered. The authors of the study concluded that they were 'encouraged' by the 'magnitude of positive change in attitude'. This was not borne out by subsequent studies. Moreover, the fact that 60 per cent of those who were sent the questionnaire did not respond to it raises questions about the validity of the study, as people with a positive attitude are more likely to respond. To date most reports have indicated that potential employers remain concerned about the reliability of people with epilepsy, their own safety and that of others in the workplace, and the potentially disruptive reaction of work colleagues to their condition.

In 1967 an editorial published in the *Canadian Occupational Health Bulletin* had identified 'lack of knowledge about the nature of epilepsy and the effect of recent medical advances' and fear of the condition as the main causes of low employability among people with epilepsy.[380] Thirty-five years later, according to the Epilepsy Foundation of America, little had changed.[381] Unemployment rates remained virtually unchanged despite decades of effort by both government and voluntary organizations such as their own foundation. They pointed out that 85 per cent of the annual cost referred to as the 'burden of epilepsy' could be accounted for by lost wages and reduced incomes. They added that the major reasons for employment problems were 'barriers of attitude and fear. It's just easier to hire someone who doesn't have a condition like epilepsy. People have concerns about the nature of the condition and its potential effect on job performance.' To counter this they launched

---

379 Hicks RA and Hicks MJ (1978) The attitude of major companies toward the employment of epileptics: an assessment of two decades of change. *American Corrective Therapy Journal* 32, 180–182.
380 Anon. (1967) Editorial: The employable epileptic. *Canadian Occupational Health Bulletin* 22, 11–12.
381 Epilepsy Foundation of America (2001) Employment of people with epilepsy: the hardest nut. *Epilepsy & Behavior* 2, 379–380.

an employment initiative called JobTech, and concluded that without employer education 'there's a substantial risk that 20 years from now very little in the employment situation of people with epilepsy will have changed'.

Their predictions seem to have been borne out. Over the last 20 years, surveys of large numbers of businesses in the UK and North America have consistently shown that less than 50 per cent of them had employed someone in the knowledge that they had epilepsy, and only 60 per cent believed that they could offer jobs that were suitable for people with epilepsy. In 2005 a study of 560 randomly selected businesses was published by Ann Jacoby and her colleagues from the Department of Public Health at the University of Liverpool, in association with the UK's Office for National Statistics and the charity Epilepsy Action.[382] Only 40 per cent of businesses that were contacted replied (presumably those that would be more likely to be sympathetic), of which around 50 per cent employed less than 20 staff. Companies admitted that around 50 per cent of their job application forms specifically inquired about health and disability issues, and that this information was generally viewed before short-listing and interviews. Around 75 per cent of employers believed that they should be informed of any history of epilepsy, even if the individual had been seizure-free for two years. Moreover, concerns about safety, insurance liability, days lost from work, and even the possible impact on business prevailed, along with more deep-seated concerns about personality, reliability, and efficiency. Consistent with these findings, only 2 per cent of employers believed that a person with epilepsy would not experience any difficulties in the employment market, whereas around 50 per cent predicted that they would encounter major problems. Employers were then asked whether, in accordance with the Disability Discrimination Act regulations (see page 243), they could make sufficient workplace adjustments to enable them to accommodate a person with epilepsy on their payroll. Around 75 per cent of employers responded that they would provide sickness cover and flexible working hours, but only 25 per cent would allow home working or provide transport to and from work. In total, 62 per cent of employers remained concerned about safety issues, and a small number were apprehensive about damage to expensive equipment or the effect on their customers of witnessing a seizure. The authors concluded that attitudes remain entrenched and that 'the need to educate employers is self-evident', but that education alone was not sufficient and that 'programmes that bring employers actively into contact with people with epilepsy are likely to have more impact than educational initiatives undertaken in the abstract'. However, they did not specify how they proposed to implement such programmes.

---

[382] Jacoby A, Gorry J and Baker GA (2005) Employers' attitudes to employment of people with epilepsy: still the same old story? *Epilepsia* 46, 1978–1987.

Realistically one might expect the business world to be more likely to respond to changes in legislation and legal accountability than to epilepsy awareness training. The main problem with short-lived education programmes for employers is their lack of sustainability. Public health messages, unless they are constantly reiterated, soon become swamped by a deluge of new information. In addition, human resources and other management staff move on to other posts and are replaced by individuals who have not undertaken the programme. Although surveys may suggest that there is some positive attitudinal change over time, the reality is that there has been no change in the levels of employability of people with epilepsy since these data were first recorded. As has already been suggested, probably the most beneficial development would be for more people in the public eye to step forward and admit to having epilepsy, thereby demonstrating to the wider public that those with epilepsy can be both successful and safe in the workplace.

Education

The majority of people who develop epilepsy do so in their formative years. The way in which children are viewed and treated by their childcarers, teachers, and peers at nursery and primary school will have a profound effect on their self-image and interpersonal skills. An unsupportive environment at this stage can cause long-term and possibly irreparable harm. It is well known that children with epilepsy are at increased risk of underachievement, mental health problems, isolation, and low self-esteem.[383] The knowledge and attitudes of childcarers and teachers will have a major influence not only on school performance and social skills, but also on post-school outcomes in areas such as higher education, employment, and the establishing of relationships. For a child with epilepsy to reach their full potential, both their interaction with their peer group and that group's understanding of the nature of their condition play a vital role. It is also important that the parents avoid becoming their child's 'stigma coach', and another influential factor relates to the attitudes of other parents to the social integration and acceptance of the child with epilepsy. The parents of other children may exclude him or her (for example, from sleepovers or birthday parties) on the basis of perceived risk or prejudiced attitudes, and this will result in the child experiencing feelings of alienation and 'being different'.

In the UK, the Equality Act 2010 states that it is unlawful for education providers to discriminate against students with epilepsy. Similar legislation exists in the USA, Australia,

---

383 Fastenau PS, Shen J, Dunn DW et al. (2008) Academic underachievement among children with epilepsy: proportion exceeding psychometric criteria for learning disability and associated risk factors. *Journal of Learning Disabilities* 41, 195–207.

and many other countries. The law applies to students of all ages, from those in nurseries and playgroups to those in higher or continuing education, including mature students. Education services therefore have a clear responsibility to ensure that teachers have an adequate knowledge of childhood epilepsy, provide the correct support, and communicate constructively with parents and healthcare professionals. There are many online aids that educators can consult when they encounter epilepsy directly in their workplace. However, their baseline level of knowledge is a critically important factor, and we shall now briefly consider a number of studies that have evaluated it.

In the early 1970s, before online information was available, a survey conducted in the UK revealed that teachers had limited knowledge of epilepsy and little or no classroom support or advice from school medical services.[384] Early studies also showed that, because of stigma and the fear of disclosure of their child's condition to the whole school, parents often chose not to inform the headteacher of their child's condition. Therefore the teaching staff would usually be unaware of the situation until a seizure occurred in the classroom. Parents also tended to conceal their child's epilepsy because they believed that any learning difficulties would be incorrectly ascribed to the condition, and then viewed by the teacher as not worth addressing because they could not be corrected.

In the early 1990s a comprehensive questionnaire survey of teachers' perceptions was conducted in the UK.[385] At that time teachers were using *Epilepsy: A Teacher's Handbook*[386] as a general reference text, and could also consult a school medical officer for specific guidance. The authors of the survey asked 142 teachers in mainstream schools about their knowledge and experience of epilepsy, and their confidence about managing it in the classroom. Most of the respondents did not feel confident about teaching children with epilepsy, and only a minority believed that their knowledge of the condition was adequate. Just four teachers had recently received any specific instructions about childhood epilepsy. However, none of the teachers agreed with the statement that 'Children with epilepsy are subnormal', although 15 per cent thought that these children were more likely to have learning difficulties. Only around 50 per cent of the respondents considered that gymnastics was a suitable activity for children with epilepsy, and two-thirds believed that teaching would not be an appropriate future career for such children. In summary, although a significant number of teachers did not regard epilepsy as an obstacle to academic success, most of them felt that they needed training and support to help them to manage epilepsy in the classroom.

---

384 Holdsworth L and Whitmore K (1974) A study of children with epilepsy attending normal schools. II. Information and attitudes held by their teachers. *Developmental Medicine & Child Neurology* 16, 759–765.
385 Bannon MJ, Wildig C and Jones PW (1992) Teachers' perceptions of epilepsy. *Archives of Disease in Childhood* 67, 1461–1471.
386 Rogan PJ (1986) *Epilepsy: A Teacher's Handbook*. Roby Educational, Liverpool.

A subsequent nationwide survey conducted in the USA and published in 2006 explored concerns that teachers' negative attitudes would affect children's academic and psychosocial development. The authors sought the opinions of elementary and middle school teachers from 11 states,[387] using a questionnaire that included the Scale of Attitudes Toward Persons with Epilepsy (ATPE). Developed by experts in epilepsy without the involvement of people with the condition, this tool contains 17 questions about knowledge and attitudes. Only 25 per cent of the 2000 teachers who were approached responded to the survey, and of these less than 7 per cent felt that they were knowledgeable about the subject. It was noteworthy that only 3 per cent of the respondents had visited an epilepsy website, despite the proliferation of online advice available. The authors concluded that 'further teacher attitude research and ongoing development and implementation of epilepsy education programmes are necessary'.

Many subsequent studies have been conducted in countries around the world, including Saudi Arabia, Thailand, Zimbabwe, South Korea, and Nigeria, among others. An ambitious study from Italy randomly selected schools in each of the country's administrative districts. A total of 582 teachers (the majority of whom were women) from 150 schools, all of whom were working with first- and second-year primary school children, were asked to complete a 28-item questionnaire. The questions covered their knowledge of epilepsy and its personal, social, and academic implications.[388] The results of the study were made available to the Italian League Against Epilepsy (LICE), resulting in their campaign 'Shed light on epilepsy at school'. The study showed that the teachers generally appeared to be well informed about epilepsy, with around 50 per cent at some time in their career having had a child with the condition in their classroom, and 25 per cent having personal experience and knowledge through a relative or friend with epilepsy. Around 60 per cent of the respondents believed that epilepsy impaired the learning process, and 50 per cent considered that mental and behavioural problems were common and that special educational support was necessary. The teachers regarded many recreational activities (for example, boxing, swimming, cycling, skiing, and even soccer) as unsuitable for children with epilepsy. More positively, only 2 per cent of the respondents believed that children with epilepsy under their care had been discriminated against by their classmates. Compared with a sample from the general population of Italy, teachers were much better informed about the condition. Only 5 per cent of them regarded it as a mental disease, compared with 36 per cent of the general public, and only 4 per cent considered it a bar to marriage, compared with 20 per cent of the general population. Although overall this study showed an improved understanding of the

---

387 Bishop M and Boag EM (2006) Teachers' knowledge about epilepsy and attitudes towards students with epilepsy: results of a national survey. *Epilepsy & Behavior* 8, 397–405.
388 Mecarelli O, Messina P, Capovilla G et al. (2014) An educational campaign toward epilepsy among Italian primary school teachers: 1. Survey on knowledge and attitudes. *Epilepsy & Behavior* 32, 84–91.

condition compared with a similar survey conducted in Italy by the same researchers around 3 years earlier, significant areas of ignorance remained. The earlier study included secondary school teachers, whose level of knowledge about epilepsy was not much better than that of the general population.[389] Thus primary school teachers appear to be better informed than secondary school teachers in Italy, so there is potential for much of the good work done by teachers at primary school to be undone when children with epilepsy move on to secondary school.

With regard to parts of the world where epilepsy remains more stigmatized, a study from Jeddah in Saudi Arabia, published in 2014, found that up to 27 per cent of primary school teachers believed that epilepsy could be caused by spirit possession or the 'evil eye', and only 17 per cent considered themselves well informed about the condition. Around 25 per cent believed that epilepsy is incurable, and around one-third thought that children with epilepsy should be managed in a special classroom or special school. The negative attitudes expressed by the teachers correlated closely with their levels of knowledge. The authors recommended that educational campaigns should be undertaken in order to develop a well-informed and tolerant teaching community. They also highlighted the need for the educational resources of epilepsy charities to be made accessible to all teachers.[390] Similar findings have been reported in many other studies from Asia and Africa.

In 2018 the findings of a systematic review conducted in the UK were published.[391] Based at Great Ormond Street Hospital and in the research department of the charity Young Epilepsy, the researchers searched medical databases for articles published between 2000 and 2017, using the keywords 'teachers', 'knowledge', 'attitudes', 'epilepsy', and 'perceptions'. They identified a total of 54 studies involving 17,256 participants from 27 different countries. It was not possible for them to accurately measure the levels of knowledge reported and the nature of the attitudes expressed, as most of the questionnaires were unique to the studies in which they were used. Consequently, no meaningful quantitative analysis of this vast amount of information could be undertaken, highlighting the need for researchers to use the same standardized questionnaires in future studies. Qualitatively, however, all of the studies showed an overall lack of knowledge and a significantly high prevalence of negative attitudes, especially with regard to the sporting activities that teachers believed were safe for children with epilepsy, and the emergency measures required when children experienced seizures while

---

[389] Mecarelli O, Capovilla G, Romeo A et al. (2011) Knowledge and attitudes toward epilepsy among primary and secondary schoolteachers in Italy. *Epilepsy & Behavior* 22, 285–292.

[390] Abulhamail AS, Al-Sulami FE, Alnouri MA et al. (2014) Primary school teachers' knowledge and attitudes toward children with epilepsy. *Seizure* 23, 280–283.

[391] Jones C, Atkinson P, Helen Cross J et al. (2018) Knowledge of and attitudes towards epilepsy among teachers: a systematic review. *Epilepsy & Behavior* 87, 59–68.

at school. Compared with other conditions, such as asthma, attention deficit hyperactivity disorder, and diabetes, epilepsy was the condition with which teachers were least familiar. Those studies that evaluated attitudes before and after educational and training interventions showed that improvements had been achieved. The authors concluded that 'better-quality research employing a more robust study design is needed to develop understanding of what negative attitudes exist and what are the most effective methods of improving both attitudes and knowledge.'

It would seem that, despite the global importance of teachers' knowledge of and attitudes toward epilepsy, researchers have generally made relatively little progress in this field over the last 50 years.

Epilepsy and sports participation

Restrictions have often been placed on children and adults with epilepsy who wish to participate in sports. In the 1970s, physical exercise was generally discouraged, and application forms for sports club membership usually contained a health declaration section that included any history of epilepsy. In fact, some studies have suggested that exercise may reduce seizure frequency and severity, and this is consistent with anecdotal evidence from many people with epilepsy.[392] Moreover, some electroencephalogram studies have found that moderate exercise can actually increase the seizure threshold.

A number of myths about sport and epilepsy need to be addressed. There is no evidence that minor head injuries can worsen the condition, so it should not be necessary to ban people with epilepsy from participating in contact sports such as rugby. Nor is there any evidence that exhaustive exercise, such as marathon running, is likely to provoke seizures. The consequences of extreme physical activity, namely dehydration, low blood sugar levels, and high body temperature, can all cause seizures, but these are just as likely to occur in a person who does not have epilepsy.

Although sporting activities should be encouraged in order to normalize life and maintain general health, there are obvious common-sense limitations to the types of extreme recreation in which people with epilepsy can safely participate. Any sport in which sudden loss of consciousness could prove fatal, such as motor sports, sky diving, or scuba diving, would clearly be unsuitable, as would sports in which there is a risk of severe repetitive head injury, such as boxing. Participation in sports such as swimming would depend on the frequency and nature of the seizures, and vigilant supervision of the activity. The International League

---

[392] Pimentel J, Tojal R and Morgado J (2015) Epilepsy and physical exercise. *Seizure* 25, 87–94.

Against Epilepsy (ILEA) has produced guidelines that categorize sports according to the level of risk involved[393] (see Table 5). However, the main message is that children and adults should not be excluded from sporting activities. and that the ILEA guidance needs to be disseminated to decision makers in schools and sports centres.

All teachers who are responsible for children with epilepsy have a professional duty to keep their knowledge about the condition up to date, by accessing the relevant educational material that is available online, much of which is provided by epilepsy charities, such as the Edmonton Epilepsy Association's *A Guide for Teachers: Epilepsy*.[394] Educational programmes have a vital role, but perhaps the most important factors are the professionalism of the teacher, the availability of easy access to educational materials when these are required, and good communication between the child's teacher and the parent(s).

Finally, there has been little research to date on the attitude of other pupils to their peers with epilepsy, and the teaching of disability issues. This would be a productive area of study and debate, as teaching young people about disability and conditions such as epilepsy may well reduce stigmatizing and discriminatory attitudes later in life.

Law enforcement and prison services

Like anyone else, many people with epilepsy will at some time engage with the law as a perceived victim, or as someone either accused or convicted of a crime. The attitudes of professionals at every level of the justice system – whether they are police officers, members of the legal profession, or those responsible for the welfare of prisoners – will influence the way in which individuals with epilepsy are treated. Therefore their knowledge of and attitudes to the condition are of fundamental importance. As was discussed in Chapter 11, the erroneous belief that people with epilepsy are inherently more likely to display aggressive behaviour than individuals without the condition persists, and has historically been perpetuated by the literature.

A relatively recent Canadian study investigated how attitudes toward epilepsy and violence had changed over a 25-year period.[395] It examined whether people with epilepsy were believed to be commonly and persistently aggressive both during and between seizures. The questionnaire, which was sent out in 1981 and again in 2006, included scenarios involving

---

393 Capovilla G, Kaufman KR, Perucca E et al. (2016) Epilepsy, seizures, physical exercise, and sports: a report from the ILEA Task Force on Sports and Epilepsy. *Epilepsia* 57, 6–12.
394 www.edmontonepilepsy.org/documents/Epilepsy%20-%20A%20Guide%20For%20Teachers.pdf
395 Collins TBK, Camfield PR, Camfield CS et al. (2007) People with epilepsy are often perceived as violent. *Epilepsy & Behavior* 10, 69–76.

and questions about epilepsy and violence. The respondents included law and medical students, care workers, people with epilepsy, and members of the general public (of whom around 50 per cent knew a person with epilepsy). Both in 1981 and in 2006 more than 50 per cent of the respondents believed that people could behave violently during a seizure, and nearly 40 per cent of all the groups surveyed gave incorrect answers to basic questions. Worryingly, law students scored lower than the general public. The results indicated that fear of violence perpetrated by people with epilepsy was prevalent, that it was contributing to the persistent stigma, and that this incorrect perception had remained unchanged over a 25-year period.

The view that people with epilepsy are more likely to end up in prison is a contentious one. In a study conducted in Scotland, 2.1 per cent of prisoners were recorded as having epilepsy, which is almost double the rate that would be expected after adjustment for the age and gender profiles of the prison population (1.2 per cent), and substantially higher than the rate for the general population (0.5–0.7 per cent).[396] Irrespective of the debate on prevalence in the prison population, some people with epilepsy will need to be cared for in prison at some point, so the training and knowledge of the prison officers will have a major influence on the experiences of those individuals while they are incarcerated. On 6 July 2009, the *Telegraph* newspaper reported the death of a 25-year-old man in HMP Belmarsh, a high-security prison in south-east London. At the Coroner's Court enquiry it was heard that he had experienced a series of epileptic seizures in the early hours of the morning, and had become confused and struggled with his guards. He was restrained, had two further seizures while held down on the floor, and subsequently died of suffocation.[397] Such tragic incidents continue to occur. For example, an account of the death of a prisoner with epilepsy in 2013 describes how 'The man suffered from epilepsy and mental health problems. He was prescribed anti-epileptic and antipsychotic drugs but often did not take them as prescribed. He suffered a number of epileptic seizures but sometimes refused to be taken to hospital. Healthcare staff made numerous references to his non-compliance with his medication in his clinical record but his prescriptions were allowed to expire with no indication of what should happen next. He was not prescribed any anti-epileptic medication for two months over the New Year.'[398] The report suggested that there should be regular medication reviews and prompt referral for hospital reviews in such circumstances. The fact that this prisoner

---

396 Graham L (2007) *Prison Health in Scotland: A Healthcare Needs Assessment.* Scottish Prison Service, Edinburgh.
397 www.telegraph.co.uk/news/uknews/law-and-order/5761839/Epileptic-prisoner-died-after-being-held-down-by-guards.html
398 Newcomen N (2013) *A Report by the Prisons and Probation Ombudsman Nigel Newcomen CBE: Investigation into the Death of a Man at HMP Stocken in March 2013.* www.ppo.gov.uk/app/uploads/2016/02/H201-13-Death-of-a-male-prisoner-Stocken-17.3.2013-NAT-31-40.pdf

received no treatment for his epilepsy over a two-month period would appear to reflect underlying prejudice and stigmatizing attitudes.

Prison officers' knowledge of and attitudes toward epilepsy have not been well studied. However, an audit of the healthcare of prisoners with the condition, conducted in the UK in 2008, reported that the term 'epileptic' was routinely used, that prisoners with epilepsy had unnecessary restrictions placed on their activities, and that when sharing a cell they were always allocated the bottom bunk, even if their seizures were well controlled with medication. Epilepsy was identified in 26 of a total of 641 inmates (4 per cent). Around 75 per cent of those with epilepsy had poor seizure control, and 50 per cent of these had not had a medical review during the previous year.[399] These observations alone suggest that the prison officers' baseline knowledge of epilepsy was low and that training was minimal, despite the fact that 4 per cent of the prisoners under their care had the condition. The Mersey Region Epilepsy Association has produced a guide entitled *Epilepsy in Prison: A Guide for Prison Staff*,[400] which concludes that it will have 'achieved its purpose if it has persuaded prison staff that epilepsy is not the fearsome affliction it is sometimes thought to be'. If we cannot gauge prison officers' views and attitudes directly, the next best thing is to find out what training they might receive to help to improve their level of knowledge and care. Given the relatively high proportion of prisoners with epilepsy, one might expect such training to be mandatory. The Freedom of Information (FOI) Act 2000 allows the reasonable questioning of public bodies. The HMP service is covered by this act, so the UK Ministry of Justice was asked whether prison officers receive epilepsy awareness training (either face to face or online), whether such training (if provided) is mandatory for all and repeated at regular intervals, and if not, whether there are any plans to introduce mandatory training at a future date, and finally whether written guidelines are available for prison officers. In July 2019, Sarah Lock from the Ministry's Learning and Development Unit responded that the foundation training programme for all new officers has one day set aside for emergency first aid, which includes epilepsy. The emergency first-aid component is valid for three years, after which re-validation is required at the discretion of each prison governor. She also mentioned that prison officers have access to Civil Service Learning (CSL), and that epilepsy is covered in the courses on 'Disability Awareness' and 'First Aid at Work', although enrolment is up to the individual and not mandatory. Finally, she stated that 'all establishments are fully equipped to support epileptic prisoners' and that 'any prisoner who discloses that they are epileptic' will be appropriately managed by healthcare professionals working alongside the prison officers to ensure that 'any

---

399 Tittensor P, Collins J, Grünewald RA et al. (2008) Audit of healthcare provision for UK prisoners with suspected epilepsy. *Seizure* 17, 69–75.
400 www.epilepsymersey.org.uk/docs/prison.pdf

reasonable adjustments are made'.[401] It is noteworthy how minimal this epilepsy awareness training is, and that the decision to enhance it is a matter of personal choice. Furthermore, the onus to 'disclose' the condition lies with the prisoners themselves, which suggests that the prison service does not actively seek medical information about those prisoners for whose welfare it is responsible during their incarceration. Clearly there is room for improvement. The use of the term 'epileptic' in the Ministry's communication is unfortunate, but sadly predictable based on the findings of the UK audit mentioned earlier.

Police officers' perceptions of people with epilepsy, and the availability of epilepsy awareness training to these professionals, have also been little studied. The press and social media contain many accounts of inappropriate treatment of people with epilepsy by the police, such as mistaking seizures for drug or alcohol intoxication, man-handling confused individuals, and lack of awareness of the importance of providing anti-epilepsy medication while the affected person is in custody. Accounts of death in custody emerge from time to time, eventually followed by an inquiry and the undertaking that 'lessons will be learned'. Following a number of cases where people with epilepsy have been tasered during or just after a seizure, the UK epilepsy charity Epilepsy Action produced a training video to help firearms officers to recognize when a seizure is occurring. However, it has not yet been confirmed whether this video will be used in the annual training of officers who are authorized to use tasers.

In the USA the Epilepsy Foundation Eastern Pennsylvania offers a Law Enforcement Curriculum to help officers to recognize seizures and provide appropriate interventions. The 45-minute course also aims to give law enforcement officers training in the needs of people with epilepsy who might be taken into custody. The course is not mandatory, but it does provide an excellent opportunity to develop positive perceptions and understanding of epilepsy. The rate of uptake of these initiatives is not known, and such training is probably only completed by highly motivated and more informed individuals. Unless training aimed at raising awareness is obligatory, it is unlikely to improve the knowledge and influence the attitudes of the majority, and it is the majority that the person with epilepsy is most likely to encounter.

Care workers

Unpaid care is often an informal arrangement whereby an individual provides help and support for a relative, friend, or neighbour who could not otherwise cope due to frailty, illness,

---

401 Personal communication in response to Freedom of Information Act request. Sarah Lock Ministry of Justice Data and Compliance Unit. July 2019.

or disability. Unpaid carers are motivated by the desire to provide care for a loved one, and are likely to have a deep understanding and empathy for that particular person's condition. In contrast, professional care is provided by a suitably qualified person who usually looks after a number of individuals with a range of conditions. Professional carers' knowledge is dependent on self-directed learning and the training provided by the organization for which they work. In the UK there is no statutory requirement for employers to provide their staff with epilepsy awareness training, although various training organizations do provide it, at a cost. A clue to the ethos of some of these training providers can be found in the claim that 'our training courses are competitively priced and we aim to beat any equivalent training quote'. It is not known what proportion of the professional carers who work with people with epilepsy have any formal training. The only published study on carers' attitudes and knowledge is based on the opinions of family members and carers on the membership list of an epilepsy charity.[402] However, the low response rate (only 600 out of 2000 individuals who were approached) raises questions about the validity of any conclusions drawn. The survey questions were aimed at family members rather than professional carers, whereas comparisons between these two groups would have been much more interesting and informative. Not surprisingly, it was found that knowledge levels were higher and attitudes were more positive among the young and the better educated. The study concluded by recommending the 'need for more effective campaigns to educate the general public', and commenting that 'it is disappointing that there are few individuals with the condition willing to act as ambassadors for epilepsy'.

With regard to professional carers' knowledge of and attitudes toward epilepsy, relevant qualifications have been introduced into their training courses, but are not mandatory. The heavy workload of care workers and the very limited resources available to fund social care have the effect of reducing opportunities for in-service training. Consequently it is difficult to ensure that epilepsy awareness and seizure response training is universally provided to those who care for people with epilepsy. The responsibility for such regulation lies with the Care Quality Commission in England and Wales, and with the Care Inspectorate in Scotland. Both of these public bodies, which are required to regulate and inspect health and social care services, including residential establishments and individuals' homes, were asked, by means of a Freedom of Information request, to outline their views on training and its monitoring. Both the Care Quality Commission and the Care Inspectorate responded that neither body set training standards, nor do they recommend that any training should be mandatory. They stated that the organization that provides care is responsible for this, and that during

---

[402] McEwan L, Taylor J, Casswell M et al. (2007) Knowledge of and attitudes expressed toward epilepsy by carers of people with epilepsy: a UK perspective. *Epilepsy & Behavior* 11, 13–19.

inspections they would expect to find adequate provision of the levels of training necessary to meet the needs of the client group being cared for. The Care Quality Commission commented that 'if a provider was responsible for the care of somebody with epilepsy, we may choose to look at the epilepsy training that is provided to staff'. There was no guidance on how training should be delivered (for example, face to face or e-learning), or how frequently it should be provided (a critical factor given the high turnover rate among care staff). Neither specified what basic epilepsy training should involve, but merely stated that where staff 'are responsible for administering [epilepsy drugs] they must have the relevant training and competence to do so'. This all suggests that regulation and monitoring are almost entirely dependent on a site visit. Such inspections are infrequent, not always unannounced, and cannot guarantee safe epilepsy care. For example, at the time of inspection an organization might have had no client with epilepsy on their books for some time, and then after the inspection acquire one.

Conclusion

Early in this chapter we quoted Rajendra Kale's comment that 'the history of epilepsy can be summarized as 4,000 years of ignorance, superstition and stigma, followed by 100 years of knowledge, superstition and stigma',[403] and it seems appropriate to end with the same quote, as it neatly sums up the situation today. The early studies of social scientists such as Goffman have provided us with working definitions of stigma and discrimination, and articulated the reality of people living with epilepsy. Meanwhile the views of educators, employers, law enforcers, and the general public seem to have remained largely unchanged. The vast majority of studies have had their validity compromised by low response rates. Half a century of research has confirmed that there is a continuing problem, but apart from recommending the collection of further data it has offered no solution. Moreover, the planning of these studies has rarely involved people with epilepsy. Many researchers have identified the important role of public training programmes, but the target groups for such training, the specific course content, and the sustainable long-term benefits have yet to be established.

The answer to the problems identified in this chapter must lie in positive awareness raising about epilepsy, especially through the media, and central to this is the need to convey the message that people with epilepsy are, apart from occasional symptoms of their condition, just like everyone else.

---

403 Kale R (1997) Bringing epilepsy out of the shadows. *British Medical Journal* 315, 2.

PART V

Epilogue

A personal account of living with epilepsy

Too much knowledge can be as damaging as too little, and in relation to epilepsy I cannot help feeling that this has become a truism within our family. After qualifying as a doctor I set my sights on becoming a neurologist, mainly because I found the complex mysteries of the brain appealing. I knew from the outset that epilepsy was one of the commonest conditions that I would encounter, but I had little specific experience or knowledge of the condition. Five years into my medical career, our 7-year-old son Tim developed epilepsy, and my wife and I found ourselves living with a condition that had hitherto been one that other people had to cope with, not us.

    I shall not describe the details of Tim's epilepsy or the emotional and physical challenges that he has faced, as that is his story to tell, as indeed he has done in his forthcoming eBook In terms of living with and adapting to epilepsy within the family, my wife and I and our two daughters have all been affected to some degree, and we have each developed our own coping strategies. Epilepsy has significantly affected our family unit, and hardly a week passes in which we are not in some way acutely reminded of it. I often ponder how different Tim's life and our own lives might have been, and wonder about all the opportunities that have been denied him as a result of the condition.

    What follows is a personal account that reflects my own views, fears, and emotions as Tim's life with epilepsy has slowly unfolded. My hope is that it will allow others who are on a similar path both to learn how to approach problems and challenges differently, and to be reassured that they are not alone in their feelings of anxiety and the constant dilemmas that they face. I hope that by reading about my own experiences, including those that have been negative and challenging, others may gain understanding and knowledge that equip them to face the daily challenges that epilepsy presents.

The early years

With the benefit of hindsight it is clear that the first hint of possible epilepsy occurred during a family summer holiday in France in 1983. In the middle of a game of tennis on a particularly hot afternoon, Tim abruptly walked off the court for no apparent reason, and without seeming to pause to check for oncoming traffic, he then crossed the busy adjoining country road. We initially thought this was a reaction to the heat, but when we caught up with him he appeared pale, confused, and scared. We assumed that this isolated episode, although odd, was a 'one-off' until we returned home and similar, apparently inexplicable episodes occurred with increasing frequency. A week later, over the course of a single day Tim experienced up to half a dozen near identical episodes, which were now accompanied by vomiting, worsening pallor, chalky white lips, and more prolonged confusion. I think that I had known from the very beginning that these episodes were caused by epilepsy, but I had pushed the condition to the back of my mind, hoping that there might be a simple alternative explanation. However, events now demanded that the truth be confronted, as the family doctor arranged an urgent hospital appointment to confirm his and my suspicion.

A diagnosis of epilepsy was soon made by the paediatric neurologist, investigations were then started to identify the cause, and possible treatments were discussed. When a CT scan of Tim's brain was planned, the possibility of a tumour was uppermost in my mind. This concern was disproportional, as only a small number of people with childhood-onset epilepsy have a tumour as the underlying cause of their epilepsy, and in those who do, it can be relatively benign and potentially curable by surgery. Despite this knowledge, parental anxiety levels were high while we awaited the findings of these potentially life-defining investigations. Added to this, the scanner had broken down on the first two occasions we attended (a fairly common event in the early days of CT technology). When the CT scan was eventually performed we were extremely relieved to hear that it was normal, although this particular cause of anxiety would soon be replaced by others.

With epilepsy confirmed, and the possibility of a minor tumour excluded, the next step was to consider drug treatment and what that might be expected to achieve. At the time, in the mid-1980s, only five or six tried and tested drugs were available, the selection of which was fairly arbitrary and based on minimizing side effects. One might expect that drugs which are powerful enough to suppress seizures could well have significant adverse effects. Physical side effects such as a rash can be easily identified, but more subtle problems, such as impaired coordination, blurred vision, and memory and behavioural changes, are very difficult to detect in a 7-year-old child. At this critical stage of development, asking them about the side effects that they might be experiencing is clearly problematic, especially as a significant number of young people with epilepsy have coexisting learning difficulties.

The information provided by drug companies in their packaging must, for legal reasons, mention every possible adverse effect, from exfoliation (skin loss) to thinning hair, coarsening facial features, and even fatal side effects. In the 1980s, apart from this documentation of side effects and a brief hospital consultation, few sources of information were available for anxious parents. Mounting concern and overprotective attitudes were inevitable if their child had to take anti-epileptic medication on a long-term basis. Today, however, user-friendly and reassuring information about the increasing number of anti-epilepsy drugs that are available, and their interactions with other medicines, can be found on epilepsy websites.

In the 1980s, the goal of effective drug treatment was to stop seizures, or at least to significantly reduce them, without causing unacceptable side effects. At the time it was generally believed that these objectives could be achieved by a single drug in 75 per cent of patients with new-onset epilepsy, and that in the remaining cases, in whom there was a minimal or negligible treatment response, it would be necessary to switch to either another anti-epileptic drug or a combination of two different drugs, with an increasing risk of side effects. In Tim's case there seemed to be a good chance of achieving an acceptable level of seizure control, but there was no discussion between us and the doctors about the social consequences of having epilepsy, or where to seek advice on how to cope with these. In that respect we were on our own, and we had no idea how the situation that we faced was going to unfold. Tim's attacks did decrease in response to drug treatment, and he seemed to be comfortably within the 75 per cent of patients with an acceptable outcome and apparently negligible side effects.

We now had the breathing space for some soul-searching questions. Why had Tim developed epilepsy? Should we have detected it earlier? What should we say to him about what was wrong? And who else should we tell? There was no paediatric epilepsy specialist, parent support group, or handbook to advise us on these issues. When parents are trying to rationalize why their child has epilepsy, with all the accompanying feelings of guilt, blame, and self-recrimination, one common question (harking back to the days when epilepsy was believed to be inherited or even contagious) must be whether there might be a family history of the condition. Memories of distant relatives are trawled for evidence of trance-like states or lapses in concentration. In fact, hereditary cases of epilepsy are relatively rare, and the vaguest possible hint of epilepsy on one side of the family may lead to the wrongful apportioning of blame. In our own case we were unable to find any concrete evidence for a family history of epilepsy.

Our next concern was that the condition might have been caused by a subtle brain injury. There can be few children who have not sustained an accidental minor head injury at some time in their formative years. Sadly, many parents of children with epilepsy come to believe that an accidental fall (for example, down some stairs or from playground equipment) was the cause of their child's condition. The parent who had been caring for the child at the time of the accident then has to cope with the additional burden of completely unjustified feelings of guilt and self-blame about a lapse of supervision. Head injuries are classified as minor, moderate, or severe, based on the presence and duration of unconsciousness. Minor head injuries only very rarely cause brain injury, and in the absence of concussion or unconsciousness, epilepsy is most unlikely to develop as a result.

Our feelings of guilt about Tim's epilepsy were linked to vaccination. The MMR vaccine, which was introduced in 1971, is a combined vaccine that protects against measles, mumps, and rubella. In recent years, without any scientific evidence to support such a view, it has been wrongly linked with the development of various forms of autism, including Asperger's syndrome. A recent study of over 1 million vaccinated children found no such relationship.[404] Tim already had eczema, and in the early days of the vaccine there were concerns that it could exacerbate this condition. We therefore decided to opt out of MMR vaccination. With advances in knowledge over time, advice about the link between eczema and MMR has changed, and today children with eczema can safely be given the MMR vaccine. However, because Tim had not received this vaccination, predictably he contracted measles at the age of 14 months, and this significantly delayed his developmental milestones. Encephalitis (inflammation of the brain) is a rare complication of measles, and although we had no objective evidence that Tim developed this, it remains the only suspected cause of his epilepsy. We shall always wonder whether, if we had been less concerned about his eczema, Tim might never have developed epilepsy. And of course we shall never know the answer to this question.

Our next concern was that if Tim's epilepsy had been identified earlier and treated sooner, both his response to therapy and his long-term outcome might have been improved. The first attacks that we observed occurred when he was seven, but Tim later told us that they had been happening much earlier in his childhood, and possibly for as long as he could remember. I can now recollect, long before the episode while on holiday in France, brief

---

[404] Taylor LE, Swerdfeger AL and Eslick GD (2014) Vaccines are not associated with autism: an evidence-based meta-analysis of case-control and cohort studies. *Vaccine* 32, 3623–3629.

night-time episodes of unexplained panic that must have been seizures, and I can recall that occasional blank stare into space. When Tim was later able to articulate his symptoms, he described feelings of inexplicable fear, terror, and panic. For a small child, the harrowing experience of being overwhelmed by such extreme emotions while having no one to turn to for reassurance and comfort, and at such a critical period of development, might well lead to the moulding of character and personality. Why had we not appreciated what was going on earlier? And had we let Tim down by failing to get help sooner? There is no clear evidence to suggest that the higher the number of seizures experienced before initiating treatment, the less likely it is that there will be a response to treatment. However, there remains the major unanswered question about the extent of long-lasting psychological damage that was caused by the untreated attacks.

By the time an official diagnosis of epilepsy was made, Tim was 8 years old, and our next dilemma was how to explain to him what was wrong and who else to tell. Clearly any individual, irrespective of age, has a moral right to be given an explanation for their illness and the rationale for and importance of taking treatment for it. However, it is no easy task to explain an illness as complicated as epilepsy to a small child, and in the 1980s few doctors made any attempt to do so. During Tim's many hospital visits we felt as if he was the bystander as we presented his seizure diary, described what side effects we thought he might be experiencing from his drug treatment, and recounted his social and academic progress.

The daunting task of telling Tim what was wrong was left entirely to us. Rather than try to explain in detail to an 8-year-old what epilepsy is and how it arises from the brain, we decided to use the unthreatening word 'feelings' to describe his attacks, and we subconsciously avoided using the term 'epilepsy' in front of Tim or his sisters. It was Tim himself who first used the term 'feelings' as the best way he could put into words what he was experiencing.

We explained that the reason for his drug treatment was to prevent the 'feelings', and that he should tell us if they had occurred without our noticing them. At this stage we did not attempt to explain why or from where they had arisen. I suspect that we had given Tim the impression that seizures were nothing unusual, in fact common to everyone, with only a few people needing to have them treated. We never discussed the idea that something unusual was happening in Tim's brain, nor did we question him in excessive detail about how he felt during his seizures. In effect we tried to normalize the problem by drawing as little attention to it as possible.

The events we observed were brief episodes of sudden pallor, chalky white lips, brief staring and a period of unawareness followed by disorientation, fear, and the need to be consoled; Tim would often run into our arms. Afterwards we all tried to get back to normal as quickly as possible, almost as if nothing had happened. We made the administering of medication as routine as tooth brushing, while unobtrusively checking that Tim was experiencing none of the side effects we had read about. The questions of when to start using the word 'epilepsy' and when to explain to him that his feelings were the result of a brain disorder were put on hold. As Tim had responded so well to his medication, we felt that we should delay this conversation for as long as possible, and indeed it was not until several years later that it took place. This procrastination was intended to make matters easier not only for him, but also for ourselves, and we shall never know how much harm this may have caused.

Today, parents have access to several thoughtful books that address how to explain epilepsy to children and their friends. Kate Lambert has produced a guide for those as young as seven,[405] as well as a fictional account of epilepsy for children in collaboration with the illustrator Rebecca Morris.[406] Such books are an invaluable aid for present-day parents, but it is regrettable that such important educational tools for explaining epilepsy to young children, their friends and parents were not available many years earlier.

Our failure to tell Tim about his epilepsy earlier on may seem bizarre by today's standards, but such reticence was very much the norm at the time. We did eventually broach the subject with him, but only after the information was long overdue, when the drugs had ceased to provide an acceptable degree of control of his seizures, and the reality of the situation had to be faced. Ironically, in later years, as a well-informed young adult, Tim regularly revisited his paediatric neurology department and, in conjunction with the newly established epilepsy specialist nurse, talked to the parents of children who had been newly diagnosed with epilepsy. Tellingly, though, he was never given the opportunity to speak directly to the children about his own experiences as a young child.

Although within the immediate family unit Tim's diagnosis was downplayed, friends, the wider family, and the authorities involved in his overall well-being had a need to know. His primary school was immediately notified of his diagnosis, as it had a duty of care to him and his schoolmates for the duration of the school day. Once the school had been informed we became keenly aware that they now knew more about the cause of Tim's 'feelings' than he himself did. We felt that this was a betrayal, albeit a necessary one.

In the 1980s, teachers had much less knowledge of epilepsy than they do today, and their attitudes to the condition were more negative. Because teachers are responsible for the welfare and safety of children under their care, parents have a duty of disclosure, but openness about a child's epilepsy can have potentially damaging consequences for him or her. Many who work in the education sector still associate epilepsy with learning disability. This association

---

[405] Lambert K (2012) *Can I Tell You About Epilepsy? A Guide for Friends, Family and Professionals.* Jessica Kingsley Publishers, London.
[406] Lambert K and Morris R (2012) *Sarah Jayne Has Staring Moments: A Fictional Children's Book for Child Absence Seizure Epilepsy.* K. Lambert.

may be correct in some cases, but a significant number of children with epilepsy have no such problems. The damage occurs when below-average performance is erroneously attributed to the condition, and teachers then lower their expectations with regard to the child's potential. In such cases, attempts to improve the child's school performance may be less proactive. In the 1980s, when school child psychology services were still in their infancy, there was a big risk that teachers would give up on a child if they erroneously believed that he or she had learning difficulties. At that time, only teachers who had undergone specialist training in the field of learning disability received any formal teaching about epilepsy. Generally little was known about the nature of seizures, trigger factors, associated anxiety, and the side effects of drugs in children of primary school age or older. In a busy classroom, subtle brief staring episodes could even go undetected by the class teacher, or be mistaken for daydreaming.

Teachers also had to consider safety issues in the classroom, in the playground, and in relation to physical education activities, such as swimming. First-aid measures at that time were not always appropriate or safe. In particular, the practice of forcing an object into a person's mouth to prevent tongue biting was considered appropriate, whereas in fact it was extremely hazardous. (I recall from an earlier era, when I was a child myself, my primary schoolteacher snatching a pencil from my desk and forcing it into the mouth of a classmate who was having a seizure.) With regard to playground settings and physical education activities such as swimming, no clear guidance was available, so the approach taken involved minimizing risk and avoiding those pursuits that other children could enjoy with impunity. This, together with the seizures or episodes themselves and the need to have medication supervised, must inevitably have induced among these children a sense of being different from others, which could potentially give rise to feelings of alienation.

The next question was what to disclose to other family members and friends, and when to do this. First we had to decide whether or not to inform the parents of Tim's school friends, bearing in mind that they were not bound by the same duty of professional confidentiality as his teachers. We opted to be guided by practical necessity in order to ensure his safety during events that were supervised by other adults, such as sleepovers, swimming activities, and trips away from home. We confided in only a small number of parents, but I suspected that the news travelled fast and that other parents, and possibly even their children, soon became aware of Tim's epilepsy. Our guardedness was not due to any feelings of shame about Tim having epilepsy. It was more a case of wanting to keep family matters to ourselves, and fearing that others would treat him differently if they knew about his condition. I suppose this fear that those who were aware of his diagnosis would become judgemental and perhaps even start to exclude him marked the point at which we started to subconsciously become Tim's stigma coaches. There is no doubt that as a result of our reluctance to discuss his epilepsy more openly, we were beginning to separate Tim and ourselves from the mainstream. What would we have done today? People's attitudes have changed since the 1980s, and we would have been more open, although we would still not have broadcast the situation. We would also have kept Tim better informed and involved him in our discussions with other people, and, importantly, in deciding the content of those discussions.

Telling our own extended family and friends also posed many problems. Older family members, perhaps tending to have outdated perceptions of epilepsy, reacted to the news more negatively, with comments such as 'It is a shame that such a thing should happen to a young child.' For this reason we tended to keep matters to ourselves in order to protect Tim from what we saw as public misconceptions of and ignorance about epilepsy. In fact, by withholding the diagnosis from some members of the wider family whom we suspected would respond negatively to the news, we were storing up problems in terms of how they would react to finding out about his epilepsy in the years ahead.

A cousin who did not learn about the epilepsy until Tim was in his twenties was surprised that he had not been told before and, clearly assuming that the subject was taboo, never mentioned it again. Had he known earlier, I suspect that his approach would have been more open, supportive, and understanding. With the benefit of hindsight it is clear that we should have taken the whole family on board from the beginning of Tim's epilepsy journey, and that had we done so this might have provided him with the long-term support network that he might come to need in later years.

Tim's two sisters, who were aged nine and two when his epilepsy first developed, became gradually aware of the seizures. Although they did not share a bedroom with him, they were conscious that he would wake in the night, become distressed, and run through to our room to be comforted. They had also observed the daytime episodes of staring, pallor, and confusion. Initially we felt that they were too young to be able to understand the problem, so as with Tim we used the unthreatening word 'feelings' rather than the term 'epilepsy' to describe the symptoms that they witnessed. We did not fully explain the condition to them for many years, and I don't know what they made of the information at the time when they received it. In retrospect I feel that we should have been more open with them from the very beginning, and given them a fuller understanding of what Tim was living with, rather than downplaying the frightening attacks that he was bravely enduring.

As Tim's seizures lessened, our confidence increased, and we became less over-protective. When he rode his bicycle or went off to the park to play football or hit a few golf balls it was no longer a worry for us. Indeed, because his seizures seemed to have become so rare, we hoped they were no longer a major problem. Towards the end of his time at primary school, Tim started to travel there and back independently, using public transport. We had our first experience with the unknowing general public when the transport police found him wandering up and down a station platform in a confused state. At that time, because Tim was so young, drug taking was not considered as a possible explanation for his state, though nowadays that possibility might not be ruled out in a child of primary school age. The police could not have been more understanding, and brought him home safe and sound. After this incident, Tim's confidence was soon restored and he resumed his independent travel. Perhaps we did not give him enough credit for the courage that this must have taken, as at the time we were mainly concerned about his safety, rather than any anxiety he might have had about returning to the scene of the incident. The reaction of the police to this childhood event contrasted starkly with the way that Tim was treated when similar episodes occurred in public places after he reached adulthood. Then it was erroneously assumed that he was either intoxicated or behaving suspiciously.

We were never entirely sure whether Tim's teachers regarded his epilepsy and its drug treatment as an explanation for any academic difficulties that he experienced, and whether this made them less proactive in addressing problems. They always denied that this was the case. As his seizures became increasingly well controlled by his medication, the need to explain to both Tim and his sisters exactly what was wrong seemed less pressing.

Although Tim appeared to be living a fairly normal life for a pre-adolescent boy, we never explored the psychological traumas that his seizures must have induced, nor did we give him full credit for the courage that he had shown in coping with these episodes. At that time doctors were much less holistic in their approach to the family with epilepsy than they are now, and there were not yet any epilepsy specialist nurses, nor were there any support groups that we could join in order to share our experiences and concerns with others in the same situation. We had, in effect, had to travel on our own without a map.

The adolescent years

For many years Tim's epilepsy seemed to be well controlled by drug treatment, and now that he was seizure-free he appeared to be enjoying a normal healthy adolescence. We were now tending to think along the lines that he 'used to have epilepsy', while at the same time acknowledging that he needed to continue to take his drug treatment three times a day. The next dilemma that we faced was whether he should remain on anti-epileptic medication after he had been free of seizures for several years. This question was particularly pertinent as the drug he was taking, carbamazepine, might be having some effect on both memory and attention, and important life-influencing exams were imminent.

In 1991 the first academic study of the risk of relapse after anti-epileptic drug withdrawal was published.[407] The results predicted the likelihood of recurrence of seizures in groups of individuals with certain common features of epilepsy characteristics, but could not provide a reliable estimate of the risk associated with drug withdrawal in a single individual. In fact, when Tim was slowly weaned off drug treatment his epilepsy soon returned, and was never again as well controlled as it had been previously. The decision to try stopping drug treatment was very much his choice. As a teenager he was aware that taking his anti-epilepsy medication set him apart from most of his peers, and he was troubled by niggling side effects such as blurred vision at what he called his 'peak dose' time. We supported his decision, concerned that the drugs were making him sleep much more than normal and that they were also affecting his concentration. The relapse of his epilepsy in these circumstances inevitably led to much soul searching, our main question being whether, if he had never stopped taking his medication, his epilepsy might have remained as well controlled as it had previously been. It is impossible to answer this question. Significantly, by this stage the word 'feelings' had been permanently replaced by the term 'epilepsy', and Tim's condition was now openly discussed within our immediate family.

The return of his seizures led to the resumption of hospital attendances, but Tim's age meant that he was now in the transition zone between child and adult healthcare services, and he was referred to the latter. In the 1990s, specialist adult epilepsy services were in their infancy and those that did exist were generally staffed by clinical pharmacologists. Here the emphasis was on trials that compared tried and tested treatments with the emerging new anti-epileptic drugs. Enrolment in such trials appeared to be a prerequisite for attendance, and while acknowledging the importance of such studies, our experience was that the wider human and social implications of having epilepsy were sadly neglected, while the seizure diary that documented the number and severity of seizures had a central role. The final straw for Tim, at that time a teenager focused on exams and gaining a place at university, was a consultation at which a young doctor, only ten years older than him, speculated that due to having active epilepsy he would be unlikely to find employment, and should resign himself to a life on state benefits. Other consultations had similarly negative effects. For example, when double vision and weight gain were cited as side effects of Tim's drug treatment, he was told that this was the price he would have to pay for an improvement in his epilepsy symptoms.

Now that Tim was back on treatment his seizures had become less frequent, but were still occurring both in the daytime and at night, and were not controlled by the various different

---

[407] Medical Research Council Antiepileptic Drug Withdrawal Study Group (1991) Randomised study of antiepileptic drug withdrawal in patients in remission. *Lancet* 337, 1175–1180.

combinations of drugs that were tried. By now, as family holidays became more adventurous and involved travelling further afield, unexpected lifestyle limitations became apparent. The first particularly memorable example occurred when Tim wanted to go snorkelling while in Turkey, and we believed that this would not be safe, despite his insistence to the contrary. One of his school friends had come on holiday with us, and the night before the planned activity we had all been kept up until the small hours by noisy neighbours. The next morning Tim knew that he was vulnerable to a seizure due to lack of sleep. This and our shared worries about the safety aspects of snorkelling resulted in him opting out of the activity. He had to sit and watch his friend snorkelling, knowing that his epilepsy had excluded him from an activity that his friend could take for granted. This seemed to mark the beginning of his acceptance that, for his own safety, there were certain activities in which he could never spontaneously participate because of the risk of having a seizure.

The next incident could have had extremely serious consequences. While staying on the fourth floor of a hotel in Rhodes, we were having breakfast when our younger daughter came down to tell us that Tim had gone out to the balcony and was attempting to climb over it into the neighbouring apartment. I rushed upstairs to find the balcony doors open but no sign of Tim. The occupants of the adjoining apartment came out into the hallway and told us that Tim had entered their apartment from their balcony and climbed into their daughter's empty bed, where they had found him sound asleep. Both the physical risk of a fall from the fourth floor, and the fact that he was an intruder in someone else's apartment, could have had very severe consequences. Fortunately, everyone was very understanding when we explained about Tim's epilepsy, although I suspect that such a reaction would have been less likely if he had been an adult travelling alone with no one to corroborate his epilepsy.

This serious incident raised many questions about future holidays. Could Tim safely go away independently, and if so, what type of accommodation would be most suitable for him? Travel would involve flights, crossing time zones (with resultant sleep deprivation) and probably staying in high-rise hotels, in a country with a hot climate. The heat, disturbed sleep patterns, and consumption of alcohol were all known risk factors for seizures to which he would probably be exposed.

Some years later we took a flight home from Chicago to Glasgow that highlighted many of the travel-related problems that are faced by people with epilepsy. Concerns about having a seizure mid-flight, with all the possible ramifications of altered behaviour, were even more stressful in the era of aircraft hijacking and armed air marshals.

The overnight flight was delayed by several hours, and before take-off Tim informed one of the cabin crew about his epilepsy in case he stood up and started wandering about when the seatbelt sign was switched on. The air hostess then loudly announced across the aisle to her colleague, and to everyone else sitting nearby, that 'This young man is an epileptic.' As if that wasn't enough, the flight was re-routed to Philadelphia to resume the journey home from there the following afternoon. Tim had enough anti-epileptic medication for the original flight home, but the rest was in his luggage in the hold, which was not to be unloaded. We were driven to a hotel and he was given a room next door to ours. I remember sleeping lightly, alert for any indication that he might have left his room. With disrupted sleep, a limited supply of medication, and in an alien environment, the inevitable happened. In the early hours of the morning I found Tim, confused and wearing only a towel, in one of the lifts. After this incident he always carried enough medication in his hand luggage to tide him over in the event of a flight delay. However, it is worth noting here that, for a person with epilepsy, a delayed flight is a hazard that undermines confidence about future travel and their ability to cope with the unexpected. Thus an experience such as this has the effect of narrowing horizons and undermining independence.

Now that Tim's seizures were relatively infrequent, there was less need to tell others about the epilepsy, as a result of which it became gradually more concealed. New friends, including girlfriends, did not know about it, and among Tim's secondary school teachers it was mentioned but not elaborated upon, and he was able to participate in contact sports such as rugby. He had no seizures while attending secondary school, and a pattern of predominantly sleep-related episodes became established. Tim prepared for exams and considered potential careers. All along we had shared an awareness that some jobs would be out of the question and that any occupations that involved travel and car driving might be unsuitable. It seemed that probably the best way forward would be for Tim to go on to higher education, as we all felt that the advantages of having a degree could offset the disadvantages of having epilepsy.

Leaving home

Now aged 18, with a place at university to study molecular biology, Tim left home for the first time. Our family doctor informed the student health service about his epilepsy, but the only support that they offered was a single appointment with the university medical officer. The information that Tim had epilepsy was not passed on to his lecturers by the health service because of a duty of confidentiality, and he was allocated a shared bedroom immediately opposite an open stairwell on the third floor of a university hall of residence. His roommate had no prior knowledge of night-time seizures until one occurred, but thereafter was very supportive. We only discovered the hazardous location of Tim's room when we visited, and to avoid drawing attention to his epilepsy and to normalize the situation, he did not wish to be relocated. However, his roommate was a smoker, and because Tim was asthmatic he did eventually request a room change, which was granted.

Because Tim was no longer living with and frequently observed by us, we had serious concerns about the risk of accidents, injury, or what became known as sudden unexpected death in epilepsy (SUDEP). As a neurologist I had first-hand experience of a very small number of patients with epilepsy who had suffered a seizure-related death. Despite its catastrophic nature, SUDEP was not defined until 1997.[408] Today physicians are obliged to inform all adults about the risk of SUDEP, which causes the death of 1 in 1000 people with epilepsy each year. This risk is higher in individuals with generalized seizures, and can be reduced by effective seizure control and adherence to anti-epileptic drug treatment.[409] When SUDEP was first identified there was debate as to whether informing patients with epilepsy about it might cause psychological harm. This paternalistic approach is no longer acceptable, as awareness of the risk gives individuals the opportunity to mitigate it by taking anti-epileptic medication regularly. Our knowledge that the type of seizure that Tim experienced was unlikely to result in sudden death was reassuring, and we did not divulge this low risk to him for some time.

With regard to giving advice nowadays to people with epilepsy who are preparing to move away from home, the small risk of SUDEP and the need to take medication regularly to reduce this risk must be explained. It is also important to point out that the risk of SUDEP is strongly linked to a relatively young age and the presence of generalized seizures that are more often than not sleep-related. Lifestyle factors that impair the effectiveness of medication, such as consumption of large amounts of alcohol and irregular sleep patterns, should also be avoided.

Another concern when a person with epilepsy flies the nest is how they will cope on their own when a seizure occurs in a public place. When Tim told me that he had had a seizure in a packed lecture theatre, what struck me most was his resilience and courage in returning to the same lecture theatre and facing the same audience on the following days. I think this kind of courage that is shown by people with epilepsy often goes unrecognized. In the 1990s, understanding of epilepsy in higher education settings was poor, and allowances were not made for seizures and medication side effects when academic performance was being assessed. Indeed, when Tim complained of medication-related double vision while using a microscope, he was asked by the lecturer in charge whether he thought being away from home and at university was a realistic choice for someone with epilepsy. Such an attitude

---

408 Nashef L (1997) Sudden unexpected death in epilepsy: terminology and definitions. *Epilepsia* 38 (11 Suppl.), S6–S8.
409 American Epilepsy Society (2017) Practice Guideline Summary: sudden unexpected death in epilepsy incidence rates and risk factors: report of the Guideline Development, Dissemination, and Implementation Subcommittee of the American Academy of Neurology and the American Epilepsy Society. *Epilepsy Currents* 17, 180–187.

would not be tolerated today, but at the time it only increased Tim's perception of being 'different' and his feelings of alienation. During the following years, as universities became obliged to provide pastoral support for students with disabilities, matters would improve beyond recognition.

Epilepsy in adulthood

Tim left university with an honours degree in molecular biology and what would become lasting friendships, but what happened subsequently is very much his story to tell. Epilepsy encroaches upon many aspects of adult potential, well-being, and quality of life, and I shall discuss these generally rather than specifically in relation to Tim, illustrating them where possible with the anonymized stories of others whom I have met travelling the same journey.

Childhood experiences and attitudes will shape the manner in which, as adults, people with epilepsy and their families adapt in the longer term. When epilepsy dates back to the formative years it will inevitably influence relationships and attitudes within the family unit, although surprisingly there have been no longitudinal studies of this that I am aware of. When one child within a family is significantly affected by illness, there is a risk of an asymmetric relationship developing, due to that child requiring more attention and different types of support compared with their siblings. One possible consequence of this is that the affected child may be empowered while their unaffected siblings feel that they are being neglected by comparison. The imbalance of attention and support can also affect parents, when one or both parents feel neglected because the child's needs are prioritized over theirs. The long-term effects of this may have a negative effect on family relationships and skew their dynamics, leading to a sea of animosity rather than a much-needed support network.

For the child with epilepsy, their earliest memories of how their parents reacted to their condition are likely to have a long-term effect on how that child will perceive him- or herself. Joseph Schneider and Peter Conrad have distinguished between the 'open' and 'closed' styles of parenting of children with epilepsy.[410] Parents who adopt the open style regard the epilepsy as 'unfortunate', but accept it and approach it in a manner that the whole family can understand and accommodate. This style of parenting minimizes the risk that the child will be treated as special, to the relative exclusion of the rest of the family. The normalizing of epilepsy by adopting this open approach should also reduce the risk of 'secondary gain', where the child with epilepsy takes advantage of their condition to manipulate others and

---

410 Schneider JW and Conrad P (1983) *Having Epilepsy: the Experience and Control of Illness*. Temple University Press, Philadelphia, PA.

take control of situations. The open style has its limitations, as it is difficult to see how the child will not be perceived at least to some extent as having additional needs to their siblings, and be treated accordingly. However, this parenting approach is still preferable to the closed approach, in which the parents seem shocked and even embarrassed by the diagnosis of epilepsy, and conceal the child's condition from their friends and family. The siblings are unable to adapt, as they do not know what is wrong. This rigid denial of the epilepsy inculcates shame in the child and resentment throughout the family unit. As Schneider and Conrad point out, this is the route to disability and dependence when the child reaches adulthood.

Balancing the needs of the child with epilepsy with those of the other children within the family is a major challenge because of all the potential situations that might arise. For example, suppose that a morning seizure coincides with exam results arriving in the post for the other sibling. Their results are excellent, but praise for the child and pride in their achievement have to be balanced with simultaneous concern and support for the affected child. This is no easy task. Adopting an open approach to the child's epilepsy, and telling their siblings about it very early on, seems to be the most effective way to prevent family dysfunction.

When providing support and advice on career choices for people with epilepsy, it is important not to dampen the person's ambitions, but at the same time to instil a sense of realism, especially if seizures are likely to persist. Clearly occupations that put the person with active epilepsy and those around them at risk due to loss of awareness should be avoided. The dilemma arises when epilepsy has been controlled for a while but is still at risk of recurring. For instance, a job that is dependent on driving may be too risky even for a person who is currently seizure-free if a relapse would result in loss of employment. Moreover, it should be borne in mind that sometimes a threat to a person's career can arise unexpectedly in what had hitherto seemed a safe choice of occupation.

The following case example illustrates this. J.P. had embarked on a postgraduate teacher training programme in the belief that this was a profession that could accommodate his epilepsy. He had declared his epilepsy both when he applied for and when he enrolled on the course, and it had not been regarded as a problem. Several weeks into his first school placement he had a seizure in the packed staffroom of a very large school just before assembly, after months of freedom from seizures. Now that his epilepsy was common knowledge, precautions had to be taken. His training as a science teacher involved the handling of chemicals, and concerns were raised about the safety of children under his care. For the pupils' safety he was provided with a teaching assistant and told that this would continue to be a requirement after he qualified and obtained a permanent teaching post. This would make him an expensive choice of job candidate for any cash-strapped education authority to which he might apply in the future. The law requires employees to make reasonable adjustments to accommodate the employment of people with medical conditions, but if an adjustment is too expensive to be affordable it is deemed unreasonable. Furthermore, the law predominantly protects individuals who are already in employment, unlike J.P., who on completion of his training would be entering the job market in competition with similarly qualified teachers without epilepsy, who would not incur costly teaching support. When J.P. weighed up his prospects, he decided to give up his course and teaching career, despite the fact that his seizures were infrequent.

The question of whether and when a person with epilepsy should disclose their condition when applying for jobs is a thorny one with no simple answer. If anything goes wrong, failure to declare their epilepsy could result in dismissal as well as refusal or reluctance of the employer to provide a reference. Conversely, being open about their condition might result in failure to get a job in the first place. Each individual has to decide what is the most suitable approach for their particular circumstances. However, failure to disclose the condition puts the person with epilepsy under stress, due to both fear of having a seizure in public and the need to conceal their medication from work colleagues, and it also has a self-stigmatizing effect.

Another case example involved M.H., an agency care worker. Because her epilepsy was well controlled, she had not disclosed it, as she did not believe that it would affect her ability to perform safely in the team, which was working with people with learning disabilities. Her managers encouraged her to apply for a permanent, pensionable post in the centre where she was working. A colleague who was applying for the same permanent job had been distressed on learning that her niece had just been diagnosed with epilepsy. M.H. then opened up about her own seizure history, in order to reassure her colleague. Management must have learned of her disclosure, as she was removed from her post and from the shortlist without explanation, and the agency offered her no further placements. When she confronted them about this, she was told that she had been dishonest in not declaring her epilepsy at the outset, and that she had placed clients at risk and made the agency liable. Shortly after this betrayal of confidence by her fellow worker, M.H. was given an incorrect diagnosis of paranoid personality disorder, as a result of which she was unable either to prove that discrimination had occurred or to find employment again. This kind of story is not uncommon, and highlights the need for caution when disclosing epilepsy to others.

Epilepsy, mental health, and social isolation

As time passes, for the young person with epilepsy the societal consequences of continuing to have seizures become increasingly apparent, especially problems with finding employment, sustaining relationships, and raising a family. By the time this stage is reached, parental anxieties are focused less on the seizures themselves and more on the lack of opportunities, inability to form relationships, escalating mental health problems, social isolation or exclusion, and the resultant despair and inherent risk of suicide.

The increased risk of suicide among people with epilepsy is well recognized, as evidenced by the awareness campaigns run by many charities and support groups. Initially studies made no reference to social factors, and instead focused on the relationship between suicide risk, type of epilepsy, and seizure control.[411] Overall the suicide rate among people with epilepsy is three times higher than that in the general population, and is highest in individuals with temporal lobe epilepsy. A more recent study did collect data on employment and marital status, but again focused on seizure type, duration, and response to treatment as well as on neuropsychiatric evaluation,[412] and concluded that a history of previous attempted suicide and a history of depression were the strongest predictors of suicide. The authors stated that 'these data reinforce the relevance of diagnosing and treating depression appropriately in epilepsy'. To reduce the risk of suicide they recommended antidepressant drug therapy, but did not mention the need to mitigate the social consequences of having chronic epilepsy, such as loneliness and social exclusion.

The establishment of relationships with friends and a long-term partnership are the best way to reduce isolation and loneliness in later life. As we have already mentioned, people with epilepsy are less likely to marry or be in a long-term partnership than those without the condition. Moreover, they have to deal with the thorny issue of how and when to disclose their condition to a potential partner with whom they would be sharing a home and bed. There is no doubt that some relationships do founder when epilepsy is mentioned. However, when working as a neurologist I encountered a great many supportive partners, and only a handful of cases where the development of epilepsy led to relationship breakdown. There is no doubt that resilience is needed when dealing with epilepsy, especially when there are young children who may witness their parent having a seizure.

People are bound together by the shared experiences of work, relationships, and parenthood. As we and our friends and family age we pass through phases of life in which we have common experiences that we can discuss, compare, and contrast. However, if a person cannot work and has no close supportive relationships, they may well start to drift away from their peers due to the lack of common experiences that they can share with each other. This results in the social isolation that poses a particular risk to people with active epilepsy.

---

411 Blumer D, Montouris G, Davies K et al. (2002) Suicide in epilepsy: psychopathology, pathogenesis, and prevention. *Epilepsy & Behavior* 3, 232–241.
412 De Oliveira GNM, Kummer A, Salgado JV et al. (2011) Suicidality in temporal lobe epilepsy: measuring the weight of impulsivity and depression. *Epilepsy & Behavior* 22, 745–749.

As the parents of a person with active epilepsy grow older they will inevitably become concerned that their child will experience increasing social isolation as they become more frail, and especially after their death. The risk of this happening can be greatly reduced by establishing a robust and informed network of supportive friends and family members early on, so that there is a network of people available to cover all eventualities.

The Epilepsy Foundation's Community Forum has recently included the following thought-provoking comments on the subject of social isolation: 'I was diagnosed with epilepsy when I was about 3 or 4 and this made my family enforcement [sic] a forced social isolation on me so "I'm not hurt" now that I'm older it's beginning to be a problem that I don't know how to interact with people cause I'm too nervous, afraid and shy' and 'I too suffer in isolation because of my epilepsy. I am always alone and on my own and have almost no friends because of it.'[413] Sociologists draw a distinction between loneliness and social isolation. Loneliness is defined as 'the subjective, unpleasant and distressing phenomenon stemming from a discrepancy between individuals' desired and achieved levels of social relations',[414] whereas social isolation is regarded as 'an imposed isolation from normal networks caused by a loss of mobility or deteriorating health'.[415] As a simple analogy, when you are in a crowded football stadium you may be lonely but you are not socially isolated. Yet the consequences of loneliness and social isolation are the same, namely a damaging effect on mental and physical health, and an increased burden on healthcare services. We need to ask how social isolation among people with epilepsy can be addressed when the majority of resources and campaigns, such as the UK's 'Campaign to End Loneliness',[416] are currently targeted specifically at older people, those with dementia, and those facing social isolation during the coronavirus pandemic.

In 2017, *The York Press* reported on a survey conducted by the UK charity Epilepsy Action.[417] One thousand people living in Yorkshire were asked how their epilepsy affected their life and emotions. In total, 60 per cent admitted to experiencing loneliness, and 75 per cent stated that epilepsy prevented them from engaging in social activities and events. One respondent commented that they did not feel 'part of the same human race as everybody else', while others mentioned feeling 'unwanted and unloved', and only 10 per cent felt that they were part of a supportive community. In the UK, government proposals such as

---

413 www.epilepsy.com/connect/forums/living-epilepsy-adults/social-isolation
414 Perlman D and Peplau LA (1981) Toward a social psychology of loneliness. In Gilmour R and Duck S (eds.) *Personal Relationships: 3. Relationships in Disorder*. Academic Press, London. pp. 31–56.
415 Windle K, Francis J and Coomber C (2011) *Preventing Loneliness and Social Isolation: Interventions and Outcomes*. Social Care Institute for Excellence Research Briefing 39. Social Care Institute for Excellence, London.
416 www.campaigntoendloneliness.org
417 Liptrot K (2017) Loneliness warning for people with epilepsy. www.yorkpress.co.uk/news/15157937.loneliness-warning-for-people-with-epilepsy

A Connected Society: A Strategy for Tackling Loneliness – Laying the Foundations for Change indicate that there is no immediate solution to this multifaceted problem, which will require the involvement of numerous separate agencies or stakeholders at significant cost.[418]

Meanwhile, what can be done for the lonely and socially isolated person with epilepsy? First, it is important to recognize the first signs of loneliness and try to intervene early on. This involves family and friends making that early intervention when they first become aware of a gradual withdrawal. Isolation and loneliness do not occur suddenly, but rather they develop as part of a process that is associated with loss of self-esteem and exacerbated by setbacks such as the loss of a job, the breakdown of a relationship, or emerging mental health problems such as depression. Family and friends should be alert for early symptoms of depression, such as loss of interest in activities that were previously enjoyed, and disrupted sleep patterns, and be ready to suggest seeking professional help sooner rather than later.

If the support of family and friends cannot prevent the situation from worsening, there are other routes for finding help. Many epilepsy charities offer befriending services, in which a volunteer (who may or may not have epilepsy) meets up with the individual on a regular basis. Volunteers are normally matched with their clients in terms of age and gender, and regularly meet with their clients in their homes or go out for coffee or to the cinema with them. Although this service undeniably provides an opportunity to have conversations and to share thoughts and experiences, it is not a friendship in the truest sense. The volunteer is advised to discourage any close personal involvement and dependency, and to avoid meeting up with the client too frequently, thus creating an artificial distance between client and befriender that would be absent in a natural friendship. Nevertheless this service is highly valued by the many people with epilepsy who use it. Support groups provide the opportunity to meet others with epilepsy and share experiences. Some have suggested that these groups create a 'ghetto' in which mainly negative experiences are shared and separation from the mainstream is exacerbated. This criticism fails to take into account the de-isolating benefits of meeting with people with whom one has much in common.

In *A Connected Society: A Strategy for Tackling Loneliness*, the potentially beneficial role of social media is highlighted. This communication tool has also been cited as a potential cause of loneliness, although most such evidence relates to young users, and there are few, if any, data for the disabled or people with epilepsy. The positive or negative effects of social media on loneliness depend on whether it is used to complement real-life contacts or to replace them, with the additional concern that some people with epilepsy may be vulnerable to Internet exploitation. Although the ability of online and social media to reduce loneliness

---

418 HM Government (2018) *A Connected Society: A Strategy for Tackling Loneliness – Laying the Foundations for Change.* assets.publishing.service.gov.uk/government/uploads/system/uploads/attachment_data/file/750909/6.4882_DCMS_Loneliness_Strategy_web_Update.pdf

among those with epilepsy remains uncertain, it is well worth engaging with the platforms of epilepsy organizations.

There are also many local community projects that aim to reduce loneliness. These are not aimed specifically at disabled people, and their details can generally be found on the Internet or in community newsletters. Some are self-funded while others have charitable status. When encouraging an isolated person to join a support group or local community project, an approach that involves gentle persuasion and perhaps even accompanying them to meetings may help them to overcome their fear of being rejected if they do engage in this way.

Because loneliness in epilepsy is the consequence of stigma, fear, lost opportunities, and loss of shared experiences with peers, a willingness to be open about the condition from its very onset will help to ensure that friends are supportive over the years. The risk of loneliness should be discussed openly within the family so that, if it does arise, it can be properly handled. A robust family network gives the best protection against isolation and loneliness in later life. For people with epilepsy who have no family or friends to support them, befriending, appropriate social media, and local community projects can be extremely helpful.

Mental illness is disproportionally common in people with epilepsy. About a third of those who experience seizures suffer from anxiety disorders, and depression is up to seven times more prevalent than in the general population. There also appears to be a link between autism and epilepsy, as around a third of people with autism have seizures, which presents a range of communication problems. Depression and mood change can occur transiently in the hours immediately before a seizure, or more commonly depression can be persistent and cyclical. It is more frequent in individuals whose epilepsy is poorly controlled, but it can also occur to a lesser extent in patients whose seizures are well controlled or in complete remission. Occasionally, depression may be precipitated by a newly prescribed anti-epileptic drug. Overdosing with these readily available drugs accounts for 80 per cent of epilepsy-related attempted suicides, so the importance of recognizing and treating depression cannot be underestimated. Not all depressed people look sad or tearful, and they often put on a brave face to mask their feelings, so family and friends should be alert for other signs. The commonest symptoms are fatigue, poor concentration, loss of interest in activities that were once enjoyed, disrupted sleep, and weight loss or weight gain, and simple enquiries will often uncover these. However, persuading the person that they may need to seek help and attend their doctor can be problematic, given the difficulties that depressed people often experience with regard to problem solving, and the conflicting views about antidepressant drugs. A 21-item questionnaire called the Beck Depression Inventory[419] is used by healthcare professionals

---

419 www.ismanet.org/doctoryourspirit/pdfs/Beck-Depression-Inventory-BDI.pdf

to detect the presence and severity of depression, and can also be easily administered by a family member or friend.

Once depression has been diagnosed and its severity assessed, the next question is how to treat it. Antidepressants are commonly used to treat moderate or severe depression, but for people with epilepsy most antidepressants are either contraindicated or used only with great caution because of concerns that they may impair seizure control. This is based mainly on evidence that one drug, sertraline, has been shown to increase seizure frequency in 4 per cent of patients treated.[420] The benefits of antidepressants also have to be weighed against their sedative effects when they are combined with anti-epilepsy drugs.

Overall the data suggest that antidepressants have beneficial effects and are an effective treatment in people with epilepsy. However, there have been no clinical studies of the effect of duration of treatment or of the incidence of recurrence of depression once drug treatment has been discontinued. As a result, the required duration of treatment for patients with depression and epilepsy is uncertain. There are many different types of antidepressant, but the newer-generation drugs such as the selective serotonin reuptake inhibitors (SSRIs) are considered to be the safest, although little is known about their long-term effect on seizure activity.[421] The treatment of depression in epilepsy remains a grey area that requires the combined expertise of psychiatrist and epilepsy specialists in order to determine the most appropriate pharmacological and non-pharmacological interventions, such as cognitive behavioural therapy (CBT) and meditation, on an individual basis.

Chronic anxiety will affect at least 25 per cent of people with epilepsy, and presents as excessive and disproportionate worrying combined with a range of other symptoms, including restlessness, disturbed sleep, rapid intrusive thoughts, over-analysing, feelings of dread, and increased irritability. The lack of an effective screening test for chronic anxiety, and the infrequent investigation of the presence of the condition, suggest that anxiety in epilepsy may be much more common than the official figures suggest. It has been proposed that increased susceptibility to chronic anxiety is a consequence of the episodic loss of self-control associated with seizures.[422] Although several different types of psychotropic drug have been shown to be effective in treating anxiety disorders, no studies have focused specifically on epilepsy to enable evidence-based treatment of the condition. However, the SSRIs are frequently used because of their assumed short-term safety in people with epilepsy. Similarly, there are few data on non-pharmacological treatments for chronic

---

420 Kanner AM, Kozak AM and Frey M (2000) The use of sertraline in patients with epilepsy: is it safe? *Epilepsy & Behavior* 1, 100–105.
421 Cardamone L, Salzberg MR, O'Brien TJ et al. (2013) Antidepressant therapy in epilepsy: can treating the comorbidities affect the underlying disorder? *British Journal of Pharmacology* 168, 1531–1554.
422 Vazquez B and Devinsky O (2003) Epilepsy and anxiety. *Epilepsy & Behavior* 4 (Suppl. 4), S20–S25.

anxiety, such as meditation, yoga, CBT, support groups, counselling, psychotherapy, and family support.

Conclusion

Although most seizures can be partially or completely controlled by drug treatment, it is important to be prepared for the possibility that active epilepsy may persist and become lifelong. In this situation, preparation for handling the challenges of restricted employment opportunities, inability to form long-term relationships, concomitant mental health problems, social isolation, and loneliness will require an open parenting approach from the outset in order to bring the wider family and friends on board. This will ensure the establishment of a robust, understanding, and supportive network for the future. It is difficult for parents to avoid becoming stigma coaches with a tendency to blame all setbacks on prejudice when the latter may more often be perceived than real. Such beliefs and misconceptions will have lasting effects on the child with epilepsy, influencing both how they see themselves and the world around them, and how they believe society perceives them. The transition from childhood and adolescence through to adulthood sees a change in the perceptions of others that is well summed up by Charles Dickens' depictions of disability in his novels, where disabled children are angels, and disabled adults are villains. It is an uncomfortable reality that a child who is having a seizure evokes sympathy, whereas the same symptoms in an adult evoke fear and mistrust.

The real meaning of having epilepsy is often misunderstood by the very healthcare professionals who care for these patients. The medical model (the control of seizures) and the social model (the mitigation of societal consequences) rarely seem to overlap, and only the medical model can be seen to be achieving some of its aims. Sadly, epilepsy remains a low-priority condition compared with cancer, childhood disorders, and many other long-term medical conditions. So long as this remains the case, to quote Rajendra Kale once again, 'the history of epilepsy can be summarized as 4,000 years of ignorance, superstition and stigma, followed by 100 years of knowledge, superstition and stigma.'[423]

---

423 Kale R (1997) Bringing epilepsy out of the shadows. *British Medical Journal* 315, 2.

Figures and tables

Table 1

ILAE 2017 classification of seizure types

Focal onset	Generalized onset	Unknown onset
Aware Unaware	Motor Non-motor	Motor Non-motor
Motor features Abnormal jerking limb movements, spasms, and stiffening **Non-motor features** Abnormal behaviour Abnormal sensory feelings: smell, taste, memory, or tingling	**Motor features** Abnormal jerking limb movements, spasms, and stiffening **Non-motor features** Absence	**Motor features** Abnormal jerking limb movements, spasms, and stiffening Non-motor features Absence and abnormal behaviour

After Fisher RS et al. (2017) Instruction manual for the ILAE 2017 operational classification of seizure types. *Epilepsia* 58, 531–542. doi: 10.1111/epi.13671

Table 2

A simple guide to the causes of epilepsy

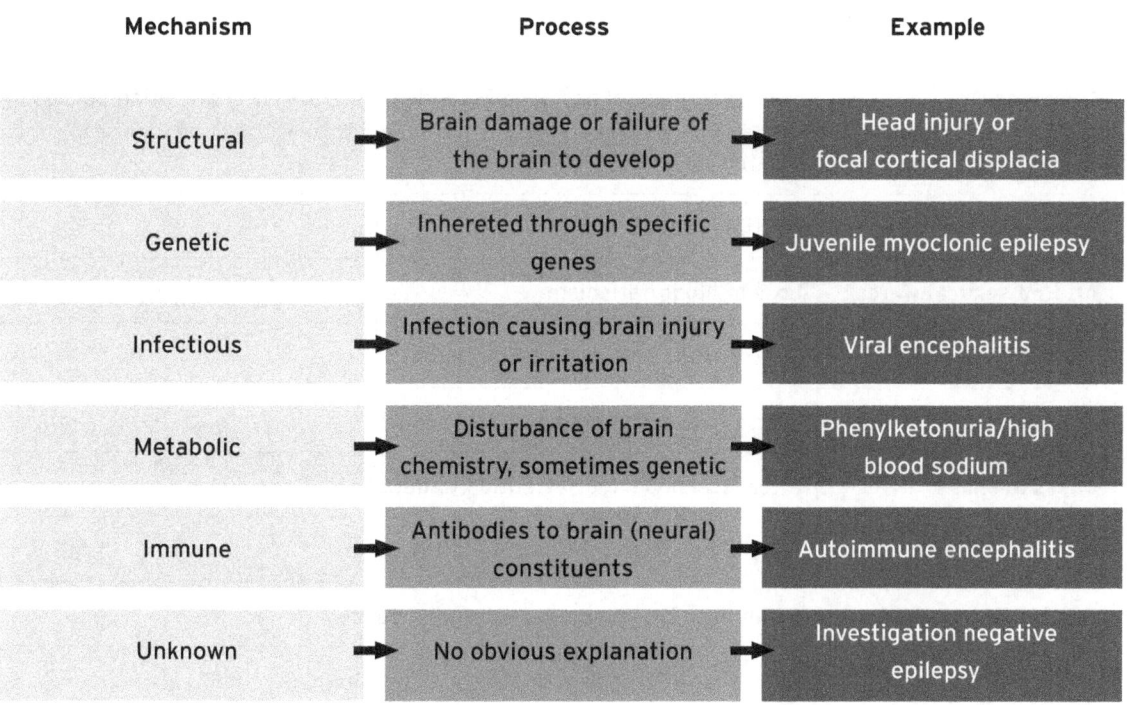

Mechanism	Process	Example
Structural	Brain damage or failure of the brain to develop	Head injury or focal cortical displacia
Genetic	Inhereted through specific genes	Juvenile myoclonic epilepsy
Infectious	Infection causing brain injury or irritation	Viral encephalitis
Metabolic	Disturbance of brain chemistry, sometimes genetic	Phenylketonuria/high blood sodium
Immune	Antibodies to brain (neural) constituents	Autoimmune encephalitis
Unknown	No obvious explanation	Investigation negative epilepsy

Table 3

Modified version of Bear and Fedio's 'epileptic personality' in people with temporal lobe epilepsy

Emotionality	Over-reactive/feelings of self-grandeur/tearful/self-deprecating/suicidal
Anger	Volatility
Aggression	Hostility/rage
Altered sexual interest	Loss of libido/fetishism
Guilt	Self-scrutiny and self-recrimination
Hypermoralism	Desire to punish perceived wrong-doers
Obsessiveness	Ritualistic behaviour/attention to detail
Circumlocution	Long-windedness/not getting to the point
Sense of destiny	Belief in personal significance/importance
Hypergraphia	Excessive writing (e.g. Dostoevsky/Van Gogh)
Religiosity	Strong religious views/involvement in cults
Dependence	Helplessness
Humourlessness	Ponderousness/lack of humour
Paranoia	Suspicion of the motives of others

Table 4

Criteria to help to determine whether or not a violent act or alleged crime was the consequence of an epileptic seizure

1. It should be established by at least two neurologists with expert knowledge of epilepsy that the person in question has the condition.
2. The person has a previous history of automatisms.
3. There is a history of aggression during previous automatisms.
4. The violent act is compatible with and characteristic of the individual's normal pattern of seizures.
5. Based on these criteria, judgement should be made by a neurologist as to whether or not the violent act or alleged crime was the result of a seizure.

*These criteria are based on the views of an expert international panel.

Table 5

Risks of sports participation in people with epilepsy

Group 1: no risk	Group 2: moderate risk excluding bystanders	Group 3: high risk including bystanders
Athletics (track)	Athletics (field)	Climbing
Most contact sports (judo/wrestling)	Archery	Diving (platform/springboard)
Baseball/hockey/football/Rugby/soccer	Canoeing	Horse riding with audience
Curling	Karate	Motor sports
Dancing	Gymnastics	Parachuting
Golf	Horse riding	Scuba diving
Tennis/squash/badminton/table tennis	Ice hockey	Solitary sailing
	Skateboarding	Wind surfing
	Snowboarding	
	Swimming	
	Water skiing	
	Weight lifting	

Modified from Capovilla G et al. (2016) Epilepsy, seizures, physical exercise, and sports: a report from the ILEA Task Force on Sports and Epilepsy. *Epilepsia* 57, 6–12.

Illustration credits

Figure 1. Image collections, National Gallery of Art, Washington, DC, USA.
Figure 2. Ralf Stephan, artist.
Figure 3. The author.
Figure 4. Dr John Greene.
Figure 5. Dr John Greene.
Figure 6. Dr Aline Russell.
Figure 7. Dr Aline Russell.
Figure 8. Dr Aline Russell.
Figure 9. British Library. © British Library Board.
Figure 10. Département Images et Prestations Numériques (Anciennement Département de la Reproduction), Bibliothèque Nationale de France, Paris.
Figure 11. Réunion des Musées Nationaux et du Grand Palais. Musée Condé, Château de Chantilly, France.
Figure 12. Museo Nacional Del Prado, Madrid.
Figure 13. Museo Nacional Del Prado, Madrid.
Figure 14. Wikimedia Commons.
Figure 15. Musée des Beaux-Arts de Nancy, Nancy, France.
Figure 16. With the acknowledgment of Stiftung Michael, Bonn, Germany.
Figure 17. Jennifer Hall.
Figure 18. Wikimedia Commons.

Acknowledgments

First and foremost I wish to thank Jo Hargreaves, development editor, without whom the translation of my jumbled thoughts into a coherent text would never have been possible. I am also indebted to the following people who, over the last three years, have provided comments and advice, and who believed in the book: Lydia Bauman, Tim Bone, Claudia Christie, Barrie Condon, Graham Cooper, Tony Fennelly, Gerard Gahagan, John Greene, Jennifer Hall, Alice Harper, Clare Harrison, Sarah Hume, Toba Kerson, Ron Lander, Gavin MacDougall, Ken McEwan, Hilary Mounfield, Janet O'Flaherty, Clare Proudfoot, Aline Russell, Bill Scott, Walter Stephen, Sir Boyd Tunnock, Nicholas Watson, Jean Williams and the late Ralph Williams, and David Wyper.

In addition I wish to thank Douglas McArthur and Ally Clark at McEwan Fraser Legal for their help with creating the website; Carol Eden; Claire Buchanan of Quarriers for support and marketing expertise; also at Quarriers, Heather Merrick, for page setting; Sharon McIntosh for graphic design; and Jan Ross of Merrall-Ross International for indexing.

The team at The Book Guild have been a pleasure to work with, and I would like to thank Jeremy Thompson, for having the confidence to publish "Sacred Lives", and Rosie Lowe, Philippa Iliffe, Hayley Russell and Jack Wedgbury for their production, editing and marketing skills.

Index

Index note: Titles of books/poems/paintings beginning with the words 'The', or 'A', are indexed under the following word, e.g. *The ABC Murders* is indexed under ABC.

1900 (1976, film) 133

Abbott, Bud (1895-1974) 214
The ABC Murders (Agatha Christie) 93
Abercrombie, Neil (1937-) 217
'absences' 52, 59
absinthe 111, 137
acceptance (by public), of epilepsy 273–274
accidents
   fatal, driving with epilepsy 189–191, 236, 239
   rates, driving 238, 239, 240
   workplace 241
accuracy of information 184
achievements, despite epilepsy 146, 177, 191, 206, 224
   see also actors; artists; famous people; musicians; writers
actors, epilepsy in 173–179
   film actors 179
   performance artist 177, 178
   stage actors 179, 180
adult epilepsy services (UK) 322
advice
   current, to people with epilepsy 325
   misplaced/wrong 84, 86

Age of Enlightenment (Age of Reason) 17–20, 21
age of onset 24
aggressive behaviour 252, 253, 269, 270
   ictal, inter-ictal and post-ictal 270
   survey, during/between seizures 304–305
   see also violence/violent behaviour
air, injecting 53
'air rage' 270
air travel, problems related to 269–270, 323–324
Akkadian texts 4
alcohol, lifestyle advice, in epilepsy 220
alcohol abuse 61, 70–71, 81, 179, 190, 214
   Alexander, Grover Cleveland 128
   Burton, Richard 179
   Hemingway, Margaux 179
   Kahlo, Frida 119
   Poe, Edgar Allan 70–71, 214, 215
   road vehicle accidents and 190
   Van Gogh, Vincent, and 111, 113
   violent behaviour/crime and 254, 264, 266
   Young, Neil 165
alcohol withdrawal, seizures 162, 179, 206, 214

Capote, Truman 216
Mussorgsky, Modest 161, 162
Peter the Great, Tsar 209
Poe, Edgar Allan 215
Swinburne, Algernon 215
alcoholism, as a disease, views of 'normals' on 280
Alexander, Grover Cleveland (1887-1950) 128
Alexander, William 28–29
'alpha wave' 51
American Breeders Association (ABA) 228
American Epilepsy Society 62
American football players 222–223
Americans with Disabilities Act (1973), USA 233
Americans with Disabilities Act (1990), USA 243
Amin, Idi 142
amygdala 95
anatomical landmarks 40–41
Andral, Gabriel (1797-1876) 79
The Andromeda Strain (1971, film) 129–130
Angelman's syndrome 126
anger 10, 24, 25, 68, 69
   Leonardo Da Vinci 110
animal magnetism 137

animal spirits, doctrine 16, 19
animals, experimental (animal models) 20, 32, 40, 49
  drug treatment testing 44, 49
'antasubbû' 4
'anthem for epilepsy' 166–167
antidepressants 332, 333
anti-epileptic drugs (AEDs)
  adverse effects 315, 322
  barbiturates *see* barbiturates
  bromides *see* bromide salts
  cessation
    in film 144–145
    in TV programme, misleading 150
  clinical trials 44–45, 322
  costs 45
  current treatment principles 45
  currently used drugs 44, 45
  development 42–43
  discovery 36, 37, 42, 49
  drug targets (receptors) 44
  failure to take, sane automatisms 273
  first used 36, 41, 42
  goals of use 315
  information availability 315
  initiation, first/second drugs 45
  lack of, in fatal prison case 305
  limited supply, in air travel 269, 270, 324
  mechanisms of action 44, 45
  need for regular use 218
  overdosing 332
  in personal account of epilepsy 315, 321, 322, 324
  relapse risk after withdrawal 322
  remission of epilepsy and driving 236, 237, 238–239
  'resistance' to 45
  selection/choice 45
  testing, animal models 43–44, 49
  see also drug treatment, of epilepsy
anti-Semitism 189, 229
antisocial behaviour 248, 267, 269, 270
anxiety
  chronic, in people with epilepsy 333–334
  of employers 296
  management 333–334
anxiety disorder 266, 267, 332, 333–334
Apollo 99
The Apprenticeship of Duddy Kravitz (1974, film) 132
  television adaptations 132

The Apprenticeship of Duddy Kravitz (Mordecai Richler) 88–89
Aretaeus of Cappadocia 7, 9
armed services/military service
  achievements, Napoleon Bonaparte 210
  Canham, Charles Edward, and 257
  invalided out, due to epilepsy 117
  prevention from joining 86, 87, 94
  prevention from taking up commission 223
  as unsuitable employment 241, 245, 283
Arnald of Villanova (1240-1311) 10–11
art 121
  advantage of epilepsy 113, 122
  see also artistic achievements, in epilepsy
  computer graphic 120
  contemporary (postmodern) 114, 122
  epilepsy depiction *see* art, works of
  interpretation, observer-dependent 122
  Metaphysical movement 116
  modern 114, 122
  public information role 122
  Renaissance 98, 99–108, 114
  Surrealist movement 116
  symbolism *see* symbolism, in art
art, works of 13, 98–122
  ancient Greek art 99
  early Christian and Renaissance 98, 99–108, 122
    Dutch/Flemish 101–102, 107–108
    German 105
    Italian 104
    Raphael's 12, 104, 107
    Rubens' 107–108
    of social commentary, precursors 107
    St Valentine associated with 105
    votive tablets, paintings 106
    wood panel painting (Bruegel) 103
  Early Latin-American art 108–110
  modern and contemporary art 114–121
  Renaissance art *vs* 114
  negative depiction of epilepsy 98, 100, 101, 102, 103, 104, 105–106, 108
  positive depiction of epilepsy 120
  realistic/graphic depictions of epilepsy 119, 120, 121
  Van Gogh's 110–113
'Art of Medicine' 9
artistic achievements, in epilepsy 113, 119, 122
  Hall, Jennifer 120–121
  Van Gogh, Vincent 111, 113
  Williams, Sir John 'Kyffin' 119
artists, with (possible) epilepsy 119, 122
  book about 120
  Chambliss, Jim 121
  Da Vinci, Leonardo 110
  de Chirico, Giorgio 116–117
  Hall, Jennifer 120–121
  Inness, George 115
  Lear, Edward 115
  Van Gogh, Vincent 110–113
  Williams, Sir John 'Kyffin' 117–118
Arts Council 178
Asclepius 99
Ashley-Cooper, Anthony 27–28
Asperger's syndrome 169, 268, 316
asthma 212
asylum(s)
  crime novels and 92
  early nineteenth century 22, 24, 25, 49
  in USA 30
  Van Gogh, Vincent in 112, 113
  Victorian era 27, 28
'Asylum for Epileptics and Epileptic Insane', Ohio, USA 30
atonic seizure 59
Atreya, epilepsy descriptions 4
attitudes to epilepsy
  in developing countries 291
  in film 123–155
  influence of literature 36
  see also public perceptions, of epilepsy
audit, healthcare of prisoners 306, 307
auditory cortex 157, 158
auditory hallucinations 112, 118, 160
  Joan of Arc 11, 207, 208
aura 6, 7, 23, 46
  in literature 76, 77, 88, 91
  seizures without 34
  types of sensations 60
  in writers 73, 74, 76, 78, 85
Australia
  discrimination legislation 243

driving accidents and guidelines 239–240
immigration to 234
Australian Disability Discrimination Act 1992 243
authors *see* writers
autism 61, 164–165, 316, 332
autobiographical accounts 85–86
　Charcot's theatre of curiosities 174
　Jobson, Richard's 218
　Waging Heavy Peace (Neil Young) 165, 166, 167
'automatic pilot' state 35, 163, 188, 248
automatisms 35, 248, 269–273
　case examples 248–249, 249–250
　　George Gershwin's 163
　　T.W. case, on a plane 269–270
　complex 248–249, 270
　　examples 248–249, 249–250
　criteria to assist courts 273, 274, 339 (Table)
　definition 35, 249
　as epileptic ecstasy 25
　false claims of, after criminal act 250, 272
　in films 124
　hystero-epilepsy *vs* 35
　ictal 270
　identification difficulties 250, 270
　inappropriate behaviour 248, 249, 250, 269, 270
　insane 271, 274
　　verdict of guilty 272–273
　lack of awareness during 35, 249, 269, 270, 272
　lack of public awareness/ understanding 250, 270
　legal classifications 271
　legal implications 25, 249
　　criminal charges 249, 250, 272, 273
　　impact on people with epilepsy 249, 250, 271
　　prosecutions for minor offences 249, 271, 272, 273
　post-ictal, homicide during 259
　prejudice and 271, 272
　range of behaviour/gestures 249
　sane (non-insane) 271, 273, 274
　simple 248, 249, 270
　sleep/other factors triggering 270, 273
　violence potential 249, 251, 252, 269, 270, 272

　danger misperception 252–253
　murders 256
autosomal dominant partial epilepsy with auditory features (ADPEAF) 118, 208
award-giving bodies, lobbying 155
awareness (during seizures)
　of imminence of attack 6, 7
　see also aura
　impaired/lack of 7
　　in automatisms 35, 249, 269, 270, 272
　　complex focal seizure 59
　　driving as hazardous 235
　　seizure classification 59
　see also confusion
awareness (public), of epilepsy *see* public awareness/understanding
Ayurvedic medicine 48
Aztecs 109
　Tlazolteotl as goddess of epilepsy 109–110, 120, 122

Babylonian cuneiform text 4
Bach, Johann Sebastian 157, 159
Bach effect 159
The Bachelors (Muriel Spark) 89
bad news, breaking 286
Baltimore Sun 253
bands, epilepsy terminology for naming 170
Barber, Ronde (1975-) 222
Barber, Tiki (1975-) 222
barbiturates 42–43
　phenobarbitone *see* phenobarbitone (phenobarbital)
　phenytoin 43, 44, 45
　barbituric acid 42
Bartholomew the English 99, 100, 330 (Fig)
baseball players, with epilepsy 127, 220–221
　film, and avoidance of term 'epilepsy' 127
Baxendale, Sallie 125, 147, 154, 169, 170, 173, 174
befriending services 331
beggars 107
behaviour
　abnormal, in people with epilepsy 267, 268
　aggressive *see* aggressive behaviour; violence/violent behaviour
　antisocial 248, 267, 269, 270
　bizarre 84
　criminal *see* criminal behaviour and

criminality
　deviant 253, 254
　disorderly 253
　involuntary *see* automatisms
　'medicalization' 58
belladonna (deadly nightshade) 118
'benefit cheats' 185, 195
benefits system, in UK 185, 194
Benin (Dahomey), attitudes to epilepsy 291
Bennett, Alexander Hughes (1848-1901) 39
bennu 4
Bentley, Derek 134–135
'Berenice' (Edgar Allan Poe) 71
Berger, Hans (1873-1941) 46, 51
Bertillon, Jacques (1851-1922) 58
'beta wave' 51
Bethel Centre, Bielefeld, Germany 29
bias, in press/news media 193
　avoidance 184
Bible, King James 13
Bicêtre Hospital, Paris 24
bicycle design, for people with epilepsy 220
The Big Sleep (Raymond Chandler) 92
bile, black, and yellow 9, 11
binge drinking 67, 71, 214
biographical accounts 91
bipolar disorder 112
birds, symbol of evil 104, 105, 114
'black blood' 69
The Black Eyed Peas 170–171
blackmail 93
Blackmore, R.D. (1825-1900) 82–83
blackouts 69, 70
Blackwell's Island Asylum, USA 30
Bleak House (Charles Dickens) 79, 80–81
blindness 137, 280
blood 9
　in brain, fatal seizures 16
blood vessels, brain, visualization 53
bloodletting 8, 9, 16, 23, 36, 73
Blunt, Nicholas 107
Blunt, Wilfred 213
body fluids 9
boiling, vapour formation 14
Bonaparte, Napoleon (1769-1821) 210–211, 251, 266
The Bone Collector (1999, film) 138–139
bone marrow donation, film 142
book(s)
　on epilepsy ix, 300
　　for parents and children 318
　　textbooks 41
　involving epilepsy *see* literature,

epilepsy in
Book of Characteristics (Bartholomew the English) 99, 100, 330 (Fig)
Book of Hours 101
Borax 37
Bosch, Hieronymus (1450-1516) 101–102, 331 (Fig)
Bouchard, Emilie Marie ('Polaire') (1874-1939) 174, 175
boxers, with epilepsy 221
'Boy in a Storm' (*Medic* TV drama) 148–149
Boyle, Susan (1961-) 169
Bragg, Melvyn 179
brain 7, 20, 57
  behaviour originating, insane automatisms 271
  development during pregnancy 57
    abnormal development 57, 61
  functional imaging, of music effect 158
  Hippocrates' theory of epilepsy 5
  infant, damage susceptibility 57, 61
  injury/damage 7, 32
    films involving epilepsy 127, 143, 147
    infants 57, 61
    personal account and self-blame 316
    Peter the Great 209
    see also head injury
  irritation, surgery 40, 41
  mapping (function localization) 26, 31–32, 33–34, 41, 327 (Fig)
    early surgery in epilepsy 38–39
    electrical stimulation during surgery 40–41, 45, 46
    Ferrier and Golzt's work 32, 38
    Horsley's work 40–41
    Hughlings Jackson's work 33–34
    Krause's work 40–41
    Macewen's work 38–39
  music processing, areas 158
  realization of origin of epilepsy in 5, 15, 16, 21
    Paracelsus' erroneous belief 14
    Tissot's view 18
    von Haller's view 19
    Willis' role 16
  scanning 50, 53, 54–58
    CT *see* computed tomography (CT)

MRI *see* magnetic resonance imaging (MRI)
scarring 47, 57
as site of seizure origin 6, 7, 11, 19, 41
surgery *see* surgical treatment
tumours 21, 35, 39, 41
  concerns about, pre-diagnosis 314
  exclusion, epilepsy diagnosis 54
  film depicting epilepsy 126–127
  Gershwin, George 163, 164
  MRI 55, 56, 57, 328 (Fig)
  in television series 151–152
  visualization techniques
    early methods 53–54
  scans *see* brain, scanning
see also specific structures/lobes
'brain pacemaker' 95
'brainstorm' 191, 254
'brainwaves' 50, 51
  measurement *see* electroencephalogram (EEG)
  Mozart effect and 158, 159
breeding, controlled 228, 229
'breeze' 6, 7, 23, 46
see also aura
British Association for Music Therapy (BAMT) 156
British Epilepsy Association 86, 140
British Eugenics Society 228
Broadbent, Sir William (1835-1907) 205, 210
Broca, Paul (1824-1880) 32
bromide salts 37, 41–42
  adverse effects 37, 42, 53–54, 73, 213
  cerebral angiography 53
  potassium bromide 36, 37, 42, 43, 112, 212
  resistance to 42, 43
'bromism' 42
Brook, Dr C 42
The Brothers Karamazov (Fyodor Dostoevsky) 77, 78, 176, 333 (Fig)
Brown, John (1735-1788) 157
Bruegel, Pieter, the Elder (1525-1569) 102, 103
Bruegel, Pieter, the Younger 103–104, 331 (Fig)
Brunonian scale 157
Brunonian system of medicine 157
Buckingham, Lindsey (1949-) 218
'burden of epilepsy', USA 297
burden on society 27, 194, 233, 234, 246

eugenics movement and 227, 228, 229, 230
burial, alive 71
Burned (Neil Young) 166
burns 73, 100
Burton, Richard (Richard Jenkins) (1929-1984) 179, 214
Byron, Lord 67

Caesar, Julius 128
campaigning 134
Canada
  driving with epilepsy 237, 238
  employment concerns 297–298
  immigration laws 233
  reporting of disability issues 193, 194
Canadian Immigration Act (1976) 233
Canadian Medical Association 237
Canham, Charles Edward 256–259
cannabidiol (CBD) oil 191–192
cannabis, medicinal 134, 191–192
Capote, Truman (1924-1984) 216
carbamazepine 137, 321
  effect on musical pitch and musicality 160
  side effects 223, 321
Care Inspectorate (Scotland) 308
Care Quality Commission 308, 309
careers
  abandonment 82, 90, 115, 220, 295, 328
  advice on choice 327
  unsuitable for people with epilepsy 220, 241, 242, 283, 300, 324, 327
  see also employment
carers/care-workers 307–309
  emotional effects on 280
  professional 308–309
    attitudes on/knowledge of epilepsy 308
    belated disclosure of epilepsy 328
    epilepsy awareness training 308, 309
  unpaid/informal 307–308
casting out evil 6, 11, 12, 13, 17
  in art 98, 104, 106
    Jesus Christ and New Testament 13, 104, 106
Castletoddy, Lord (in *Vanity Fair*) 69
catamenial epilepsy 8
cataplexy 71
catatonic state 257, 258
categories of epilepsy 34

Arnald of Villanova's 10–11
Cullen's 20
Esquirol, Jean-Étienne,
  observations 23–24
John of Gaddesden's 11
St Hildegard of Bingen's 10
see also classification of epilepsy
Catholic Church 10, 140, 217
  exorcism 108
Caton, Richard (1842-1926) 50–51
Causae et Curae (St Hildegard of Bingen) 10
causes, of epilepsy 21, 60–61
  acquired 60–61
  alcohol abuse *see* alcohol abuse
  brain tumours *see* brain, tumours
  classification of seizures and 59–60, 336 (Table)
  developmental 57–58, 61
  drugs of abuse 165, 168
  in films 126, 127, 128, 138, 139, 147
  head injuries *see* brain, injury/damage; head injury
  historical views/studies
    ancient Greek beliefs 99
    Cullen's views 20
    early nineteenth century studies 24
    Galen's views 6, 7
    Haller's views 19
    Hughlings Jackson's work 34
    Middle Ages 99–100, 102
    Paracelsus' views 14
    phlegmatic humour 9–10
    Victorian era views 26–27, 49
  investigation of *see* investigation of epilepsy
  in literature 81
  mechanism and process 337 (Table)
  neurocysticercosis 55
  parental questions 315–316
  proximate or remote 20
  unidentified 61
causes, of illnesses 5
cauterization 16, 100
Cave, Nicholas (1957-) 171
Caveness, William (1909-1981) 281
celebrities, present-day 216–217, 218, 223, 224
  'coming out', stigma reduction 294, 299
Celsus, Aulus (*c.* 25 BCE - *c.* 50 CE) 8

cerebral angiography 53, 54
cerebral cortex, development 57
Cerebri Anatome (Thomas Willis) 15–16
Cesalpino, Andrea (1519-1603) 14
Chalfont Epileptic Colony 28, 41
Chambliss, Jim 121
Chandler, Johanna (1820-1875) 28
Chandler, Raymond (1888-1959) 92
Charcot, Jean-Martin (1825-1893) 36, 40, 173–174, 174–175
'The Charge of the Light Brigade' (Tennyson) 69
charities, epilepsy x, xii, 63, 86
  actors not needing 178
  befriending services 331
  information on driving with epilepsy 236
  prize for best-informed epilepsy new story 193
  promoting message for high achievement 224
  responsible reporting, promoting 184, 193
  websites 198
  see also specific charities
Charyton, Christine 159
Chelsea Flower Show, RHS 213
Chesterton, G.K. (1874-1936) 228–229
child abuse 143
childbirth 12, 24, 30
childhood trauma 24
children
  carers of, attitudes 299
  deaths due to epilepsy 5, 15
  dietary treatment 48
  experiences shaping adulthood 326
  explaining/telling about epilepsy 317
  failure to tell about epilepsy 317, 318
  health problems in, father with epilepsy 166, 168
  Hippocrates' observation 5
  individuals with epilepsy fearful of having 70, 84, 120, 122
  individuals with epilepsy not allowed to have 18, 27, 52, 228
  personal account 313–334
  sibling relationships 320, 326, 327
China
  disability discrimination legislation 243–244
  marriage legislation 232

  stigmatization of disabled people 243, 244
  university application and medical test 243–244
Chirico, Giorgio de (1888-1978) 116–117
chloral hydrate 37, 83
chloroform 26, 39, 40, 51, 257
Chopin, Frédéric (1810-1849) 161–162
chorea 13
Christian church
  art 12, 98, 99–108
    casting-out of demon 99, 104, 106
  stigma metaphors 278
  views on epilepsy 10, 12
  see also Catholic Church
Christie, Agatha (1890-1976) 92–93
Christina the Astonishing (Christina Mirabilis) (*c.* 1150) 171–172
chronic epilepsy 7, 8, 25
Churchill, Winston (1874-1965) 229
Cider with Rosie (Laurence 'Laurie' Lee) 86
cinema films *see* film(s)
cinematography 123, 124
circumcision 18
Civil Aviation Authority 241
Clark, Leon Pierce (1870-1933) 266–267
classification of disease 58
classification of epilepsy 58–60
  Cullen's 20
  see also categories of epilepsy
classification of neurological disorders 26
classification of seizures 58–60
  key features for 59, 60
Clayton, George 69
Cleopatra (1934, and 1963, film) 128
Cleopatra, Queen, of Egypt 128
Clignet, Marion (1964-) 219–220
clinical investigation 23
clinical trials, anti-epileptic drugs 44–45, 322
The Closet Hanging (Tony Fennelly) 94
cloves, oil of 257
coaches (sports), epilepsy and 196
Cobb, Stanley (1887-1968) 43, 47
Code of Hammurabi 4
Coelho, Tony (1942-) 217
cold baths 23
Colet, Louise 74
Collins, Willkie (1824-1889) 78–79
Colony for Mercy of Epileptics 28
colony movement, epilepsy 27–36, 62
colour, use/perception, Vincent Van Gogh 113

Commission for the Control of Epilepsy and its Consequences (USA) 31
Commissioners in Lunacy 25
compassion 11, 14, 28, 52
　for disabled people with visible disabilities 194, 195
　in films 134, 135
compensation, for miscarriage of justice 187
complex focal seizure 59
complex partial epilepsy *see* temporal lobe epilepsy
composers, with epilepsy 160–173, 180
　autism and, Hikari Ōe 164–165
　Chopin, Frédéric 161–162
　Gershwin, George 163
　John, Elton 168
　Mussorgsky, Modest 162–163
　see also songwriters, with epilepsy
computed tomography (CT) 47, 54–55
　applications/uses 55, 56, 58
　development 53, 54
　MRI comparison 55, 56–57
　in personal account of child's epilepsy 314
　spatial resolution 54, 55
computer graphics 120
concealment, of epilepsy 27, 30–31, 75, 81
　by artists 116, 122
　by composers/musicians 161, 180
　Connecticut court ruling 231
　to employers 288, 295–296, 328
　by family/parents 287, 288, 289, 300
　felt stigma resulting in 287
　in films 128, 129, 130, 139, 141
　in India 232
　to overcome felt stigma 288
　by parents 287, 289, 300
　to partners/spouses 287, 288–289
　by present-day celebrities 216, 223
　in Royal Family (UK) 139
　by songwriter 168–169
　in TV drama 149, 151
　by writers 75, 81, 87, 88, 97
concentration
　drugs affecting 322
　lapse in 315
confidentiality, driving and 235, 237–238
confusion 7, 59, 124, 248, 270
　alcohol withdrawal seizures 214
　complex focal seizure 59
　in film, after seizure 145

in personal account 314, 317
　see also awareness (during seizures)
Conklin, Hugh William (1877-undated) 47–48
A Connected Society: A Strategy for Tackling Loneliness 331
Conqueror's syndrome 210
Conrad, Peter 253, 278–279, 289, 290, 326
consciousness
　level, classification of focal seizures 59
　loss 7, 12, 16
　　cause, electrical overactivity 35
　　driving hazard 235
　　in literature 69
　　recovery from 16
　　seizures without 13
　　unilateral seizures not progressing to 33
contact sports 219, 221, 222, 303
contagious nature, of epilepsy 6, 12, 23, 282, 285
Control (2007, film) 142, 168
controlled epilepsy
　driving and 235–236
　　Canada 237
　　UK 236
　　USA 238
　reporting of seizures and 240
Convulsionists of Saint Médard 16–17
convulsions *see* seizure(s)
coping strategies 289, 313
coping with epilepsy and stigma 279, 313
　parents influencing 289
Cormack, Alan (1924-1998) 54
Coronation Street (1960- , TV programme) 152, 155
cortical dysplasia 57
Costello, Lou 214
'Counterfeit Cranks' 107
courage 219, 321, 325
court cases 187–188
　automatisms and 249, 250, 270, 271, 272, 273
　　criteria for assessing 273, 274, 339 (Table)
　　sane automatism, defence of 273
　　see also automatisms
　convictions, guilty act and guilty mind 272
　defence, medical issues used 187–188, 189, 273
　fees, increase and impact 247

　insanity and defence of automatism 272
　intent to commit crime 272
　see also criminal behaviour and criminality
Cox, Henry 28–29
Craig Colony (New York) 62
'Creative Sparks' website 121
Crichton, Michael (1942-2008) 94–95, 130
cricketers, with epilepsy 219
crime
　false claims of automatisms after 250, 272
　intent to commit 272
Crime and Punishment (Fyodor Dostoevsky) 77
crime novels 92–96
criminal behaviour and criminality
　automatisms and 249, 250, 272–273, 274, 339 (Table)
　characteristics of criminals 252
　epilepsy relationship
　　epileptic equivalent theory 254
　　evidence refuting 252–253, 262
　　Goring's studies 251–252
　　low frequency 260
　epileptic, insane, and born, as criminal types 251
　historical descriptions 250–251
　'not guilty by reason of insanity' (NGRI) cases 265–266, 272–273
　petty criminal behaviour 266
　television programmes 150, 152
　see also court cases; murder and homicide; violence/violent behaviour
criminal degenerates 92, 251
criminology 251
'cripple', use of term 195
Critchley, MacDonald (1900-1997) 159
crows 114
The Crucible (1996, film) 129
Cullen, William (1712-1790) 19–20, 26
The Cure of Folly (Hieronymus Bosch) 101–102, 331 (Fig)
Curtis, Deborah 168–169
Curtis, Ian (1956-1980) 142, 168–169
Cushing, Harvey (1869-1939) 45
custody, deaths in 307
Cuyp, Benjamin 102
cybercrime 200
cyclists, with epilepsy 219–220

Da Vinci, Leonardo (1452-1519) 110,

216
Daily Beast (US), vehicle accident report 190
Dalhousie University, Nova Scotia, studies 199, 201, 202, 203
Damadian, Raymond (1936-) 55
The Dance of St John or St Vitus (Pieter Bruegel) 103
dancing mania 103–104
dancing over a bridge 103
Dando, Jill 186, 187
Dandy, Walter (1886-1946) 53
dangers, of epilepsy 90
  to others, misperception 252, 261, 266, 273–274, 305
    epileptic personality and 268–269
    excessive restrictive regulations 230
    murder and homicide 261, 262, 263, 265
    see also violence/violent behaviour, and epilepsy
'dark illness' 74
Darwin, Leonard (1850-1943) 228
Davenport, Charles (1866-1942) 228
David B 96
David Copperfield (Charles Dickens) 81
DDA *see* Disability Discrimination Act 1995 (UK)
de Chirico, Giorgio (1888-1978) 116–117
De Epilepsia (Arnald of Villanova) 10
Deadwood (2004-2006, TV programme) 151–152
death(s)
  causes, in epilepsy 15
  children, due to epilepsy 5, 15
  in custody 307
  in prison, after seizures 305
  transient in seizure, link to Christ's resurrection 104–105
  see also murder and homicide
death metal 172
death penalty 12
debauchery 18, 24
Deceiver (1997, film) 137–138
definition of epilepsy
  Hughlings Jackson's 34, 58
  in media/press 197
degeneration theory 251
degenerative diseases 61
deities 106, 109, 110
déjà vu 46, 60, 175
Delasiauve, Louis Jean (1804-1893) 259–260

delirium tremens 162, 214, 215
Dell, J.L. 278
delusional state 255
dementia 173, 195
'the Demon' (Lear's reference to) 82
'demonic', word in news stories about epilepsy 193
demons, possession by *see* possession, by gods/demons
denial of epilepsy 91
depersonalization 70
depression 266, 272, 329, 331, 332
  detecting 332–333
  symptoms 331, 332
  treatment and duration of 329, 333
  Vincent Van Gogh 111, 112, 122
derealization 70
derogatory language *see* pejorative language
descriptions of epilepsy
  Galen's 7
  historical *see* history of epilepsy
  Priscianus' 7
desertion of family, due to epilepsy 177
despair 177, 329
destigmatizing epilepsy *see* stigma/stigmatization, reducing
DeToledo, John 30
developing countries
  discrimination 277
  inaccurate perceptions of epilepsy 227
  incidence of epilepsy 290, 291
  teachers' knowledge 301
developmental disorders 57–58, 61
deviant behaviour 253, 254
devil, epilepsy association, in art 105–106, 109
Deyn, Agyness 143, 145
diabetes mellitus 7, 271
diagnosis of epilepsy
  confusion about 290
  disclosure *see* disclosure of diagnosis
  early, improved outcome 316–317
  impact of 84, 85, 279, 286
    patients' feelings 290
  in literature 90
  personal account 314, 316–317, 318
  relief on 222, 286, 290
  re-negotiating/uncertainty 286
Dickens, Charles (1812-1870) 36, 67, 76, 79–81, 107, 334
  source of knowledge on epilepsy

79
Dickinson, Emily (1830-1886) 83–84
dietary therapy 10
  fasting, history of 11, 47–48
  foods avoided 48
  ketogenic (starvation) diet 43, 47–48
  'water diet' 47
Different Strokes (1978-1986, TV drama) 150–151
'differentness' 277, 278, 299, 326
digitalis 13, 112, 113
dilantin 216
diminished responsibility, plea 252, 262
disability, and disabled people 11–12, 36, 79, 80
  in age of austerity in UK (2007-2008) 194
  as burden on society 246
  Charles Dickens' depictions 334
  definition 243, 244, 245, 246
  discrimination prevention legislation 243
  disenfranchized, by digital communications 198
  eugenics movement and 227, 228
  'hidden' x, 193, 195
  legislation impact 227
  misrepresentation in films/TV 155
  negative perceptions/reporting in press 185, 193
  press articles on, numbers 194–195
  reduced derogatory language over time 185
  reporting, Israel *vs* Canada 193, 194
  state benefits for those living with 185
  'unseen', lack of empathy/support for x, 193, 195
Disability Discrimination Act 1995 (UK) 243, 244
  claims made, number 245
  Equality Act 2010 replacing 242, 243, 245
  limitations 244, 245, 246
  medical evidence to prove disability 244
  obstacles in making a claim under 244, 245
  occupations not covered by 245
  workplace adjustments 298
Disability Rights Commission (DRC)

245
discharge, seizures 20, 34
  music therapy effect 48–49
disclosure of diagnosis
  to colleagues, caution 328
  failure to, employment 288, 328
  felt stigma reduced by 290
  to friends/partners 287, 329
  in job applications 296–297, 298, 328
  by prisoners 307
discrimination x, 279
  by education providers 300
  in employment 242, 243, 244–245, 326
    enforcement of Equality Act 2010 245, 247
    obtaining/keeping work 242–243
    proving, and misunderstanding of risks 244
    see also Disability Discrimination Act 1995 (UK)
  immigration and 233
  in India 277
  institutional 245
  interviewee comments 279
  legislation preventing 243, 244
  overt, hidden, indirect or legal 279–280
  prevention, in film/TV 155
  in recreational activities 233
  reducing, in South Africa 219
  sportsmen/women 219, 220
  stigma and social isolation linked to 278
  see also prejudice
disease transmission, prevention 228
disempowering, people with epilepsy 278
disfigurement 80, 90
The Disquieting Muse (Giorgio de Chirico) 117
dissocial behaviour 268
distraction strategies 48
'divine evil' 13
divine intervention 11, 13, 14
divine origin, of epilepsy 5, 9
  Hippocrates rejection of 5
divorce 232
doctors, reporting to driving authorities 236, 237, 240
dogs, seizure alert 142
domestic abuse 259
dopamine 159
Dostoevsky, Fyodor (1821-1881) 36, 76–78, 163, 176, 268, 333 (Fig)
Doussin-Dubreuil, Jacques-Louis (1762-1831) 24
Doyle, Joe (1939-2009) 217
Dr Kildare (1961-1966, TV programme) 149, 155
dramatic presentations see theatre, epilepsy in
'dreamy state' 34
drive, right to 235–241
Driver and Vehicle Licensing Agency (DVLA) 189, 236
  classes/groups of drivers 237
  guidelines for medical practitioners 236–237
  informing about epilepsy 236
driving (people with epilepsy)
  accident rates 238, 239
    Australia 239–240
    Canada 238
    UK 237, 239
    USA 239
  bad, epilepsy association illogical 190
  commercial vehicles 237, 283
  controlled epilepsy, safe to drive 235–236
  dangerous 235, 236
    not due to epilepsy 189
  employment requiring 236, 244–245, 283, 327
  fatal/serious accidents 189–191, 236, 239
  film depiction 132
  guidelines
    Australian 240
    British 236–237
    Canadian 237, 238
  hazardous activity 235
  legal aspects and public perceptions 189
  legislation/regulations 191, 230, 235–236
    Australia 240
    Canada 237, 238
    time since last seizure 236, 237, 238
    UK 189, 236, 237
    USA 238
    variation between countries 230
  poorly controlled epilepsy 238–239
  press and public perceptions of risk 189, 190, 235
  prevention/licence loss 219, 222
  responsible attitude of people with epilepsy 190, 238
  right to drive 235–241
  sportsmen/women with epilepsy 219, 220, 222
  of trains 241
  TV depiction 152
  uncontrolled epilepsy 236
driving licence
  Australia 239, 240
  Canada 237
  in job descriptions, and discrimination 244–245
  loss 219, 220, 222
  UK 236, 237
drop attacks 59
drug development, process 44–45
drug resistance 45
drug treatment, of epilepsy
  current treatment principles 45
  seizure number before and impact 315
  twentieth century 41–45
  Victorian era 36–37
  see also anti-epileptic drugs (AEDs)
drugs of abuse 165, 168, 214
Drugstore Cowboy (1989, film) 129, 147
Du Camp, Maxime 74
DVLA see Driver and Vehicle Licensing Agency (DVLA)

earthquakes 14
Eastenders (1985-) (TV programme) 153, 154, 155
Eastman, George 124
Echeverria, Gonzalez 256
'ecstatic aura' 78
Edison, Thomas (1847-1931) 124
Edmonton Epilepsy Association of Northern Alberta 216
education 299–303
  of children with epilepsy 299–303
  discrimination unlawful in 299–300
  at Epilepsy Centre Bethel, Bielefeld, Germany 29
  poor, demonic possession belief 17
  of prison officers 306
  of public see public education
  of teachers, about epilepsy 300, 302, 303, 304
  see also schools; teachers
Edwards, John Passmore (1823-1911) 28
EEG see electroencephalogram (EEG)

eggs 12
egotism 266
Eichenwald, Kurt 200
'El Bosco' (Hieronymus Bosch) 101–102
electrical activity of brain 50
  measurement *see*
    electroencephalogram (EEG)
electrical discharge *see* discharge, seizures
electrical inhibition 35
electrical overactivity, concept 34, 35
  anti-epileptic drug action 44
electrical stimulation, of brain 40–41, 45, 46
Electricity (2014, film) 90, 143–146, 147, 177
Electricity (Ray Robinson, novel) 90–91, 143
electrodes, insertion in brain, novel 95
electroencephalogram (EEG) 46, 50–52, 54
  diagnosis of epilepsy by 52
  driving safety/ability 238
  in focal, and general epilepsy 329 (Fig)
  George, Barry 186
  history of development 51–52, 51–53
  music effect on temporal lobe epilepsy 158
  recent advances 52–53
  Ruby, Jack 188
  seizure classification/types 58–59
  violent/deviant behaviour and 254
    murderers 254, 261–262
  Young, Neil (songwriter/musician) 166
Elementa Medicinae (John Brown) 157
Eliot, George 72
embarrassment x, 139, 196, 250, 290, 295, 327
Emery, John 68
emetics 8, 16
Emmerdale (TV programme) 154
emotion(s) x
  cause of epilepsy 10, 20, 24, 34
  response to visual images, Vincent Van Gogh 113
emotional arousal, musicogenic epilepsy 160
employers
  of care staff, epilepsy awareness training 308, 309
  concerns about employees 297, 298, 299
  education programmes 298, 299
  liability 241

prejudice by 295, 297
employment 295–299
  1950s (UK) 295
  1960s (UK) 295–296
  2000s (UK and North America) 298
  application/appointment process 296–297, 298, 328
  barriers to 295, 296, 297, 298
  in China 243
  concealment of epilepsy 288, 295–296, 328
  conference in UK (1985) 296–297
  declaration of epilepsy in applications 242, 243
  difficulties in obtaining/keeping 241, 279, 280, 296, 297, 328
    nursing profession case 242
    in personal account 322
  discrimination in *see* discrimination
  dismissals due to epilepsy 295, 328
    protection against 242, 328
  entrenched attitudes 298
  hazards (genuine, perceived and anxiety) 296
  improving attitudes 298, 299
  law *see* legislation
  prejudice against people with epilepsy 241, 295–296, 297
  requiring driving 236, 244–245, 283, 327
  as teacher, concerns 326–327
  tribunals 245
  types of 295, 296
  unsuitable occupations for people with epilepsy 220, 241, 242, 283, 300, 324, 327
  USA study (1978), and improved attitudes 297
  see also unemployment
encephalitis 60–61, 209, 316
energy, abnormal, in brain 19
entertainers, mimicking seizures 174
environmental factors, seizure trigger 61
epilepsy
  causes *see* causes, of epilepsy
  definition *see* definition of epilepsy
  diagnosis *see* diagnosis of epilepsy
  as disability 230
  as a disease, history of 5–6, 13, 22
    Paracelsus 14
    Van Swieten, Gerald 18
  as disease of grey matter 34–35

as lifelong 334
not a single disease 35
origin of term 3
as a symptom, causes 34, 35, 50
when to tell a child 317
Epilepsy, Leaving Behind the Nightmare (Eduardo Urbano Merino) 120
Epilepsy Across the Spectrum (IOM document) 183
Epilepsy Action 154, 184, 191, 217
  driving with epilepsy and 236
  survey on loneliness/social isolation 330–331
  training video for firearms officers 307
Epilepsy Action Australia 219
Epilepsy Association of Scotland 193
Epilepsy Centre Bethel, Bielefeld, Germany 29
epilepsy cerebralis 20
epilepsy colony movement 27–36
  Chalfont Epileptic Colony (UK) 28
  USA 30–31
Epilepsy Foundation (of America) 149, 150, 190, 223, 282, 297
  Community Forum 330
  cyberattack 200
  Epilepsy Hall of Fame 214
Epilepsy Foundation Eastern Pennsylvania 307
'epilepsy metaphors', Peter Wolf's research 97
'epilepsy movement' 62, 63
epilepsy occasionalis 20
Epilepsy Scotland 222
epilepsy societies, development 62–63
Epilepsy Society (UK) 145, 152, 153
  cyberattack and GIFs 200
  Embroidered Minds Epilepsy Garden 213
Epilepsy Society of Australia 240
Epilepsy South Africa 219
epilepsy sympathetica 20
Epilepsy Today (newsletter) 153–154
Epileptic (David B) 96
'epileptic', pejorative use 185, 187, 189, 190, 191, 192, 193, 204
  about sportsman 221
  by Ministry of Justice (UK) 307
'epileptic boy', casting out unclean spirits 13, 104, 107–108
epileptic ecstasy 25
'epileptic equivalent' theory 253–254
epileptic equivalents 254
'epileptic furor' 250–251, 260

'epileptic homicide', term 258, 260
'epileptic insanity' 24–25
'epileptic mania' 251, 258
'epileptic personality' 10, 24, 73, 266–269, 338 (Table)
  de Chirico, Giorgio 117
  features 266–267, 268
  lack of evidence for 268
  negative perceptions of 267, 268–269
  origin and criteria of concept 266–267
  Poe, Edgar Allan and 215
  Swedenborg, Emanuel 116
  Van Gogh, Vincent 113
epileptic singers (*gommeuses épileptiques*) 174, 175
Epilepticus Sic Curatubitur 100, 330 (Fig)
l-epileptique sauteuse (the epileptic leaper) 174
episodic dyscontrol syndrome 254
Equality Act 2010 (UK) 242, 243, 245, 247, 299
  funding and enforcement limitations 245, 247
Equality and Human Rights Commission (EHRC) 245, 246
ergot 16
Ernst, Max (1891-1976) 116
erroneous beliefs 14
Esquirol, Jean-Étienne (1772-1840) 22–23, 23–24, 25
'essential epilepsy' 18
Eugenical Sterilization Law (1914) 30
Eugenics and Other Evils (G.K. Chesterton) 228–229
eugenics movement and eugenicists 27, 227–230
  conferences 228
  criticisms and defence of 228
  development and early eugenicists 27, 228
  eugenics definition 227–228
  false claim of inherited disease 228, 229, 230
  Galton (Francis) and 27, 228
  Germany 27, 52, 185, 228, 229, 230
  sterilization (compulsory) 30, 185, 229, 230
  USA 52, 61, 229
Eugenics Record Office 228, 229
The Eugenics Review 228
Eugenics Society 228
eulogy 91
Euripides (Greek playwright) 67

Europe, epilepsy centres 29
euthanasia 151, 152, 193
Evans, Margiad (1909-1958) 85–86
Evans, Mary Ann (George Eliot) (1819-1880) 72
excitability of cells 44
excitation, nervous system 26
excitement, seizures triggered by 87
execution 135
exercise, seizure frequency reduction 303
exhaustion 75–76
exorcism 4, 10, 12, 13
  Catholic Church 108, 140, 141
  in film 140, 141
  paintings/art 100, 106, 108
  see also casting out evil
The Exorcism of Emily Rose (2005, film) 140–141
'expert patients' 284
expert witnesses 188, 189
  murder/homicide cases, disagreements 188, 255, 256, 258, 261
  unchallenged power in court cases 258
experts, on epilepsy xi
  advice/support for films 145, 147, 155
  disability discrimination cases 244
  see also psychiatrists
extermination of people 229
The Extraction of the Stone of Madness (The Cure of Folly) (Hieronymus Bosch) 101, 102, 331 (Fig)

Fabing, Howard 277
Facebook 197, 198, 199, 204
facial tic 209
'falling evil' 12
The Falling Sickness (Owsei Temkin) 3–4, 106
falling sickness/disease 4, 12
  in literature 67, 77, 90
  St Valentine, false link 105
familial epilepsy 24, 61, 83
family
  asymmetric relationship with children 326, 327
  burden of epilepsy 212–213, 326
  concealment of diagnosis 287, 288, 289
  loneliness risk discussions 332
  needs of all children within 326, 327
  relationships explored in literature 91

  social isolation/loneliness intervention 331
  stigmatization/discrimination 279–280
  what/who/when to disclose to 318, 319–320
  see also parents
famous people, with epilepsy 110, 205–224
  Americans 217
  erroneous claims 205, 206, 224
  historical figures 206–216, 224
  myths surrounding 216
  politicians and governors 217
  popular musicians/song-writers 218
  present-day 'celebrities' 216–217, 218, 223, 224
  sportsmen/women 218–223, 224
  unsubstantiated 'famous names' 206, 211, 212
  see also actors; artists; poets; writers
Fascism, Spain 87
Fascist Party, Italy 133
'Father of the American Landscape' (George Inness) 115
fear
  of child being treated differently 319
  of epilepsy and other conditions 85, 146
  of having children with epilepsy 70, 84, 120, 122
  inexplicable, feelings, personal account 317
  of public reaction 31
  of stigma, in TV programme 149
  sudden, Vincent Van Gogh 112
  of violence, stigma persistence 305
  in witnesses of seizures 276
febrile convulsions 57, 61, 211
'feeble-minded'/'feeble-mindedness' 69, 228, 229, 230
  criminals, and reproduction regulation 252
  definition 229
  marriage prevention 31, 230, 231
'feelings', term for attacks 317, 318, 320
Fennelly, Tony (1945-) 94
Fenton, George 261
Fenwick, Peter 206
Ferrier, David (1843-1928) 32, 38, 39
Fight for Life (1987, film) 134
film(s) 123–147, 154
  actors with epilepsy 178–179, 180

advice/support of experts 145, 147, 155
biographical 142
development/invention 123–124
epilepsy charity input for 145
filming of seizures, *Involuntary Dances* 177–178
independent 146
industry, lobbying 155
public information 146
television *see* television films, depicting epilepsy
film depiction of epilepsy/seizures 126, 147, 154
concealment of epilepsy 128, 129, 130, 139, 141
for criminal gain 129
driving with epilepsy 132
employment and 130, 132
faked death 137–138
false seizures 129, 147
first depiction of fit
in animated film 126
in silent film 124
impact of epilepsy on lifestyle 142, 143, 144
in *Involuntary Dances* show 177, 178
loss of right to control over body 141
male *vs* female characters 147, 154
murder or homicide in 132, 137, 138
negative depiction 89, 128, 131–132, 139, 147
abandonment 133, 144
attitudes in East Africa 142
dysfunction of young man 137, 138
hopelessness 127
impedance of career 128, 130
as personality flaw and burden 131, 132
possession by demons/devil 129, 140, 141, 147
prejudices 125, 130, 138, 142
psychiatrist's opinion 138
relationship failure 127, 131–132, 142
separation from community/family 139, 140
as sign of impurity 136
as victim of condition 142

vulnerability 128, 136, 137, 144, 145, 147
organization to campaign for rights 132
from patient's perspective 139
of poorly controlled epilepsy 142, 143, 145
positive depiction 132, 281
accurate depiction 126–127, 136, 143, 145
compassionate 134, 135
education of public 145
empathy, redemption 138–139
musical talent and lasting impression 142
'people power' and campaigning 134
as role model 146
reviews 125, 146–147, 154
seizure experience shared by viewers 143
seizures as vehicle to shock viewer 133, 146, 154
social aspects of epilepsy 131, 146
stereotypes 125, 138, 154
surgery, and overcoming disability 133–134
of temporal lobe epilepsy 126, 137–138, 140, 141
financial costs, of immigrants with epilepsy 233, 234
firearms officers 307
firemen 220, 241, 283
first aid 68
ictal aggressive behaviour and 270
inappropriate practices 89, 148, 177, 281, 319
in schools 319
in television programmes 148
training of care workers 308
training of prison officers 306
First Lines of the Practice of Physic (William Cullen) 20
Fishelson, David (1956-) 176
A Fitful Life (Tim Bone) 313
fitness, question of, for US Supreme Court 196–197
fitness to drive 230, 237
fits *see* seizure(s)
FLAIR image 57
Flaubert, Gustave (1821-1880) 73–76, 206
George Sand's friendship 75–76
flights, problems related to 269, 270, 323, 324

flying and pilot's licence 240–241
focal cortical dysplasia (FCD) 57, 61, 328 (Fig)
focal epilepsy 59, 60
EEG 329 (Fig)
management 60
focal seizures 26, 34, 59
classification 59, 336 (Table)
complex 59
in literature 70, 72, 80
with secondary generalization 59, 80, 209
simple 59
symptoms 34
in writers 74
Foerster, Otfrid 46
"folk devil" 195
Fontana, Abbé Felice (1730-1805) 20
foods, avoidance 48
footballers, with epilepsy 217, 223, 224
Forbes, Leslie 212, 213
Ford Motor Company 241
Forster, Frank 188
'the Fourth Estate' 184
Frame, Janet (1924-2004) 88
France
attitude to epilepsy in cyclist 220
epilepsy centre 29
'fraudsters', use of term 195
Freedom of Information (FOI) Act 2000 246, 306, 308
freedom of movement 233–235
between countries 233–235
within USA 233
see also immigration, legislation
Freud, Sigmund 36
Friedlander, Walter 68
friends
school 318, 323
social isolation/loneliness intervention 329, 330, 331, 332
telling, about epilepsy 318
friendships 329, 330
'From the Storm' (artwork collection) 120
frontal lobe epilepsy, murderer 262
fugue state 71
funding/funds
epilepsy centres/charities 28, 178
Equality Act 2010 enforcement 245, 247
lack, developing countries 291, 292
public education about epilepsy 285, 286

research 43, 217
'funny turns' 50, 289
'furor epilepticus', concept 250–251, 260
fury, epileptic 24

Galen (*c.* 130-210 CE) 6–7, 9
Galium album (lady's bedstraw) 29
Gallup, George (1901-1984) 280–281
Galton, Francis (1822-1911) 27, 228
gambling 214–215
Gastaut H 113
Gauguin, Paul 111
Geigerfeld, Hans Georg 105
gender imbalance, epilepsy 24
generalized epilepsy 59, 60
  EEG 329 (Fig)
  management 60
  SUDEP linked to 325
generalized (bilateral) seizures 33, 34, 59, 336 (Table)
  features 59–60
  Napoleon Bonaparte 210–211
  in writers 85
genetic factors 18, 61, 83, 315
genius 78, 205, 210, 224, 251
George, Barry 186–187
George Sand (Amantine Lucile Aurore Dupin) (1804-1876) 75–76
Germany
  epilepsy centres 29
  epilepsy surgery 41
  eugenics movement 27, 52, 185, 228, 229–230
Gershwin, George (1898-1937) 163–164
Geschwind, Norman 267
Geschwind's syndrome 267
ghosts 175
Gignoux, Régis (1816-1882) 115
global campaign 62, 291–292
global problem 290–292
Glover, Danny (1946-) 179
glucose 43, 48
glycerine 83
Godlee, Sir Rickman (1849-1925) 38–39
Goffman, Erving (1922-1982) 278, 280, 284, 309
Gogh, Vincent van *see* Van Gogh, Vincent
Golda's Balcony 176
Goldberg Variations (Johann Sebastian Bach) 157
Golzt, Friedrich (1834-1902) 32
la gommeuse épileptique (the gummy epileptic) 174

gommeuses épileptiques (epileptic singers) 174, 175
Goring, Charles Buckman (1870-1919) 251–252
Gospels, of New Testament 13, 104, 106
Gowers, Sir William (1845-1915) 35, 251
'grand mal' 6, 7, 23, 59
  in literature 77
  in rugby player 222
Grant, Colin (1961-) 91–92
graphic art 120
graphic books 96
graphic interchange format (GIF) 200
'Great Disease' 6
Great Expectations (Charles Dickens) 81
Greek tragedies 173
Greeks, ancient 5–9
  art 99
  history of epilepsy 5–6
  treatment of epilepsy 6–7
  trepanning (trephining) 37–38
Green, Anne 15
green, colour symbolizing hope 104
Greene, Dai (1986-) 220
Greene, Graham (1904-1991) 84–85
Greig, Tony (1946-2012) 219
grey matter
  epilepsy as disease of 34–35
  focal cortical dysplasia 57
  insanity as impairment of 26
  instability/lesions, seizures due to 34
  MRI 57
Grove, Valerie 86, 87
Guardian newspaper 191–192
guilt, feeling about child 316
Gunn, John 260, 261
gymnastics 300

Habans, Jean-Paul ('Paulus') (1845-1908) 174
Hall, Jennifer 120–121, 333 (Fig)
Hall, John (Shakespeare's son-in-law) 68, 69
Haller, Albrecht von (1708-1777) 20
hallucinations 207
  auditory *see* auditory hallucinations
  de Chirico, Giorgio 116, 117
  musical 118
  olfactory *see* smell, seizures and
  Prince (Prince Rogers Nelson) 167
  Van Gogh, Vincent 111, 112
  visual *see* visual hallucinations
Hamlet (William Shakespeare) 69
'Hammer of Witches' 11, 12

hand movement, brain mapping 46
handwriting 73–74
Harle, Jonathan 17
Harman, Thomas (*fl.* 1547-1567) 107
Harvard Epilepsy Commission 43
Hauptmann, Alfred (1881-1948) 42–43
Having Epilepsy: the Experience and Control of Illness (Joseph Schneider and Peter Conrad) 253, 278–279, 289, 290
Haward, Dr F 42–43
head injury
  boxing and 220
  cause of epilepsy 20, 21, 24, 34, 38, 40, 60
  empathy increase (USA) 281
  in literature 79, 93
  in rugby 220, 303
  in sportsmen 219, 220, 303
  in TV programme 150
  of writer 82, 86
  see also brain, injury/damage
headaches, George Gershwin's 163, 164
health information 183
  on Internet 197–198, 199, 204
  on social media, limited 198, 199, 200, 204
  Twitter 199, 200
  YouTube 201
healthcare insurance, USA 234
healthcare professionals, 'wish list', developing countries 292
'healthy immigrant effect' 234
Hemingway, Margaux (1955-1996) 179
herbal remedies 11, 16, 23
  ancient Greek and Roman period 6–7
  Aztec use 109
  European Renaissance 100
  at French epilepsy centre 29
  for Williams, Sir John 'Kyffin' 118
Hereditary Genius (Francis Galton) 27
hereditary nature of disease 5
  epilepsy 16, 18, 61, 83, 84, 315
  false claims 84, 228, 229, 230
Heredity in Relation to Eugenics (Charles Davenport) 228
Hermeticism, theory of 14
hidden disability x
'high evil' (epilepsy) 94
The High Evil (Georges Simenon) 94
Hill, Sir Denis (1913-1982) 261
Hippocrates 5–6, 8, 9
history of epilepsy 1–63, 277
  Age of Enlightenment 17–20
  ancient civilizations 3–4

ancient Greeks 5–9
ignorance, superstition and stigma 277
medieval period (c. 500-1500 CE) 9–17, 99–100, 102
  religious beliefs 9, 10, 11
  scientific (humoral) view 9, 10
  witchcraft and 10, 11–12
nineteenth century, early 22–26
Roman period 6
twentieth century 41–49
Victorian era see Victorian era
Hoenheim, Philippus von (Paracelsus) (1493-1571) 13–14
holidays, in personal account 323
Hollyoaks (TV programme) 154
Homage to Vincent Van Gogh (painting) 114
homeless person with epilepsy 93
homicide see murder and homicide
'homunculus' 46, 327 (Fig)
hope, with understanding 177
Hopkins, Anthony 285, 286
Hopkins, Katie (1975-) 223–224
Horovitz, Adam (1966-) 218
Horsley, Sir Victor (1857-1916) 40
hospital(s), epilepsy 27–36
  in Ohio, USA 30
  in Pennsylvania, USA 31
  Victorian era (UK) 27–28
hospitalization, of patients 22, 23
hotels 233
Hounsfield, Sir Godfrey (1919-2004) 54
House M.D. (television programme) 148
Hughes, John 206, 209, 211, 216
human rights 235, 246
  concerns, in developing countries 291
  to drive a vehicle 235–241
    see also driving
  to freedom from discrimination 243
    see also discrimination
  to freedom of movement 233–235
    see also freedom of movement; immigration, legislation
  to marry 230–232
    see also marriage
  to work 241–246
    legislation in UK 243, 244, 245, 246
    see also employment; legislation
humanist view 121
humiliation 86
'humoral constitutionalism' 9, 13

humoral theory of disease 9, 10, 21
humorism 9
humours, four 5, 9, 10, 13
hurdler, with epilepsy 220
Huxley, Julian (1887-1975) 228
Huys, Pieter 102
hyacinth 99, 100–101
Hyakinthos 99
hypergraphia (excessive writing) 112, 113, 116, 117, 267, 268, 333 (Fig)
hypersensitiveness 266
hypnosis 137
hyposexuality 73, 267
hysteria 8, 17, 18, 35, 175
  epilepsy coexistence 35, 205
  epilepsy confused with 74, 171, 175
    Flaubert, Gustave 73, 74
    paintings 103, 106, 108, 122
  epilepsy distinguished from 26, 35
    by Charcot 36, 174, 175
  features of 36
'hysterical epilepsy' 210
'hystero-epilepsy' 35

iconography 12
idiopathic epilepsy 20, 26
The Idiot (Fyodor Dostoevsky) 77, 176
illiteracy, in China 243
Illness as Metaphor (Susan Sontag) 275
illustrations, of books 107
  Aztec drawings in codices 109
image, importance for celebrities 223
imagery, confused, in early film of seizure 124
imaging see brain, scanning
immigration, legislation
  to Australia 234
  to Canada 233
  to UK 235
  undesirability of people with epilepsy 233, 234
  to USA 234–235
Immigration Act (1903), USA 234
Immigration Health Surcharge (IHS), UK 235
impulse control disorder 254
impulsive behaviour 263
Incas, names for epilepsy 108
incidence of epilepsy
  Esquirol's studies 24
  Scotland, Victorian era 28
  USA 31, 52
  see also prevalence of epilepsy
indecent behaviour 249–250
India

disability discrimination legislation 243
discrimination 277
marriage legislation 232
Indian Epilepsy Association 232
infant brain, damage susceptibility 57, 61
infections
  after surgery 39
  epilepsy cause 60–61
information dissemination, by social media 197–198, 199
inheritance, of epilepsy see hereditary nature of disease
inhibition, nervous system 26
injuries
  head/brain see brain, injury/damage; head injury
  seizure-related 86
injustices 72
Inness, George (1825-1894) 115
The Innocents, film adaptation of novella 175
insanity 8, 23, 25, 26, 205
  epilepsy as, decrease in perception (1949-1979) 281
  homicide associated 255, 257, 258, 265, 266
  not guilty by reason of 265–266, 272
insomnia 157
Institute of Medicine (IOM) 293, 294
institutions, for people with epilepsy
  asylums see asylum(s)
  early nineteenth century 22, 23, 25
  Europe 29
  USA 29–30, 31, 62
  Victorian era 27
  see also hospital(s), epilepsy; residential care
The Insulted and Injured (Fyodor Dostoevsky) 77
insurance 130, 234
'inter-ictal activity' 51
inter-ictal antisocial behaviour 270
'interictal dysphoric disorder' 73
'inter-ictal personality disorder' 267–268
inter-ictal state, personality traits 267
International Brigades 87
International Bureau for Epilepsy (IBE) 62, 291–292
International Hygiene Exhibition 228
International League Against Epilepsy (ILAE) 59, 62, 147, 154, 291–292
  guidelines on sports 304

Mexican branch, logo 110
prize for best-informed epilepsy news story 193
Internet 197–203
  health information 197–198, 199, 204
  key messages for public education 294
  as news source 184
  use related to epilepsy 198–199
  see also social media
interviews, with people with epilepsy
  developing countries 292
  UK (Scambler & Hopkins) 285–288
  USA (Paschal et al) 284–285
  USA (Schneider & Conrad) 278–279, 289
  see also surveys
investigation of epilepsy 50–58
  aims 50
  brain scanning 53–58
    CT 54, 55, 56, 58
    MRI 56, 57, 58
  brain visualization, early methods 53–54
  EEG *see* electroencephalogram (EEG)
  resource-rich countries 54
involuntary behaviour *see* automatisms
Involuntary Dances (show) 177–178
iodide, contrast agent 54
Iphigenia among the Taurians (Euripides) 173
Irish moss 118
The Irish Times, vehicle accident report 189–190
irritability (personality) 25
'irritability', as concept (of nervous system) 19, 20, 21
Islam, founder of 206–207
isolated life *see* social isolation; solitary life
Israel, reporting of disability issues 193
Italian League Against Epilepsy (LICE) 301
Italy, teachers' knowledge of epilepsy 301–302

Jackson, Elizabeth Dade 35
Jackson, John Hughlings (1835-1911) 33–34, 40, 58, 59, 176, 251
Jacksonian epilepsy 59
Jacksonian march 34
Jacksonian seizure 25, 34, 39, 51
Jacoby, Ann 282–284, 298

Jager, Talia 96
jamais vu 46, 60
James, Henry (1843-1916) 175
Jasper, Herbert (1906-1999) 46–47
jerking, episodes 59
Jesus Christ 11, 12, 13, 17, 101
  art depicting, driving out unclean spirits 106
  'casting out', epileptic boy 13, 104, 107–108
  Transfiguration of Christ (Raphael) 12, 104
  The Transfiguration of Christ (Rubens) 107–108
Joan of Arc (1412-1431) 11, 206, 207–208
job application process 296–297, 298, 328
Jobson, Richard (1960-) 218
JobTech 298
John, Duke of Berry 101
John, Elton (1947-) 168
John, Prince (son of King George V) 139
John of Gaddesden (1280-1361) 11
Josephine, Empress 210
journalists, information service for 184
Joy Division (band) 168
Joyner, Florence Griffith (Flo Jo) (1959-1998) 196, 218
judgement, questioning 196–197, 219
Julius Caesar (William Shakespeare) 3, 67–68, 69, 173
Jung, Carl 101
justice
  disabled people pursuing 242, 243, 244, 247
  evasion, by possibly faking epilepsy 258
justice system, attitudes of professionals in 304

Kahlo, Frida (1907-1954) 119, 122
Kaiser Family Foundation 183
Kale, Rajendra 277, 309, 334
Kellogg, Abner Otis (1818-1888) 260
Kennedy, John F (1917-1963) 187
Kepler's malt extract 84
Kerner, Justinus (1786-1862) 17
Kerson, Jenny 125
Kerson, Lawrence 125
Kerson, Toba 125, 146–147, 154, 196
Kesey, Ken (1935-2001) 89, 132
Kill, Jerry 196
King James Bible 13
Kiss Yourself Goodbye (Tony Fennelly) 94
Kollonitsch, Cardinal 209
Kork Epilepsy Centre, Kehl-Kork,

  Germany 29
Kraemer, Heinrich 11–12
Krause, Fedor (1857-1937) 40–41
Krishna, paintings of 106

La Spirale (Gustave Flaubert) 73, 74
La Teppe, Tain-l'Hermitage, France 29
Lamb (Bernard MacLaverty) 89–90
lamotrigine 193
language, brain mapping 38–39
Laos, attitudes to epilepsy 291
"larval" epilepsy 260
The Last King of Scotland (2006, film) 142
law(s) *see* legislation
law enforcement 304–307
  training of officers 307
Lear, Edward (1812-1888) 81–82, 115
learning disability 58, 134, 135, 191, 224, 300, 318
Lee, Laurence 'Laurie' (1914-1997) 86–88
leeches 10
Legge, Leon (1985-) 223
legislation 227–247
  disability 227, 230, 243
  discrimination prevention 243–244
    China 243–244
    employment 243–244, 245, 327
    enforcement limitations (UK) 244, 245, 247
    results/effects of laws in UK 244
    UK 243, 244–245, 247
    USA and Australia 243
    see also Disability Discrimination Act 1995 (UK)
  flying/pilot's licence 240–241
  freedom of movement
    between countries 233–235
    denial of venue access, in USA 233
    see also immigration, legislation
  marriage *see* marriage
  right to drive a vehicle 235–236
    see also driving (people with epilepsy)
  rights of disabled people 243
Lennox, Margaret 206
Lennox, William (1884-1960) 52, 104, 108, 211
Leonardo Da Vinci (1452-1519) 110, 216
leprosy 12
Les Très Riches Heures du Duc de Berry 101, 330 (Fig)

Let Him Have It (1991, film) 134–135
Letchworth, William (1823-1910) 62
'Let's Get Retarded' (The Black Eyed Peas) 170
Lexicon Medicum (John Quincy) 72
LexisNexis database 192, 194, 195
licence
  driving (vehicle) *see* driving licence
  pilot's 240–241
  train drivers' 241
Lichtenthal, Peter (1780-1853) 157
lifestyle
  after concealment of epilepsy, TV 149
  causes of epilepsy 18, 24
  impact of epilepsy, in film 142, 143, 144
  of person with epilepsy 90–91
    in personal account 323
    sportsmen/women 220
    Williams, Sir John 'Kyffin' 118
  'rock-star' 166, 168
lifestyle advice
  ancient Greek and Roman period 6–7, 8
  for de Chirico, Giorgio 116
  epilepsy in films 127
  seizure control 220
  in television medical drama 149
lifetime risk, of epilepsy 217
Lister, Joseph 38
literature, epilepsy in 67–97
  books/poetry 67, 69, 70, 71, 72, 75, 79, 87, 88
    autobiographical accounts 85–86
    biography 91, 96
    catalogue of how epilepsy is used 97
    contemporary 90, 91, 96, 97
    crime novels 92–96
    Dickens' books 36, 79–81
    Dostoevsky's novels 36, 77–78
    graphic books 96
    injustice due to epilepsy 72
    musicogenic epilepsy 159
    negative features symbolized by 69, 71, 75, 88, 89, 90, 91, 94, 95–96
    poetry 70, 84
    positive portrayal 75, 78, 97
    science fiction 94–95
    sympathetic view 93, 94, 96
    violent stereotype 95, 96
    young adult fiction 96

  see also writers; *specific writers/poets*
  'epileptic' character 26
  influence on attitudes to epilepsy 36
  sources of information for writers 72
  Victorian 36
  writers affected by epilepsy *see* writers
litigious, person viewed as 243
Livingstone, Samuel 262
lobbying, of movie industry 155
local community projects 332
Locock, Sir Charles (1799-1875) 37
The Lodging Woman (Fyodor Dostoevsky) 77
Lombroso, Cesare (1835-1909) 92, 210, 251
The London Practice of Physick (Pordage) 16
loneliness 330
  early signs and intervention 331
  interventions 331, 332
  prevention 329, 330–331
  social media effects 331–332
  UK government proposals 331
  see also social isolation
Lorna Doone (R.D. Blackmore) 82–83
Los Angeles Times 196, 216
The Lost Prince (2003, film) 139
lumbar air encephalogram (LAEG) 53, 54, 166
lumbar puncture 53
Lumière, Auguste 123
Lumière, Louis 123
Luminal (phenobarbitone) 42
'lunacy' 12
Lunacy Commission 25, 28
Lunacy/Lunatics Act 1945 27
lunar influence 5, 6, 10, 12, 17–18

Macbeth (William Shakespeare) 69
Macewen, Sir William (1848-1924) 38–39
MacLaverty, Bernard (1942-) 89–90
'mad pig disease' 291
Madame Bovary (Gustave Flaubert) 73, 74
Maghull Home for Epileptics 28–29
magnetic resonance imaging (MRI) 47, 55–58, 328 (Fig)
  clinical applications 55, 56–57
  CT comparison 55, 56–57
  development 55
  FLAIR image 57

  functional (fMRI) 56, 158
  scanners 56
magnetic treatment 79
Maid of Orléans (Joan of Arc) (1412-1431) 11, 206, 207–208
Maisonneuve, Jacques Gilles (1745-1826) 23
Malevolent Creation 172–173
malingering 258
Malleus Maleficarum 11, 12
mania 112
  dancing 103–104
  'epileptic' 251, 258
manifestations of epilepsy
  Aretaeus of Cappadocia's observations 7
  Galen's observations 7
  Prichard's description 25, 26
  Priscianus's observations 7
  Van Swieten's description 18
  in writers 73, 74
  see also seizure(s); symptoms
manipulation, seizures for
  film depictions 129
  Napoleon Bonaparte 210
Mansfield, Sir Peter (1933-2017) 56
Manuel, Peter 253, 261–262
Marcalo, Rita 177–178, 180
marital status 24
marriage
  annulment 84, 231–232
  avoidance (voluntary) 84, 89, 122, 329
  considerations before 84
  disclosure of diagnosis prior to 287
  legislation 230–232
    China 232
    India 232
    UK 231–232
    USA 230–231
  prevention 230
    eugenics and 27
    historical 4, 27, 30, 31
    USA 30, 31, 230–231, 277
  right to 230–232
Marriage Law (USA) 30, 31
Marsh, Terry (1958-) 221
Marshall, Fiona 174
Martin Chuzzlewit (Charles Dickens) 81
'masked epilepsy' 25
Massie, Robert 209
masturbation 18, 24, 27
Matrimonial Causes Act (1937), UK 232
A Matter of Life and Death (1946, film)

126
Maudsley, Henry (1835-1918) 251, 258, 260
Mayas, names for epilepsy 108
Maynard, Paul (1975-) 217
McKinley, Ida Saxton 30–31
McKinley, William 30–31
Mead, Richard (1673-1754) 18
Mean Streets (1973, film) 130–131
measles 316
media 183–204
  influence of, and responsibility 195
  key messages for public education 293–294
  mobile 183
  negative coverage *see* negative perceptions of epilepsy
  news *see* news media
  online sources 184
  platforms, news sources 183–184
  printed/press *see* press, the
  reports of antisocial behaviour 270
  seizure, coverage 196, 197
  social *see* social media
medical model, of epilepsy 334
medical soaps/dramas (television) 148–149, 154
medical statistics 24
medicinal plants *see* herbal remedies
Medics (television drama) 148–149, 155
medieval period (Middle Ages) 9–17
melancholy 119
Méliès, Georges (1861-1938) 123–124
Member of Parliament, UK 217
memory
  brain mapping 46
  loss/impairment 4, 7
    behaviour on plane, automatism 270
    criminal behaviour 260
    homicides and 23, 259, 260, 261, 263
    in literature, or writers 70–71, 72, 93, 94
    Poe, Edgar Allan 214, 215
    in rugby player with epilepsy 222
meningitis 39, 61
menstruation 8, 24
mental health 328–334
  music impact 156–157
mental health problems 266, 332–334
  see also anxiety; depression
mental illness
  admitting, increased numbers 217

epilepsy perceived as 175, 271, 277, 286
present-day famous people with 217
press/news broadcast, miscarriage of justice case 187
prevalence in epilepsy 332
mental tasks 48
mercy killing 52, 152
Merino, Eduardo Urbano (1975 -) 120
Merritt, Hiram Houston Jr (1902-1979) 43–44
Merton, Robert (1910-2003) 280
mesial temporal sclerosis (MTS) 57, 328 (Fig)
Mesmer (1994, film) 136–137
Mesmer, Anton (1734-1815) 136–137
Mesopotamia, epilepsy descriptions 4
Metro newspaper article 191
Mexicans, in USA 235
Michael Foundation, Bonn, Germany 114
Michelangelo (1475-1564) 110
microgyria 58
Middle Ages (medieval period) 9–17
migraine 116, 117
'mild', use of term for epilepsy 244
military genius 210
military service/career *see* armed services/military service
mimicry 23
mind, the 7, 271
miniature painters 101
Ministry of Justice (UK) 306
The Miracles of St Ignatius of Loyola (Rubens) 108, 122
miscarriage of justice 187
misconceptions xi
  in crime novels 92
  most common (2007) 285
  violence and epilepsy *see* violence/violent behaviour, and epilepsy
  see also negative perceptions of epilepsy
misdiagnosis, of epilepsy 35
MMR vaccine 316
M'Naghten Rules 188, 272
mobile media 183
A Moment of War (Laurence 'Laurie' Lee) 86, 87–88
Moniz, Egas (1874-1955) 53–54
monosodium glutamate (MSG) 48
Montgomery, David 255–256
Montreal Neurological Institute 46
moon, link with epilepsy 5, 6, 10, 12, 17–18

morality, cause of epilepsy 10, 24, 27
morbid curiosity 174
morbus comitialis 6
morbus major 6
Morel, Bénédict Augustin (1809-1873) 24–25
Morris, Jane 212, 213
Morris, Jenny 212, 213
Morris, William (1834-1896) 212–213
motor cortex 39
  mapping 41, 46
movement
  abnormal/excessive, disorder classification 26
  absent, disorder classification 26
  brain mapping 46
moving screen 123–147
  see also film(s); television programmes
Mozart, Wolfgang Amadeus 158, 159
Mozart effect 118, 158, 159
MRI *see* magnetic resonance imaging (MRI)
Muhammad (570-632) 206–207
Munn, Michael 179
Munthe, Axel (1857-1949) 174–175
murder and homicide 251
  EEGs, neurological/psychological abnormalities 254, 263
  epileptic basis, concept 260, 263
    typical features of murder 263
  during 'epileptic mania' episode 258
  in films 132, 137, 138
  impossible during a seizure 253
  in literature 69, 71, 77, 90
    crime novels 92, 93, 94
  motive lacking 257, 258, 260, 261
  by people with epilepsy 255–266
    Canham, Charles Edward 256–259
    EEGs changes 254, 261–262, 263
    evidence against link 253, 254, 263–264
    famous cases 255–266
    historical cases 259
    Kellogg (Abner Otis)'s patient 260
    literature review 259, 265
    Manuel, Peter 261–262
    Maudsley's criteria to guide the law 260, 261
    Montgomery, David 255–256
    Mr A, case 260–261

Podolsky (Edward)'s cases 263
Ruby, Jack 262
statistical studies 263–264
temporal lobe epilepsy diagnosis 259, 261, 264
Walker (Arthur Earl)'s patient 259
reporting on news/in the press 186
in TV programme 151
see also violence/violent behaviour
The Murder on the Links (Agatha Christie) 92–93
'museum of living pathology' 174
music 49, 156–180
appreciation 156
bidirectional relationship with epilepsy 156–157
brain activity affected by 158, 159
brain areas for processing 158
effect on spatial reasoning 158
epilepsy in musicians *see* musicians
physiological relationship with epilepsy 156–157
pitch, anti-epileptic drug or surgery effect 160
popular, depiction of epilepsy in 169–170
negative perceptions 170, 172–173
song lyrics referring to 170, 172–173
positive impact on epilepsy 156, 157, 158–159
effects on mental health 156–157
effects on physical health 157
mechanisms 159
social benefits 156
as trigger for seizures 118, 159–160
see also composers; musicians
music therapy 48–49, 156–157
active and receptive types 157
The Musical Doctor (Peter Lichtenthal) 157
musical savant 165
musicians, epilepsy and 156–160, 160–173, 180
absence of epilepsy among 161
Chopin, Frédéric 161–162
contemporary popular musicians 218
epilepsy impact on 156
lasting impression by, despite epilepsy (film) 142
reticence about epilepsy 161, 180
as role models 173
see also music
musicogenic epilepsy 118, 159
Joan of Arc 207
management 160
psychological cause 160
Musicophilia (Oliver Sack) 156
Mussorgsky, Modest (1839-1881) 162–163, 214
My Sister's Keeper (2009, film) 142
myelin 57
myoclonic seizure 59
The Mystery of Edwin Drood (Charles Dickens) 79
myths x, 27
aggression and crime due to epilepsy 253, 258–259, 268–269, 273–274
in crime fiction 92
'epileptic personality' 268–269, 274
famous people *see* famous people, with epilepsy
history of epilepsy *see* history of epilepsy
possession by demons *see* possession, by gods/demons
sport and epilepsy 303
violence and epilepsy *see* violence/violent behaviour

Napoleon I (Napoleon Bonaparte) (1769-1821) 210–211, 251, 266
National Association for Music Therapy (NAMT) 157
National Epilepsy Awareness Month 200
National Health Service (NHS), UK 235
National Hospital, Queen Square, London 37
National Hospital for the Paralysed and the Epileptic, London 28, 33, 35, 37, 39, 41
National Society for the Employment of Epileptics 28
Nature and Its Symbols 100
Nazi Germany 27, 52, 185, 228, 229
negative perceptions of disability 193
in Israel *vs* Canada, review 193
in UK, during/after age of austerity (2007-2008) 195
negative perceptions of epilepsy 98, 274, 278
in 1980s and 1990s (USA) 282
in books/poetry 69, 71, 75, 88, 90, 91, 94, 95–96
in developing countries 227, 291
in films *see* film depiction of epilepsy/seizures
increased by the defence in US court case 189
in music 170, 172–173
in newspapers/media 192–193, 196
Chief Justice John G Roberts' seizure 196–197
Dando murder case (UK) 186
in/after UK age of austerity (2007-2008) 194
Israel *vs* Canada review 193
Jack Ruby court case (US) 188
review/survey (1991-1996) 192–193
road vehicle accidents 189–191
in US newspaper reports 195–196, 197
by patients and public, questionnaire 285
in songs 170–171, 173
in theatre 174, 175, 176, 180
on Twitter/tweets 199–200
in UK (2004) 283, 285
violence *see* violence/violent behaviour
in works of art 98, 100, 101, 102, 103, 104, 105–106, 108
in YouTube videos 201, 202
see also public perceptions
negative stereotype 278
Neighbours (TV programme) 154
Nelson, Prince Rogers (1958-2016) 167–168
Nemesis (Agatha Christie) 93
'nervous hallucinations' 74
'nervous sickness' 73, 74, 76
nervous system sensitivity 19, 20
neurocysticercosis 55, 328 (Fig)
neurological disorders
classification 26
in murderers/violent criminals 254
reporting errors and stigmatization 196
neurology 15–16, 175
neuromusicology 49
neurostimulation 95
neurosurgery 39
neurotransmitters 44
music effect on seizures 159
New Testament, casting out demons 13, 104, 106

New York, epilepsy institution 62
New York Times 125, 177, 188, 196, 220
news information 183–184
news media 183–184, 184–197, 203
  current trends 184
  Dando murder case 186
  Jack Ruby trial (US) reporting 188
  lack of understanding about epilepsy 197
  manipulation of 183
  power of, and need for accuracy 184
  prize for best-informed epilepsy new story 193
  television 184
  vehicle accident reporting 189–190
  see also newspapers; press, the
newspapers 184
  accuracy of reporting about epilepsy 192, 196
    ensuring by epilepsy charity 184, 193
    inaccuracies 193, 196
  articles about epilepsy forms and approaches 185
    number and review 192, 195, 196
  articles involving people with epilepsy
    cannabidiol oil need 191–192
    Chief Justice John G Roberts Jr. 196–197
    Dando murder case 186
    Jack Ruby trial (US) 187–188
    Jerry Kill (sports coach) 196
    road vehicle accidents 189–191
  best and worst of reporting 193
  campaign for medicinal cannabis 191–192
  disability issue reporting
    in/after age of austerity (2007-2008), UK 194
    increase in article number (2010-2011), UK 194–195
    Israel *vs* Canada 193
    US survey on neurological conditions 195
  editorial slant 184, 185
  epilepsy definition (what constitutes epilepsy) 197
  improvements in reporting 191, 193, 194

  influence wielded by 195
  negative perceptions/reports *see* negative perceptions of epilepsy
  pejorative language *see* pejorative language
  positive reporting/stories 191–193, 196
  stigmatization of people with epilepsy 195–196
  see also press, the
Newton, Isaac 17–18
Night Mother (Marsha Norman) 176–177, 180
Night Unto Night (1949, film) 127
nihilism, medical 19, 31
No Thoroughfare (Charles Dickens) 79
Nobel, Alfred (1833-1896) 211, 216
non-epileptic attack disorder (NEAD) 8, 36, 129
  in film 137
non-hereditary epilepsy 16
non-pharmacological treatments 47–49
non-profit organizations 199
  see also charities, epilepsy
normal life, in epilepsy 283, 284
normalizing seizures/epilepsy 317, 326
Norman, Marsha (1947-) 176
North American Epilepsy Foundation 179
'not guilty by reason of insanity' (NGRI) 265–266, 272–273
Nullity of Marriage Act (1971), UK 232
nursing home, for people with epilepsy 29
nursing profession, employment difficulty 242

Obamacare 197
observation, power of 9
observations, on epilepsy *see* manifestations of epilepsy
obsessiveness 118
occupations, unsuitable *see* careers
Ōe, Hikari (1963-) 164–165
offensive terminology 170–171
  see also pejorative language
'officialdom' 227–247
oil of vitriol 14
The Old Curiosity Shop (Charles Dickens) 81
olfactory cortex 163
olfactory hallucinations *see* smell, seizures and
Oliver Twist (Charles Dickens) 79, 80
On the Sacred Disease (Hippocrates) 5
One Flew over the Cuckoo's Nest (1975, film) 132
One Flew over the Cuckoo's Nest (Ken Kesey) 89
Online Harms Bill 200
online information 184
opium 14, 37, 78
opportunities, loss 279, 280
Orphan Homes of Scotland 28
Osler, Sir William (1849-1919) 39–40
Oswald, Lee Harvey (1939-1963) 187, 188
Othello (William Shakespeare) 68, 69, 173
Our Mutual Friend (Charles Dickens) 79, 80
'out of control' x
Owls do Cry (Janet Frame) 88
ownership, of epilepsy 290

pain, insomnia due to, music effect 157
paintings *see* art, works of
pallor 314, 317
'palming' 102
panic, in child 317
Paracelsus (Philippus von Hoenheim) (1493-1571) 13–14
paralysis 32, 33
parents
  campaigning, cannabis access 134, 192
  concealment, of epilepsy by 287, 289, 300
  concerns over adult child 329, 330
  as 'felt stigma coaches' 287, 289, 299, 319, 334
  impact of child's epilepsy on 326–327
  information sources (present-day) 318
  lack of information/support for 315
  letting child down 315, 316, 317
  negative attitudes to child's seizures 84, 139, 287, 288, 289
  'open' and 'closed' approaches to epilepsy 289, 326–327
  overprotective attitudes 84, 315
  reaction to child's epilepsy, impact on child 326–327
  shielding role 289
  see also family
parietal lobe, mapping 45

Parker, Robert B. (1932-2010) 92
partners/spouses 329
    concealment of epilepsy to 287, 288–289
    disclosure of diagnosis to 287, 329
Paschal, Angelia, study 284–285
pathology of epilepsy
    The Enlightenment 18, 19, 20
    medieval period 15–16
    see also brain
patients, on display 174
patron saints, of epilepsy (St Valentine) 13, 105
pejorative language 170–171, 185
    'epileptic' see 'epileptic', pejorative use
    in the media/press 185, 190, 193
        in Canada vs Israel reporting 193
        in UK, during economic downturn 195
        in US newspaper reports 195–196
Penfield, Wilder (1891-1976) 46
Pennsylvania Epileptic Hospital and Colony Farm, USA 31
peony/peony root 6, 16
'people power' 134
perceptions on epilepsy see public perceptions, of epilepsy
Perchance to Dream (Robert B. Parker) 92
performance art 177–178
Perr, Irwin (1928-2018) 241
personal account of living with epilepsy 313–334
    adolescent years 321–324
    adulthood 326–328
    early years 314–321
    leaving home and university 324–326
Personal Independence Payments (PIP) 185
personality
    changes due to epilepsy 73, 266–269
        Gershwin, George 164
    descriptors 9
    'epileptic' see 'epileptic personality'
    manipulative, in film 137, 138

phlegmatic type 9
    psychotic 262
    traits, in epilepsy 266–267, 268
    of Van Gogh, Vincent 111, 267–268
'personality defect' 266–267
pessimism, about epilepsy 77
Peter the Great, Tsar (1672-1725) 208–210
'petit mal' 23, 59, 121
    EEG 52
Pfeiffer's syndrome 168
phenobarbitone (phenobarbital) 42–43, 45
    adverse effects 86, 216
    clinical results, and benefits 42, 43
    overdose 179
phenytoin 43, 44, 45
    adverse effects 89
    in literature 89
philanthropists 28, 62
philosophy, about epilepsy 121
phlegm 5, 8, 9, 10, 11
phlegmatic humour 9–10
phlegmatic personality type 9
photographic records, women with seizures 175
photosensitive epilepsy 129–130
    Curtis, Ian 169
    Horovitz, Adam 218
    targeted on Twitter 200
physiognomy 251
Picard, Fabienne 112
pictorial art see art; art, works of
Pictures at an Exhibition (Mussorgsky) 162
Pilcher, Rosamunde (1924-2019) 90
Pilgrimage of the Epileptics to the Church at Molenbeek (Pieter Bruegel) 103, 104, 331 (Fig)
pilocytic astrocytoma 164
pilot's licence 240–241
placebo 45
plants, medicinal properties 14
plays see theatre, epilepsy in
Pliny 6
pneumoencephalography 54
Podolsky, Edward (1902-1965) 263
Poe, Edgar Allan (1809-1849) 67, 70–71, 214–215
poets
    Dickinson, Emily 83–84
    Lear, Edward 81–82, 115
    Lee, Laurence 'Laurie' 86–87

    Tennyson, Alfred Lord 69–70
'Polaire' (Emilie Marie Bouchard) 174, 175
police officers
    confused child, understanding response 321
    inappropriate treatment of people with epilepsy 307
    perceptions and training on epilepsy 307
politicians
    with epilepsy 217
    eugenics movement influence 227
poorhouse 22, 28, 30, 79
Porgy and Bess (George Gershwin) 163
Portrait of my Father (Frida Kahlo) 119
positive perceptions of epilepsy 280, 283
    in books/poetry 75, 78, 97
    on film see film depiction of epilepsy/seizures
    'future in-depth studies' 283
    in the press/media 191–193, 196
    in UK 283
    in works of art 120
    of young people 282
    see also public perceptions, of epilepsy
positron emission tomography (PET) 158
The Possessed (Fyodor Dostoevsky) 77
possession, by gods/demons 4, 9, 10, 12, 15, 16, 17
    in art 98, 101, 105–106, 108
    casting out see casting out evil
    in films 129, 140, 141, 147
    in literature 68, 73, 76, 90
    news reporting and 193
    release, by trepanning 15
    Saudi Arabia, teachers' attitudes 302
post-ictal antisocial behaviour 270
post-ictal state 248
potassium bromide 36, 37, 43, 112, 212
prayers 11, 13
    answered, votive tablets, paintings 106–107
    in Book of Hours 101
pregnancy, witnessing a seizure during 18
prejudice
    against disabled people 230
    Dostoevsky's defence of people subjected to 78

insane *vs* sane automatisms
(epilepsy *vs* diabetes) 271
against people with epilepsy
273, 274, 279, 280
    despite seizure control
277
    by employers 295–296
    in employment 241
    freedom of movement
233
    increased with more
disclosure 288
    reduction (1949-1979)
281
see also discrimination; stigma/
stigmatization
press, the 183, 184–197
    accuracy of reporting 184,
193
    campaign for medicinal
cannabis 191–192
    charity collaboration 184
    debate over what constitutes
epilepsy 197
    derogatory/negative language
185–186, 190
        see also pejorative language
    fatal accident, driver with
epilepsy 236
    improved reporting on people
with epilepsy 191
    Jack Ruby case (US) reporting
188
    Jill Dando murder case
186–187
    negative aspects of coverage
185
    positive impact on epilepsy
191–193, 196
    power of, and need for
accuracy 184
    power to bring change 192
    reporting on healthcare issues
192–193
    right-wing *vs* left-wing,
reporting and 185
    road vehicle accident reporting
189–191, 236
    UK financial crisis, image of
disabled people 194
    see also newspapers
prevalence of epilepsy 217, 290–291
    in Scotland 246

Prichard, James Cowles (1786-1848) 25
priest, solace from 85
Prince (Prince Rogers Nelson) (1958-
2016) 167–168
'The Princess' (Tennyson) 70
printed media *see* newspapers; press, the
Priscianus, Theodorus 7
prison(s) 24, 27, 30, 36, 49, 79
    audit of healthcare in 306
    characteristics of persons in
252
    deaths in, after seizures
305–306
    prevalence of people with
epilepsy in 252, 253, 305,
306
    restrictions on activities 306
prison officers, training/knowledge 305,
306–307
prison services 304–307
progressive myoclonic epilepsy 61
Prophet, the (Muhammad) 206–207
prophylaxis (prevention) of epilepsy 16
pseudo-seizures 8, 36
psychiatrists
    early nineteenth century 23,
24
    expert opinions 188, 261
    in films 138
    in science fiction 95
psychiatry 175
'psychogenic attacks', Napoleon
Bonaparte 211
psychogenic non-epileptic seizures 36,
208–209
psychological damage, of seizures 321
    pre-diagnosis 317
psychomotor epilepsy
    Ruby, Jack 187, 188
    see also temporal lobe epilepsy
psychopathology, and epilepsy 267
psychotic personality 262
public awareness/understanding
    1949-1979, and 1979-1989
281, 282
    inadequate/lack of 273, 274,
276, 293
        of automatisms 250, 270
        by teachers/child carers
299, 300
    negative impact
        of court cases 189, 197
        of news media 196, 197
    raising 178
        editorial belief in 195

        by films/film actors 145,
146, 178, 179
        by present-day celebrities
223–224
        press and charity
collaboration 184–185
        by show *Involuntary
Dances* 178
        by sportsmen/women
219, 222
    see also public perceptions, of
epilepsy
public education 273
    of employers 298, 299
    by exposure of patients 174,
175
    key messages for public
(IOM) 293–294
    need for, in USA 282, 293
    opinions of epilepsy patients
on 284–285, 286
    to reduce stigma 293, 294
    by social media and Internet
use 199, 201
    strategies, and funding
limitations 285
    by television films depicting
epilepsy 134, 155
    training *see* training
    by YouTube, on epilepsy and
first aid 201
public opinion, analysis 273
    advances in 281
    'future in-depth studies'
283–284
    UK surveys/research 282–284
    USA surveys/research
280–281, 284
public perceptions, of epilepsy 273–274
    of childhood event, *vs* adult
event 321
    in developing countries 291,
292
    impact on employment/
careers 283
    misconceptions, most
common 285
    negative *see* negative
perceptions of epilepsy
    popular music impact 173
    positive *see* positive
perceptions of epilepsy
    protecting from, in personal

account 318–319
  of risk of driving 189
  stigmatization/discrimination due to 278, 279
  in UK 282–284, 286
    present-day 319
  of university lecturer 325–326
  in USA *see* USA
  of violence *see* violence/violent behaviour
  see also prejudice; public awareness/understanding
punishment
  for crime, by boy with epilepsy 135
  for sins/misdemeanours 9, 10, 21
pupils, attitudes to peers 304, 318
purgation 7, 9, 16, 36
Putnam, Tracy Jackson (1894-1975) 43–44
Pynchon, Thomas (1937-) 88

Qasim, Abul (936-1013 CE) 250–251
The Quack (Benjamin Cuyp) 102
quacks 101, 102
Quarrier, William (1829-1903) 28
Quarriers (charity) xii
A Quiet Passion (film, 2016) 83
Quincy, John 72

radio waves 56
rage 68, 69
randomized controlled trials (RCTs) 44–45, 191
Raphael (Raffaello Sanzio da Urbino) (1483-1520) 12, 104, 122
Rauscher, Frances 158
A Ray of Darkness (Margiad Evans) 85
Reagan, Ronald (1911-2004) 127
recreational activities/facilities 233
The Red Curtain (*c.* 1965) (painting) 114, 333 (Fig)
refusal to be defined by epilepsy 90
regulations *see* rules and regulations
rehabilitation 277
relationships
  burden of epilepsy, in film 127, 131–132
  to reduce isolation/loneliness 329
religious treatment 10, 11, 12, 13
remedies 16
  ancient Greek and Roman period 6–7, 8, 86

  herbal *see* herbal remedies
  Paracelsus' views 13, 14
Renaissance, art 98, 99–108, 114
reporting, in press *see* newspapers; press, the
reporting to driving authorities
  Australia 240
  Canada 237, 238
  UK 236, 237
reproduction, regulating *see* marriage; sterilization
Requiem (2006, film) 140, 141
residential care
  epilepsy studies in 23
  UK and Europe 28–29
  in Victorian era 28–29
'respectability' of epilepsy, in literature 79
restaurants 233
'retarded', pejorative use 170–171
'retarded', song lyrics and pop group 170–171
reticence to confirm epilepsy 216
  see also concealment, of epilepsy
Reynolds, Sir John Russell (1828-1896) 26
Rhazes (*c.* 854-825) 102
Rhodes, Jonathan (Jonty) (1967-) 219
Richler, Mordecai (1931-2001) 88–89
Ries, Janet 280
right and wrong, distinguishing between 188, 256
rights *see* human rights
risk factors 19
risk-adverse culture 241
road vehicle accidents *see* driving (people with epilepsy)
Roberts, John G 196–197
Robinson, Ray (1971-) 90–91
role models 217
  lack, football players 224
  musical artists 173, 224
  sportsmen/women 218, 220–221
Roman Catholic Church *see* Catholic Church
Romper Stomper (1992 and 2018, films) 135–136
Roosevelt, Theodore (1858-1919) 212, 216, 229
Roosevelt Island, USA 30
Rosa Medicinae (John, of Gaddesden) 11
Royal College of General Practitioners (RCGP) 295–296
Rubens, Sir Peter Paul (1577-1640) 107–108, 122, 332 (Fig)

Ruby, Jack (1911-1967) 187–188, 262
rugby and rugby players 220–221, 303
rules and regulations 230–246
  basis for, and misperception 230
  inconsistencies between countries 230
  see also human rights; legislation
'rum fits' 214
Rushdie, Salman (1947-) 90
Rutter, Henry 30

Sabuncuoglu, Serefeddin (1385-1468) 100
Sack, Oliver 156
sacred disease/illness ix, 5, 12, 21, 90
sadness 24, 82, 83, 115
St Hildegard of Bingen (1098-1179) 10
St Ignatius of Loyola (1491-1556) 108
St Paul (Paul of Tarsus) 152
St Severein 105
St Valentine 12, 13, 105, 327 (Fig)
St Vitus 13, 105
'St Vitus' dance' 13
sainthood 141
Sakikku 4
Salem Witches Trial 16
Salpêtrière Hospital, Paris 22–23, 36, 174
Sand, George (1804-1876) 75–76, 161
Sandys, Laura (1964-) 217
'sanitizing' of epilepsy 78
Sanzio da Urbino, Raffaello (Raphael) (1483-1520) 12, 104, 122
Sartre, Jean-Paul 74–75
The Satanic Verses (Salman Rushdie) 90
Saudi Arabia, teachers' knowledge of epilepsy 302
Savage, Michael 197
scalp stimulator, electric 163
Scambler, Graham 285, 286
Schachter, Steven 120, 122
schizophrenia 108, 207, 208
Schneider, Joseph 253, 278–279, 289, 290, 326
schools
  activities unsuitable for children 300, 301, 303, 319
  attitudes at, towards epilepsy 299, 318–319
  notifying about epilepsy in child 318
  pupil attitudes to peers with epilepsy 304
  safety issues at 318, 319
  see also education; teachers

Scola, Kathryn 127
Scotland
   EHRC responses and role 246
   insanity, and automatism 272
   prison and people with epilepsy 305
Scottish Human Rights Commission 246–247
'scroungers', use of term 185, 195
seasons, humours and 9
sedatives 42, 43
seizure(s) 34
   aborting, mental tasks 48
   alcohol causing *see* alcohol abuse; alcohol withdrawal, seizures
   in art
      European Renaissance 100–101
      Jesus casting out unclean spirits 13, 104, 106
      Raphael's painting, epileptic boy 12, 104, 107
   associated features 60
   benign idiopathic 197
   classification 58–60
   complex focal 59
   in composers/musicians 162, 163, 165, 166, 167, 168, 169
   control, music impact 156, 157, 158–159
   as 'demons', news report 193
   description 7, 25, 59
      in newspaper/TV news 186
      in song lyric 172
      see also individual famous people
   discharge causing *see* discharge, seizures
   drugs of abuse causing 165, 166
   EEG 52
   exercise beneficial effects 303
   in films *see* film(s)
   focal *see* focal seizures
   frequency 24
   functional 36
   generalized (bilateral) *see* generalized (bilateral) seizures
   lack of control after, murders and 256
   lack of support by public during 276
   in literature 68, 69, 70, 71, 80, 81, 88
   localizable 34
   mechanisms/causes *see* causes, of epilepsy
   medicinal cannabis effect 192
   metaphorical/joke use of term, on Twitter 199–200
   as multiple understanding of self (J Hall) 121
   petit mal, *vs* temporal lobe 121
   in plays/theatre 173, 177
   progression, observations on 5, 7, 25
   psychogenic 36
   psychologically based episodes resembling 35
   in public place 276
      in personal account 325
   reduction, by improved health/care 31
   simple focal 59
   singer-dancers mimicking 174
   site of origin *see* brain, mapping
   sleep-related, driving and 236–237
   solitary, driving in UK and 237
   stereotypic form in individual 59
   threshold 44
   tonic–clonic *see* tonic–clonic seizures
   triggered by GIF files 200
   in TV programmes 148, 149, 151, 153
   on Twitter, portrayal 199–200
   types 16, 336 (Table)
      with/without aura 34
   unilateral (one-sided) 33, 34
   of unknown onset 336 (Table)
   as vehicle to shock viewer
      films 133, 146, 154
      TV programme 150
   violence linked *see* violence/violent behaviour
   witnessing 281
      public reaction 274, 276
      triggering epilepsy 18, 23
   in writers 70, 71, 73, 74
   on YouTube 201–202, 203
Seizure: The Story of Kathy Morris (1980, film) 133–134
'seizure disorder' 290
selective serotonin reuptake inhibitors (SSRIs) 333
Selene 5, 99
self-employment 236
self-esteem 241, 272
   loss 272, 331
self-management 290
self-promotion, using epilepsy for 223
self-strangulation 27
'senile dementia' 25
sensitivity of nervous system 19, 20
sensory cortex, mapping 46
serial killers 261
sertraline 333
Seventh International Medical Congress (1881) 32
sex drive, alterations 267
sexual abuse 137, 254
sexual arousal, as trigger 68
sexual excess 18, 69, 70, 215
sexual intercourse, prevention 231
sexual promiscuity 27
sexuality, withdrawal from life due to 82, 84
Shakespeare, William (1564-1616) 3, 67–69, 173
shaking episodes, famous artists 110
shame x, 5, 26, 68, 70, 279
   concealment of epilepsy *see* concealment, of epilepsy
   epilepsy in literature 75
   felt stigma and 287, 288, 290
   Lear's (Edward) 81, 82, 115
   Lee's (Laurence 'Laurie') 88
   Morris, Jenny and William's 213
   parents'/family sense of 287, 327
Shaw, George Bernard (1856-1950) 228
The Shell Seekers (Rosamunde Pilcher) 90
siblings, relationship with person with epilepsy 320, 326, 327
Sieveking, Sir Edward (1816-1904) 37
Silas Marner (George Eliot) 72–73
Silesia, epilepsy centre 29
Simenon, Georges (1903-1989) 94
simple focal seizure 59
Simple Men (1992, film) 136, 137
singer-dancers, epileptic 174
singers, with epilepsy 165–166, 168, 169, 175, 218
   gommeuses épileptiques (epileptic singers) 174
sins, epilepsy as punishment for 9, 10
skull
   curative powers of 15, 38
   foreign bodies inside, epilepsy and 101, 102
   injuries 7
   opening, epilepsy cure 15, 37, 40
skull shavings 15
slaves 4, 6
sleep deprivation 76, 177, 189, 220, 239, 270, 273
   in personal account 323
sleep-related episodes 59, 126, 218, 220, 222, 244, 324

driving and 236–237
Sloane, Sir Hans (1660-1753) 100
Sloop, Gregory 163, 164
smartphones 198, 199
smell, seizures and 60, 91, 126, 141
   George Gershwin 163
A Smell of Burning (Colin Grant) 91
smelling salts 16
Smith, Dr R. Percy 256, 258
Smith, Preacher (Reverend Henry Weston Smith) 151–152
Smith, Tom (1971-) 220–221
Snelling, Jason (1983-) 222–223
snorkelling 323
Snow White and the Seven Dwarfs (1937, film) 126
soccer players 223
social acceptability 62
social class, in Victorian era 27
social consequences of epilepsy
  early nineteenth century 24
  in literature 90
social disadvantages of epilepsy, in book, Renaissance 107
social engineering 27
social isolation 26, 328–334
  alleviated by social media 198
  causes 329
  concerns by parents 330
  definition 330
  depiction in play 177
  interventions 331
  prevention 329, 330, 331
  stigma and discrimination linked 278
  writers 74–75, 83, 84, 88
  see also loneliness
social marketing 294
social media 197, 198, 203–204
  alleviation of social isolation 198
  campaign for medicinal cannabis 191–192
  inappropriate treatment of people by police 307
  key messages for public education 294
  loneliness cause/reduction 331–332
  misleading/inaccurate information 202, 204
  missed opportunity for positive information 200, 204
  seizures triggered by GIFs 200
  use related to epilepsy, extent 198, 199

viewer response to TV programme (*Eastenders*) 153
  see also Twitter; YouTube
social model, of epilepsy 334
social responsibility
  of drivers with epilepsy 238
  eugenics and 228
societies, epilepsy 62–63
society, 'normal', shunning of people with epilepsy 278
socioeconomic factors, young offenders and criminals 253
sodium valproate (Epilim), film 134
solitary life
  artists 115, 118
  writers 74–75, 82, 83, 88, 97, 115
  see also social isolation
songs, popular, epilepsy depiction 169–170, 172, 218
  1890s 174
  of Christina the Astonishing 171–172
  discriminatory/negative 170–171, 173
  seizure depiction 172
The Songs of Love (Giorgio de Chirico) 117
songwriters, with epilepsy 165–169, 180
  Curtis, Ian 168–169
  Horovitz, Adam 218
  Jobson, Richard 218
  John, Elton 168
  Prince 167–168
  Young, Neil 165–166
Sontag, Susan 275–276
The Sopranos (television programme) 151
soul, seat of 7
South Korea, violence and epilepsy review 264
Spanish Civil War 86, 87, 88
Spark, Muriel (1918-2006) 89
'spastic', use of term 185, 204
spatial awareness 159
spatial reasoning 158
'specialized factories' 295
'spike and wave' burst of activity 52
spiritual world, interest in 116
spiritus vitae 14
spitting 6
sports participation 303–304
  myths about, addressing 303–295
  risk levels, groups of sports 304, 340 (Table)
  unsuitable sports/activities 303, 323, 340 (Table)
sportsmen/women, with epilepsy 127,

217, 224
  coaches 196
spouses *see* partners/spouses
Sprenger, Johann 11–12
'squills' (medicinal plant) 6–7
staring episodes, in personal account 317, 319
stars, effects on human body 18
state benefits, reporting about 185
statistics, medical 24
status epilepticus 23
  in literature 80–81
  TV programme 152
sterilization 27, 30, 228
  compulsory 27, 30, 52, 230
  eugenics movement and 30, 185, 229, 230
  US legislation 229, 230, 231
  voluntary 61, 230
stigma/stigmatization xi, 3, 17, 74, 277–290
  affecting writers 74, 83, 87
  in book *Visions: Artists Living with Epilepsy* 120
  in China 243, 244
  coaches
    doctors 290
    parents 287, 289, 299, 319, 334
  definition/origin of word 'stigma' 195, 277, 278
  in developing countries 291
  discrimination and social isolation linked 278
  employment and 288
  enacted stigma 278, 287, 288, 290
  epileptic equivalent theory 254
  exacerbated by concealment 289
  of fear, television programme 149
  felt stigma 287, 288, 290
  in film 146
  global problem 290–292
  incidence 285
  internalized stigma 277
  interpersonal stigma 277–278
  in literature 68, 75, 97
    Morris, Jenny (daughter of William Morris) 212, 213
  in *Othello* (Shakespeare) 68
  perceived stigma 277
  in the press/media 186, 187
    in newspaper articles 193
    in US newspaper/media reports 195–196
  reducing 264, 292–294

effectiveness, assessment 294
IOM's key messages 293–294
by present-day celebrities 223–224
public and patients targeted 294
by sportsmen 219
by writers 94, 97
singer (Boyle, Susan) 169
on social media/Internet 204
on Twitter 200
on YouTube 202
survey of public perceptions, UK (Scambler & Hopkins) 286–288
survey/interviews with people with epilepsy 286–288
impact of diagnosis 286
meaning of 'being epileptic' 287
on public education 284–285
UK study (Scambler & Hopkins) 286–288
USA study (Schneider & Conrad) 289
'victim', 'normal' and 'wise' categories 278, 284
Young, Neil 166
'stone of folly/madness' 101, 102, 122
Strathclyde Centre for Disability Research 194
strobe lighting, seizures and 168
stroke (apoplexy) 18, 60, 173
strychnine 37
'substitution splicing' 124
sudden unexpected death in epilepsy (SUDEP) 8, 138, 192, 325
in literature 91
risk, and advising patients of 325
suicidal ideation 84, 85, 125, 139
suicide
after indecent behaviour (automatism) 250
attempted 213, 332
court cases over automatisms 249–250, 272
Curtis, Ian 168
predictors of 329
risk/rate among people with epilepsy 329
Van Gogh, Vincent 113
support groups 331
The Surgeon (Van Hemessen) 102, 331 (Fig)
surgical treatment 15, 18–19, 37–41
in art/paintings

Renaissance 100, 101, 102, 103
stone removal, sham operations 101, 102
development and history 29, 38–39
early history 15, 18–19, 37–38, 100
twentieth century 45–46
Victorian era 37–41
electrical stimulation of brain during 40–41
epileptic focus removal 41
in Germany 41
Hopkins, Katie 224
Horsley's work 40
localization of tumour/lesion 39, 40
Macewen's work 38–39
in science fiction novel 95
social media use on 199
temporal lobe epilepsy 47
murderer 259, 264–265
TV programme 150
see also trepanning (trephining)
surveys
of aggression and epilepsy link 304–305
of employment in UK (1950s) 295–296
of epilepsy patient views 284–285
about public education (Paschal et al) 284–285
on seizure sensation (Schneider & Conrad) 289–290
on stigma (Scambler & Hopkins) 286–288
see also stigma/stigmatization
of public attitudes to epilepsy 273
developing countries 291
UK (Jacoby's study) 282–284
UK (Scambler & Hopkins) 286–288
USA (Gallup's study) 280–281
WHO campaign study 291–292
see also interviews
Sutherland, Allan 178
Sweden, violence and epilepsy not associated 263–264
Swedenborg, Emanuel (1688-1772) 116
swimming, risks 149, 303, 319
Swinburne, Algernon (1837-1909) 215
symbolism, in art 98, 114, 122
of evil 105, 106, 114
of rebirth 99
of seizures 100–101

sympathy, YouTube videos of seizures 202, 203
'symptomatic epilepsy' 20
symptoms 34
correlation with brain anatomy 33, 34
initial, in epilepsy attack 60
'march' of 34
recognized by the public 283
seizure-related 34
temporal lobe seizures 34
warning *see* aura
see also manifestations of epilepsy
syphilis 33, 34, 73, 74, 77–78

tapeworms 55
taste, seizures and 60
Taxil, Jean (1564-1618) 15
teachers
attitudes/perceptions 300–301
academic difficulties and 319, 321
improved by interventions 303
UK 300, 302, 318, 319
USA 301
knowledge of epilepsy
African/Asian/Middle East countries 301, 302
educating on 300, 301, 302, 303, 304
inadequate 300, 301, 302, 318–319
Italy 301
surveys 300
systematic review (UK) 302–303
up-to-date, professional duty 304
responsibilities 318
teaching, as career, concerns 326–327
Teagan's Story: Her Battle With Epilepsy (Talia Jager) 96
Telegraph newspaper 186, 220, 305
television films, depicting epilepsy 134, 148, 154
Prince John, concealment 139
television programmes 148–154
accurate portrayal of epilepsy 148–149, 153, 154
expert advice to improve 149, 152, 153, 154, 155
activities limited by epilepsy 149, 153
concealment of epilepsy 151
disabled actors for disabled characters 153

driving with epilepsy (*Coronation Street*) 152
epilepsy as divine intervention 152
first-aid inaccuracy 148
inaccuracies in 148, 150
industry, lobbying 155
negative stereotype prevention 154, 155
news
  driving with epilepsy, fatal accident 236
  primary source of information 184
prejudice against epilepsy 151
public educational role 148, 149, 150, 151, 152, 153, 154
seizures/epilepsy for dramatic effect 151, 154
undesirable characters with epilepsy 150, 151, 152, 155
viewer reaction, social media 153
Temkin, Owsei 3–4, 6, 38, 106, 206
temporal lobe
  abnormal behaviours arising from 268, 338 (Table)
  auditory cortex 157, 158
  memory as function 46
  mesial temporal sclerosis 57
  scarring 47, 57
  surgery 47
    effect on musical skills/appreciation 160
  tumour 328 (Fig)
temporal lobe epilepsy 4, 11, 46, 57, 59
  artists with 120
    de Chirico, Giorgio 116–117
  auditory hallucinations 160
  automatisms 248, 270
  in biography (of Christopher Grant) 91
  brain visualization, early methods 53
  Chopin, Frédéric 162
  'epileptic personality' in 338 (Table)
  in famous people, disputed 206
  in films 126, 137–138, 140, 141
  Gershwin, George 163–164
  hallucinations in 207
  in *The Innocents*, stage adaptation 176
  left *vs* right lobe, behaviours 268
  Mozart effect 158–159

murder and homicide association 264–265
music effect 158–159, 160
personality traits associated 267, 268
Ruby, Jack 187, 188
seizures
  complex automatisms 270
  MRI, brain tumour 328 (Fig)
  symptoms 34
  suicide risk 272
  surgery 47
  in TV programme 150
  violent behaviour 251, 264
  writers with 78
Tennyson, Alfred Lord (1808-1892) 69–70
The Terminal Man (Michael Crichton) 94–95, 130
tesla (magnetic field intensity unit) 55
Tesla, Nikola (1856-1943) 55
Thackeray, William Makepeace (1811-1863) 69
The Big Sleep, film adaptation 92
theatre, epilepsy in 173–179, 180
  actors with epilepsy 178–179
  Greek tragedies 173
  The Innocents 175
  negative perceptions/portrayal of epilepsy 174, 175, 176, 180
    destructive effects on life 176, 177
  patients on display, Charcot's 174, 175
  plays based on Dostoyevsky's novels 176
  reviews 174
  seizure depiction 173, 174, 177
  Shakespeare's 173, 180
  understanding and dignity 177
therapeutic nihilism 19
threatening behaviour, misperceptions 230, 268–269
  see also violence/violent behaviour
timing of seizures
  epileptic fury 24
  stars/moon significance 10, 17–18
Tissot, Samuel-Auguste (1728-1787) 18
Tlazolteotl 109–110, 120, 122
Tlazolteotl Healing a Child of Epilepsy (Eduardo Urbano Merino) 120
To What Red Hell (1929, film) 125
Tolstoy, Leo 216
tongue biting 7, 36
  prevention 89, 112, 145, 177, 319
  Williams, Sir John 'Kyffin' 117–118
tonic–clonic seizures 6, 59
  in art 106
  in sportsmen/women 220
  in writers 85
torture 12
Toulouse-Lautrec, Henri de 174
toxins, gut 47
track and field athletes, with epilepsy 196, 218
train drivers 241
training, epilepsy awareness
  care workers 308, 309
  law enforcement officers (USA) 307
  police officers 307
  prison officers 306–307
  teachers 300, 302, 303, 304
trances, in literature, or writers 70, 71, 72, 73
Transcending (Jennifer Hall) 120, 333 (Fig)
Transfiguration of Christ (Raphael) 12, 104, 107, 122
The Transfiguration of Christ (Rubens) 107–108, 332 (Fig)
transmission of epilepsy, Aztec beliefs 110
traumatic event, seizures after 24, 36, 71, 150, 208
travel-related problems 269–270, 323
Treatise on Epilepsy (Samuel-Auguste Tissot) 18
treatment of epilepsy 16, 49
  by Aztecs 109
  dietary *see* dietary therapy
  drugs *see* drug treatment
  history
    ancient Greeks 6–7, 8, 99
    early nineteenth century 23
    The Enlightenment 18–19
    John of Gaddesden's 11
    medieval period 10, 14, 15, 100
    Paracelsus' treatments 14
    Roman period 6, 8
    Willis' approach 16
  inadequate, developing countries 291, 292
  in literature 87, 88, 89
  music, role 159
  negative beliefs about (nineteenth century) 23
  newspaper articles 192, 196

non-pharmaceutical, twentieth
  century 47–49
religious 10
surgical *see* surgical treatment
symptomatic, Paracelsus 13, 14
trepanning (trephining) *see*
  trepanning (trephining)
in USA, in Victorian era 29–30
Victorian era *see* Victorian era
trepanning (trephining) 15, 18–19, 37,
  100
  history of 15, 18, 37–38, 100
  eighteenth century 38
  painting of, Renaissance 100, 101
triggers, of epilepsy attacks 5, 11
  Cullen's views 20
  electrical 20, 34, 35
  environmental factors 61
  epileptic fury and 24
  in literature 68, 69
  moon association 5, 6, 10, 12, 18
  music 118, 159–160
  proximate or remote 20, 61
  removal/prevention 16
  sane automatisms and 273
tuberculosis 234
tuberous sclerosis 58
Turkey, epilepsy due to supernatural
  causes 277
The Turn of the Screw (Henry James)
  175–176, 180
Turner, William Aldren (1864-1945)
  41–42
The Twelve Chairs (1970, film) 129
twins, with epilepsy 222
Twitter 198, 204
  metaphorical/joke use of seizure
    term 199–200
  seizure portrayal 199
  seizures triggered by GIF 200
  treatment/care of people with
    epilepsy 199
types of epilepsy *see* categories of epilepsy

UK
  disability discrimination laws *see*
    Disability Discrimination Act
    1995 (UK)
  driving licence 236, 237
    see also driving (people with
      epilepsy)
  economic crisis/age of austerity
    194
  government minister with
    responsibility for the disabled
    246
  immigration legislation 235
  'not guilty by reason of insanity'
    (NGRI) cases 265–266,
    272–273
  pilot's licence 240–241
  public perceptions of epilepsy
    282–284
  teachers' attitudes 300
UK Civil Service model, employment
  296–297
unconsciousness *see* consciousness, loss
underachievement 206
understanding about epilepsy *see* public
  awareness/understanding
undressing, attempt, on early film 124
unemployment 280, 295
  automatism on plane, case 270
  detrimental effects/impact of 280
  level in USA 281
  prejudice by employers 295–296
  rates 241, 295, 297
  see also employment
'unintended consequences' 280
university
  mandatory medical test in China
    243–244
  personal account 324–325
University of St Andrews, qualifications
  33–34
unpredictability of epilepsy 178
USA
  compulsory sterilization 229, 230,
    231
  discrimination legislation 243
  driving with epilepsy 238
  epilepsy centres and treatment
    29–30
  eugenics movement in 229
  famous Americans with epilepsy
    217
  freedom of movement and 233,
    234–235
  immigration legislation 234–235
  marriage legislation 230–231
  marriage prevention in people with
    epilepsy 30, 31, 230–231,
    277
  pilot's licence 240
  prevalence of epilepsy 52
  public perceptions of epilepsy
    1949-1979 280–281
    1980s and 1990s 282
  reducing stigma 293–294
  stigmatization in the press/media
    195–196, 196
  Supreme Court 196–197
  teachers' attitudes 301
uterine epilepsy 8, 26, 35
  drug treatment 37

vaccination, epilepsy link 316
vagal nerve stimulation 45
Valentine of Terni 105
Van Gogh, Theo 110–111, 112, 268
Van Gogh, Vincent (1853-1890)
  110–113, 114–115, 122, 267–268
  biographical facts 110–111
  evidence for (possible) epilepsy
    112–113
  psychiatric conditions 112–113
Van Hemessen, Jan Sanders 102, 331
  (Fig)
Van Swieten, Gerald (1700-1772) 18
Vanity Fair (William Makepeace
  Thackeray) 69
vapours, harmful 15, 21
  release by trepanning 15, 37
verbal output, excessive 267
'victim', stigma 278
Victorian era 26–41, 50
  drug treatments 36–37, 49
  epilepsy hospitals and colony
    movement 27–36
  history of epilepsy in 26–41
  surgical treatment 37–41
violence/violent behaviour, and epilepsy
  27, 248, 249, 250–254
  automatisms link 249, 251, 252,
    269, 270
  Canadian studies (1981/2006),
    changing attitudes 304–305
  criteria to guide law process 260,
    261, 339 (Table)
  deliberately planned 256, 258
  EEGs of individuals 253, 254
  evidence refuting link 252–253,
    254, 263–264, 265
  extreme nature of violence 265
  fear of, and stigma persistence 305
  in films 137, 138
  Goring's studies 251–252
  historical suggestion of link
    250–251, 259
  ictal and inter-ictal 251, 270,
    304–305
  increased violence with treatment
    failure 264
  literature reviews of 259, 265

in literature/writers 67, 68, 80, 95–96
misperception perpetuation 230, 253, 265, 266, 273–274, 305
  cases 261, 262, 263
  'epileptic personality and 268–269
Napoleon Bonaparte 210
in newspaper articles 193
over-estimation of link 265
psychiatric illness/abuse/alcoholism associated 254, 264
during seizures 252, 256, 257
  in absence of signs of seizures 254
  Canham, Charles Edward's case 257, 258
  evidence against 252–253, 265
  murders, features associated 258, 263
  rarity 253
South Korean study 264
Swedish study refuting link 263–264
timing of seizures and 264, 265
in TV programme 151
see also criminal behaviour and criminality; murder and homicide
vision, double 322, 325
Visions: Artists Living with Epilepsy (Steven Schachter) 120, 122
visual hallucinations 74, 112, 116, 117
  Chopin, Frédéric's 161–162
  in films 143, 144
  Joan of Arc's 11, 207, 208
  in *The Innocents* 175–176
vital fluids (humours) 5, 9
vivisection experiments 32, 40
volunteers 331
von Baeyer, Adolf 42
von Haller, Albrecht (1708-1777) 19
von Hoenheim, Philippus (Paracelsus) 13–14
votive tablets 106–107
vulnerability, in epilepsy
  in films 128, 136, 137, 144, 145, 147
  in literature 73, 75, 80, 90, 93
  sportsmen 219

Waging Heavy Peace (Neil Young) 165
Walker, Arthur Earl (1907-1995) 259
Walker, Greg (1959-) 220–221
walking 82, 84

warlocks 10, 12, 17, 21
'water diet' 47
Watts-Dunn, Theodore 215
Waxman, Stephen 267
Wayne, Lil (1982-) 218
welfare burden, in UK 194
'Welfare Island', USA 30
Wells, H.G. (1866-1946) 228
West Riding Lunatic Asylum, reports 32
What's the Time, Mr Wolf? (2011, film) 146
Wheat Fields with Crows (Vincent Van Gogh) 114–115
Whistler, Peggy (Margiad Evans) 85–86
white matter 57–58
Whitney, Leon 229
William Quarrier Scottish Epilepsy Centre xi–xii
Williams, Peggy (Margiad Evans) 85–86
Williams, Sir John 'Kyffin' (1918-2006) 117–118, 122
  obituaries 119
Willis, Thomas (1621-1675) 15–16, 54
Wilson, Woodrow (1856-1924) 229
The Winning Team (1952, film) 127–128
'wise', stigma category 278
witches and witchcraft 10, 11–12, 16, 17, 21
Wolf, Peter 76, 97
women, epilepsy in 8
  hysteria and 17, 35
  musicogenic epilepsy 159, 160
  seizures, photographic record 175
work, right to 241–246
  see also careers; employment
workplace 299
works of art *see* art, works of
World Health Organization (WHO) 62, 291–292
wormwood 7
worthlessness 133, 177
writers
  affected by (possible) epilepsy 67, 70, 73–74, 97
    Blackmore, R.D. 82–83
    Dickinson, Emily 83–84
    Dostoevsky, Fyodor 76, 77–78
    Evans, Margiad 85–86
    Flaubert, Gustave 73–75
    Greene, Graham, diagnosis 84
    Lear, Edward 81–82, 115
    Lee, Laurence 'Laurie' 86–87
    Poe, Edgar Allan 67, 70–71
    Pynchon, Thomas 88
    Tennyson, Alfred Lord 69–70
  describing epilepsy with candour 85–86
  sources of information on epilepsy 72
  use of epilepsy for vulnerability/ weakness 73, 76
  see also literature, epilepsy in
writing, excessive (hypergraphia) 112, 113, 116, 117

X-ray 54, 56
contrast agents 53–54
injected air, brain visualization 53

Young, Neil (1945-) 165–167
young adult fiction 96
The Young and the Restless (1973-) 149–150, 155
Young Epilepsy 220, 223, 302
YouTube 197, 201, 203–204
  educational potential 201, 203
  epilepsy search/review results 201, 202–203
  inaccuracy of video information 202, 203
  indiscriminate use 203
  seizure depiction 201, 203
    accuracy of diagnosis/ classification 203
  negative comments on 201–202

Zach: A Film about Epilepsy (2009) 146
The Zahir (Paul Coelho) 159
Zeitbloom, Bartholomäus (1455-1515) 105
zinc salts 37